# Trust Carol J. Buck and Elsevier
## to take you through the levels
## of coding success

## Step 4: Professional Resources

## Step 3: Certify

With the resources you need for every level of coding success, Carol J. Buck and Elsevier are with you every step of your coding career. From beginning to advanced, from the classroom to the workplace, from application to certification, the Step Series products are your guides to greater opportunities and successful career advancement.

**Keep climbing with the n...coding**

...hor and Educator
...ol J. Buck, MS, CPC, CPC-H, CCS-P

# Step 3: Certify

***Congratulations on reaching the certification step in your career!*** As you know, certified coders are in top demand in today's marketplace. That's why, as a lifelong coder and educator, I have dedicated myself to providing the most up-to-date, comprehensive, and user-friendly certification review books on the market. I update this book every year so you will have the best tool possible when studying for your certification exam. It's time to hit the books. ***You can do it! I know you can!***

— Carol J. Buck, MS, CPC, CPC-H, CCS-P

## Track your progress!

**See the checklist in the back of this book
to learn more about your next step toward coding success!**

# 2012
# CPC® CODING EXAM REVIEW

## The Certification Step

# 2012

# CPC® CODING EXAM REVIEW

## The Certification Step

## Carol J. Buck

MS, CPC, CPC-H, CCS-P

Former Program Director, Medical Secretary Programs
Northwest Technical College; East Grand Forks, Minnesota

ELSEVIER

http://evolve.elsevier.com

**ELSEVIER**
SAUNDERS

3251 Riverport Lane
St. Louis, Missouri 63043

CPC® CODING EXAM REVIEW 2012: THE CERTIFICATION STEP                    ISBN: 978-1-4557-0659-4

NOTE: *Current Procedural Terminology, 2012,* was used in updating this text.

Current Procedural Terminology (CPT) is copyright 2011 American Medical Association. All rights reserved. No fee schedules, basic units, relative values, or related listings are included in CPT. The AMA assumes no liability for the data contained herein. Applicable FARS/DFARS restrictions apply to government use.

**Library of Congress Cataloging-in-Publication Data**

Buck, Carol J.
   2012 CPC coding exam review : the certification step / Carol J. Buck.—2012 ed.
      p. ; cm.
   Rev. ed. of: CPC coding exam review 2011 / Carol J. Buck, Cynthia Stahl. c2011.
   Includes index.
   ISBN 978-1-4557-0659-4 (pbk. : alk. paper)
   I. Buck, Carol J. CPC coding exam review 2011.   II. Title.   III. Title: CPC coding exam review.
   [DNLM: 1.   Classification—Examination Questions. 2.   Clinical Coding—methods—Examination Questions.   3.   Terminology as Topic—Examination Questions.  WB 18.2]
   LC classification not assigned
   616.001′2076—dc23
                                                                                    2011034417

*Publisher:* Jeanne R. Olson
*Developmental Editor:* Diane Chatman
*Publishing Services Manager:* Pat Joiner-Myers
*Senior Project Manager:* Joy Moore
*Senior Designer:* Amy Buxton

Printed in the United States of America

Last digit is the print number:  9  8  7  6  5  4  3  2  1

# Dedication

*To coding instructors,*
*who each day strive to enhance the lives*
*of their students and provide the next generation*
*of knowledgeable medical coders.*

**Carol J. Buck**

# Acknowledgments

There are so many, many people who participated in the development of this text, and only through the effort of all of the team members has it been possible to publish this text. **Jackie Grass,** who has assumed enormous responsibilities for development of this text.

**Sally Schrefer,** Executive Vice President, Nursing and Health Professions, who possesses great listening skills and the ability to ensure the publication of high-quality educational materials. **Andrew Allen,** Vice President and Publisher, Health Professions, who sees the bigger picture and shares the vision. **Jeanne R. Olson,** Publisher, who maintains an excellent sense of humor and is a valued member of the team who can always be depended upon for reasoned judgment. **Diane Chatman,** Developmental Editor, who assumed the responsibility of shepherding this project to production with steady fortitude. **Kate Mannix,** Production Editor at Graphic World, who assumed responsibility for many projects while maintaining a high degree of professionalism. The employees of Elsevier, who have participated in the publication of this text and demonstrated exceptional professionalism and competence. **Arlene Scher,** Senior Program Coordinator at Augusta State University Division of Continuing Education for her sharp eye and help regarding the organization of the CPC exam questions.

# Preface

Thank you for purchasing *CPC® Coding Exam Review 2012: The Certification Step,* the latest guide to the outpatient physician coding certification exam. This 2012 edition has been carefully reviewed and updated with the latest content, making it the most current guide for your review. The author and publishers have made every effort to equip you with skills and tools you will need to succeed on the exam. To this end, this review guide presents essential information about all health care coding systems, anatomy, terminology, and pathophysiology, as well as sample examinations for practice. No other review guide on the market brings together such thorough coverage of all necessary examination material in one source.

## ORGANIZATION OF THIS TEXTBOOK

Following a basic outline approach, *CPC® Coding Exam Review 2012* takes a practical approach to assisting you with your examination preparations. The text is divided into four units—Anatomy, Terminology, and Pathophysiology; Reimbursement Issues; Overview of CPT, ICD-9-CM, and HCPCS Coding; and Coding Challenge—and there are several appendices for your reference. Additionally, examinations are provided on the companion Evolve website to help assist you in your preparation.

**Unit I, Anatomy, Terminology, and Pathophysiology** Covers all the essential body systems and terms you'll need to get certified. Organized by body systems to follow the CPT codes, the sections also include illustrations to review each major anatomical area and quizzes to check your understanding and recall.

UNIT I   Anatomy, Terminology, and Pathophysiology

Figure **1-18** Internal view of heart.

**Unit II, Reimbursement Issues** Provides a review of important insurance and billing information to help you review the connections between medical coding, insurance, billing, and reimbursement.

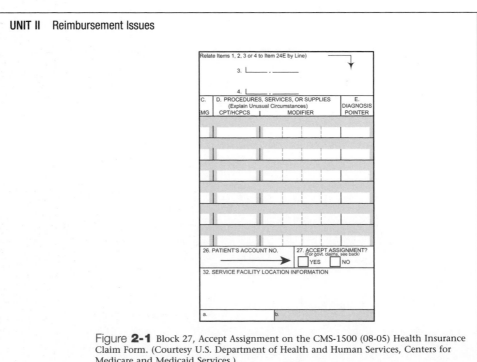

UNIT II   Reimbursement Issues

Figure **2-1** Block 27, Accept Assignment on the CMS-1500 (08-05) Health Insurance Claim Form. (Courtesy U.S. Department of Health and Human Services, Centers for Medicare and Medicaid Services.)

## Unit III, Overview of CPT, ICD-9-CM, and HCPCS Coding

Contains comprehensive coverage of the different coding systems and their applications, making other references unnecessary! Simplified text and clear examples are the highlights of this unit, and illustrations are included to clarify difficult concepts.

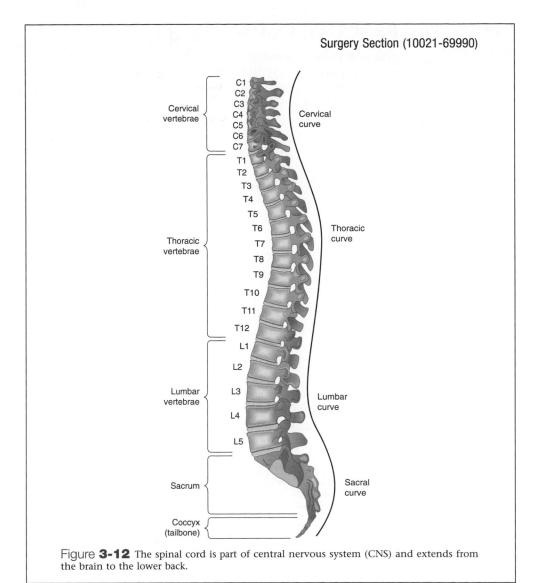

Surgery Section (10021-69990)

Figure **3-12** The spinal cord is part of central nervous system (CNS) and extends from the brain to the lower back.

## Unit IV, Coding Challenge

Contains a Final Examination modeled after the actual CPC® examination, to be taken at the end of your complete program of study. To help you quantify the examination, this is meant to be taken using paper and pencil.

Final Examination

# FINAL EXAMINATION

**Direction: Report only the professional component unless specifically directed to do otherwise within the question.**

**Subject Area: Medical Terminology**

1. This term means the surgical removal of the fallopian tube:
   A. ligation
   B. hysterectomy
   C. salpingostomy
   D. salpingectomy

2. This combining form means "thirst":
   A. dips/o
   B. acr/o
   C. cortic/o
   D. somat/o

## ABOUT THE PRACTICE EXAMINATIONS

The companion Evolve website contains valuable resources to assist you with your preparation for the CPC® coding certification examination. (See *Additional Evolve Resources* for more information on how to access this website.) It includes two timed and scored 150-question practice examinations (the same examination is taken twice) modeled after the actual format of the CPC® examination. The Pre-Examination on the Evolve website should be completed at the start of your study, and the Post-Examination, also on the Evolve website, should be taken after your study is complete. By comparing the results of these examinations, you can see your improvement after using the review guide! Once you check your scores, you are ready to take the Final Examination in Unit IV of the text.

### Summary Screen

When using the program, the Exam Sessions screen serves as home base. Here you can find information relating to your progress and performance in different subject areas. From this screen, you can choose an examination mode, submit an examination, check your progress, review your results, and access the Final Examination scoresheet and answers.

In addition to displaying your scores for completed sections and tracking the total elapsed time, this screen also shows the total, attempted, and correct questions in each subsection. You can return to the Exam Sessions screen at any point while taking or reviewing an examination, and all information related to your answers and position is saved.

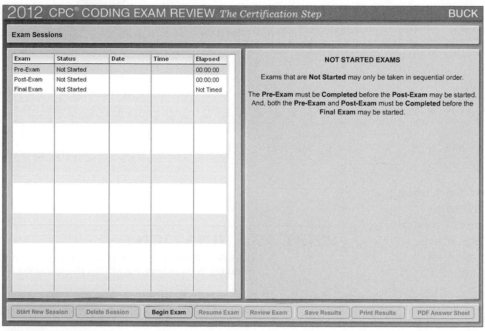

**Summary screen.**

### Taking the Examination

While taking the examination, click on the circle beside the letter of your answer choice, and the circle will appear orange. Click on the "Next" button at the bottom of the screen to proceed to the next question. At the top of the screen, the Quick Jump feature displays the current question number and doubles as a pull-down menu that allows you jump to any question in the current section. Additionally, the Bookmark button at the top of the screen allows you to mark questions for later reference.

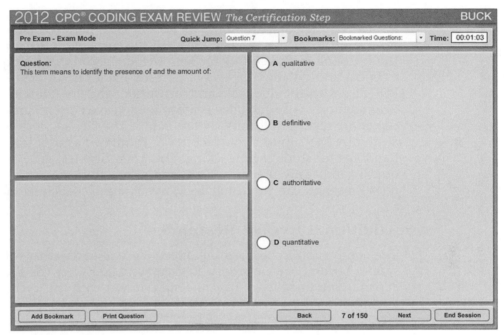

**Question screen.**

## Reviewing Your Results

Once you have taken the Post-Examination on the companion Evolve website, you have the option to review all the Pre- and Post-Examination questions with rationales, even the ones you answered correctly, by clicking the "Review Exam" button at the bottom of the screen. The correct answer is shown for each question, and a rationale is given for each answer option. Or, if you prefer, you can review the answers and rationales using a PDF answer sheet. You can also compare your results on the Pre- and Post-Examinations by clicking on each exam on the Exam Sessions screen and viewing your results in the "Completed Exams" on the right or by printing out your results.

Once you have completed the Final Examination in Unit IV, you will access the electronic score sheet on the Evolve website and enter your answers. The software will then provide you with the answers and rationales.

## SUPPLEMENTAL RESOURCES

However you decide to prepare for the certification examination, we have developed supplements designed to complement the *CPC® Coding Exam Review 2012*. Each of these supplements has been developed with the needs of both students and instructors in mind.

### Instructor's Electronic Resource

No matter what your level of teaching experience, this total-teaching solution, located on the companion Evolve website, will help you plan your lessons with ease, and the author has developed all the curriculum materials necessary to use the textbook in the classroom. This includes additional unit quizzes, a course calendar and syllabus, lesson plans, ready-made tests for easy assessment, and PDF files with the questions and answers for the Pre-/Post- and Final Examinations. Also included is a comprehensive PowerPoint collection for the entire text, and ExamView test banks. The PowerPoint slides can be easily customized to support your lectures or formatted as overhead transparencies or handouts for student note-taking. The ExamView test generator will help you quickly and easily prepare quizzes and exams from the ready-made test questions, and can be customized to your specific teaching methods.

### Additional Evolve Resources

The companion Evolve website offers many resources that will extend your studies beyond the classroom. Related WebLinks offer you the opportunity to expand your knowledge base and stay current with this ever-changing field, and additional material is available for help and practice.

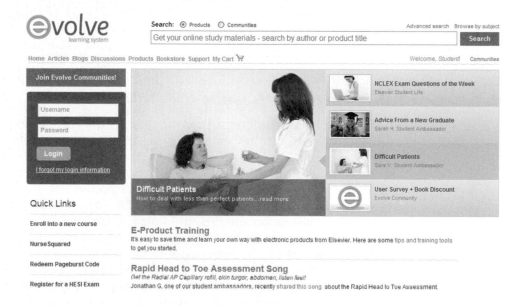

A Course Management System (CMS) is also available free to instructors who adopt this textbook. This web-based platform gives instructors yet another resource to facilitate learning and to make medical coding content accessible to students. In addition to the Evolve Resources available to both faculty and students, there is an entire suite of tools available that allows for communication between instructors and students. Students can log on through the Evolve portal to take online quizzes, practice examinations, participate in threaded discussions, post assignments to instructors, or chat with other classmates, while instructors can use the online grade book to follow class progress.

To access this comprehensive online resource, follow the instructions located on the inside front cover of this book. You will need the Course ID number provided by your instructor. If your instructor has not set up a Course Management System, you can still access the free Evolve resources at http://evolve.elsevier.com/Buck/cpc/.

# Development of This Edition

This book would not have been possible without a team of educators and professionals, including practicing coders and technical consultants. The combined efforts of the team members have made this text an incredible learning tool.

**LEAD TECHNICAL COLLABORATOR**

**Jacqueline Klitz Grass, MA, CPC**
Coding and Reimbursement Specialist
Altru Health System
Grand Forks, North Dakota

**SENIOR CODING SPECIALIST**

**Lindsay-Anne Jenkins, CRNA, CPC, CPC-H, CIRCC, CPC-I, CANPC**
Coding and Auditing Specialist
St. Louis, Missouri

**SENIOR ICD-9-CM AND ICD-10-CM CODING SPECIALIST**

**Karla R. Lovaasen, RHIA, CCS, CCS-P**
Coding and Consulting Services
Abingdon, Maryland
—Coauthor of *2012 ICD-9-CM Coding: Theory and Practice with ICD-10,* St. Louis, 2012, Saunders.

—Coauthor of *ICD-10-CM/PCS Coding: Theory and Practice,* St. Louis, 2012, Saunders.

**SENIOR COLLABORATOR AND ICD-10-CM CONSULTANT**

**Nancy Maguire, ACS, CRT, PCS, FCS, HCS-D**
Physician Consultant for Auditing
   and Education
Universal City, Texas

## CODING SPECIALISTS

**Robert H. Ekvall, PhD, CCS, CPC-H, CPC, CPMA**
Coder/Biller
Scripps Green Hospital
La Jolla, California

**Jody Klitz, CPC**
Coding and Reimbursement Specialist
Cancer Center of North Dakota
Grand Forks, North Dakota

**Debra Kroll, RHIT**
Denial and Billing Compliance
  Supervisor
Altru Health System
Grand Forks, North Dakota

**Danielle Laitres, CPC**
Owner
Coastal Billing Solutions
Stuart, Florida

**Nancy Maguire, ACS, CRT, PCS, FCS, HCS-D**
Physician Consultant for Auditing
  and Education
Universal City, Texas

**Sylvia Partridge, CPC**
Coding Instructor
Athens, Georgia

**Joan E. Wolfgang, MEd, CPC, CPC-H, CPC-I, CHCA**
Independent Consultant
Milwaukee, Wisconsin

## QUERY MANAGER

**Patricia Cordy Henricksen, MS, CHCA, CPC-I, CPC, CCP-P, PCS**
Approved PMCC Instructor
Education Director, Lexington Local
  Chapter of AAPC
Bluegrass Medical Managers
  Association
Lexington, Kentucky

## QUERY TEAM

**Debra Kroll, RHIT**
Denial and Billing Compliance
  Supervisor
Altru Health System
Grand Forks, North Dakota

## EDITORIAL REVIEW BOARD

**Bonnie Blazevich, CPC, RMC**
Medical Billing/Coding Instructor,
  Independent
Coding/Billing Specialist
Compass Career College
Hammond, Louisiana

**Andrea D. Potteiger, CCS, CCS-P, CPC, CMAA, CBCS, CHI, NR-CAHA, NR-CMA, NR-CPT, NR-CEKG**
Lead Healthcare Instructor
New Horizons, Harrisburg
Mechanicsburg, Pennsylvania

# Contents

Contents

# Success Strategies

This review was developed to help you as you prepare for your certification examination. First, congratulations on your initiative. Preparing for a certification examination can seem like a daunting and formidable task. You have already taken the first and hardest step: you have made a commitment. Your steely determination and organizational skills are your best tools as you prepare to complete this exciting journey successfully.

How do you prepare for a certification examination? The answers to that question are as varied as the persons preparing for it. Each person comes to the preparation with different educational, coding, and personal experiences. Therefore, each must develop a plan that meets his or her individual needs and preferences. Success Strategies will help you to develop your individual plan.

## THE CERTIFICATION EXAMINATION

This text has been developed to serve as a tool in your preparation for the outpatient (physician-based) **CPC®** (Certified Professional Coder) certification examination offered by the American Academy of Professional Coders (AAPC). The CPC® certification examination consists of a total of 150 multiple choice questions covering medical terminology, anatomy, pathophysiology, CPT, ICD-9-CM, HCPCS, and coding concepts. You have 5 hours and 40 minutes to complete the examination. Exam results are reported with scores and your top three areas of weakness. Visit the AAPC website (www.aapc.com/certification/cpc.aspx) for the latest information on the CPC® examination.

To be successful on the CPC® certification examination, you will have to know how to assign medical codes to patient services and diagnoses. This textbook focuses on providing you with that coding practice as well as anatomy, terminology, pathophysiology, reimbursement, and coding concepts in preparation for the CPC® examination.

### Date and Location

Although every journey begins with the first step, you have to know where you are going to make a plan to get there.

- Choose the **date and location** for taking the certification examination. The AAPC's website (www.aapc.com/certification/locate-examination.aspx) contains detailed information about the examination sites and dates.

- The American Academy of Professional Coders has information that can be downloaded from their website at www.aapc.com or sent for by contacting:

American Academy of Professional Coders
2480 South 3850 West, Suite B
Salt Lake City, UT 84120
Telephone: 800-626-2633

- After you have obtained the examination materials, read all the information carefully. Review all competencies outlined in the material to ensure that your study plan contains strategies to address each of these competencies.

- The questions within this textbook are not the same questions that are in the certification examination, but the skill and knowledge that you gain through analysis, coding, and recall will increase your ability to be successful on examination day.

## MANAGING YOUR TIME

Role strain! That is what you get when you have so many different roles in your life and you cannot find time for all of them! Know that feeling? Are you a daughter/son, mother/father, wife/husband, student, friend, worker, volunteer, hobbyist—the list is endless. Each takes time from your schedule, and somehow you now need to fit into the role of successful learner. Because you have only 24 hours in your day, being a successful learner requires a time-balancing act. Maybe you will have to be satisfied with dust bunnies under your bed, dishes in your kitchen sink, or fewer visits with your friends. Whatever you have to do to juggle the time around to give yourself ample time to devote to this important task of examination preparation, you must do and make a plan for in advance; otherwise, life just takes over and you find you do not have adequate study time.

If you are planning a big event in your life—moving, a trip, and so on, think about postponing it until after the examination. Your focus right now has to be on yourself. Make your motto **"It's All About Me!"** Sounds self-centered, I know, and most likely very different from who you are, but just this once, you need to carve out the time you need to accomplish this important goal. This time is for yourself. Make it happen for yourself. Move everything you can out of the way, focus on this preparation, and give this preparation your best effort.

## SCHEDULE

Each person has an individual learning style. The coding profession seems to attract those most influenced by logic and facts. The best way for a logical and factual person to learn is to problem-solve and apply the information. Hands-on practice is how you will build your skill and confidence for the examination.

- Choose a location to be your Study Central.

- Gather into Study Central the following study resources:

  - Certification packet or handbook from the certifying organization

  - CPT, current edition

- ICD-9-CM, current edition

- HCPCS, current edition

- *Official Guidelines for Coding and Reporting* (Can be accessed by following the Evolve Resources link provided in Appendix A of this text)

- Medical dictionary

- Coding textbooks, professional journals, and magazines

- Terminology, anatomy, or pathology text, as needed

- See Appendix G for Further Text Resources

Make Study Central your special place where you can get away from all other responsibilities. Make it a quiet, calm getaway, even if it is a corner of your bedroom. In this quiet place have a comfortable chair, adequate lighting, supplies, and sufficient desktop surface to use all your coding books. This is your place to focus all your attention on preparation for the examination, without distractions.

- Plan your **schedule** from now until the certification examination using a calendar. Make weekly goals so that you have definite tasks to accomplish each week and you can check the tasks off—a great feeling of accomplishment comes from being able to check off a task. In this way, you can see your progress on your countdown to success.

- Choose a specific **time** each day or several times a week when you are going to study and mark them on your calendar. Make this commitment in writing. After each study session, you should check off that date on the calendar as a visual reminder that you are sticking to your plan and are one step closer to your goal.

- You should plan your study time in advance, know what you are going to be studying the next session, and **be prepared** for that upcoming study session. This will greatly increase the amount of material you are able to cover during the session. At the end of each session, decide what you are going to study next session and ensure that you have all the material and references you will need readily available. At the end of each session, you should be ready for the next study session.

- Your plan should include those areas where you know you will need improvement. For example, when is the last time you read, not referenced or reviewed, but really read, the CPT Anesthesia Guidelines? You probably do not code anesthesia services often, if ever, and as such are not familiar with the information in these guidelines. That is an area of improvement, and your plan should include a thorough reading of all the CPT section guidelines.

- **DO THIS BEFORE YOU BEGIN YOUR STUDY: Assess** your strengths and weaknesses. By making this assessment, you will know where to concentrate your efforts and where to focus your study schedule. You know those areas where you already have strong skills and knowledge and will not need to spend as much time preparing in these areas. The **Pre-Examination,** found on the Evolve website, is an examination that you can use as a tool to assess your current skill level. This examination should be taken before you begin your study and then again immediately after you have completed your entire study schedule. Do not analyze the questions by reviewing the rationales (located on the Evolve website); rather, wait until after you have completed your studies and have taken this same examination a second time. If you review the rationales after the first time you take the examination, you will know the answers too well to provide a valid comparison between examinations. See Unit IV of this textbook for further information.

- After you have completed your course of study, take the **Post-Examination** on the Evolve website. You should plan to cover the examination in the same amount of time as will be given for the certification examination you are going to take. Compare your scores to those from the first time you took this examination. Note the areas where you did not demonstrate sufficient skills and knowledge.

- Develop a **second plan** to improve the specific areas where you believe you need further study.

- You are now ready to take the **Final Examination** that is located in Unit IV of this text. Take the examination in the same amount of time that will be allocated for the certification examination. It is best if you do this final in one sitting, thereby mimicking the actual examination. If your schedule does not allow for taking the examination in one sitting, plan to take it in several sessions, but always keep track of the time used to ensure that you take the examination in the same amount of time allowed for the official examination. Learning to work within the time allocated is part of the skill you are developing. Remember the certification examinations assess not only your coding knowledge but also your efficiency in completing the examination within the allocated time.

## USING THIS TEXT

This text is divided into:

- Success Strategies

- Unit I, Anatomy, Terminology, and Pathophysiology

- Unit II, Reimbursement Issues

- Unit III, Overview of CPT, ICD-9-CM, and HCPCS Coding

- Unit IV, Coding Challenge

- Appendix A, Resources (Web-Based)

- Appendix B, Medical Terminology

- Appendix C, Combining Forms

- Appendix D, Prefixes

- Appendix E, Suffixes

- Appendix F, Abbreviations

- Appendix G, Further Text Resources

Appendices B-F are combined lists of Medical Terminology, Combining Forms, Prefixes, Suffixes, and Abbreviations used within Unit I, Anatomy, Terminology, and Pathophysiology.

The material in this review features the following:

- Comprehensive guide in outline format

- Photos and drawings to illustrate key points

- Pre-/Post-Examination (on the Evolve website)—150 questions

- Final Examination (in Unit IV of this text)—150 questions

- **Unit I** is a review of the anatomy, terminology, and pathophysiology by organ systems designed to provide you with a quick review of that organ system. In addition, there is a list of combining forms, prefixes, suffixes, and abbreviations that are often used in that organ system. At the end of each organ system, there is a quiz that will give you an opportunity to assess your knowledge.

- **Unit II** is a review of reimbursement issues and terminology. A quiz is located at the end of the unit to assess your knowledge.

- **Unit III** is a review of CPT, HCPCS, and ICD-9-CM. The CPT and ICD-9-CM material follows the order of the manuals. There is no quiz at the end of this unit because you will be applying this material in the practice examinations and in the Final Examination.

- **Unit IV** contains the examinations. The Pre-/Post-Examination is a 150-question examination located on the companion Evolve website. This same exam should be taken twice—once before you begin your study and the second time after you have completed your study. You should allow 5 hours and 40 minutes (340 minutes) to complete each examination because this is the amount of time you will have for the CPC® examination. The computer software stores your scores and compares the results from the first and second time you took the examination; so you can see not only your score on each section but also the improvement from the first to the second examination. The Final Examination is also a 150-question examination, but located in the text with answers on the Evolve website.

> NOTE: To enable the learner to calculate an examination score, the minimum of 70% has been identified as "passing" within this text; however, this may or may not be the percentage identified by the American Academy of Professional Coders as a "passing" grade. It is your responsibility to review all certification information published by the American Academy of Professional Coders as they are the definitive source for information regarding the CPC® certification examination.

There are many ways you could use this text. However you decide to prepare, you should take the examination before you begin your study to ensure that you develop a study plan that includes time and activities that will increase your knowledge in those areas where your test scores indicate areas of weakness. You could then take the units in the order they are presented, or you may want to review the anatomy, terminology, and pathophysiology for a body system and then review the CPT material for that body system. There is no one best way to approach the use of this text because each individual will have a personal learning style and preferences that will direct how the material is used. Your skills may be very strong in one or more coding or knowledge areas and you will want to delete those areas from your individual study plan.

This text is not meant to be the only study source, but only one tool of many that you will use. For example, if your terminology skills need a complete overhaul, the brief overview in this text may not meet your needs. You may want to supplement this text with a terminology text and an in-depth study of terminology.

- **Appendices** are a resource for you as you prepare your study plan.

  - **Appendix A,** Resources, is an Evolve Resources link (web-based) to the *Official Guidelines for Coding and Reporting*. This link provides the rules for use of ICD-9-CM codes and will be referenced in Unit III when reviewing the use of ICD-9-CM codes.

- **Appendix B,** Medical Terminology, is a complete alphabetic list of all the medical terms listed in the Medical Terminology portion of the organ system reviews used in Unit I.

- **Appendix C,** Combining Forms, is a complete alphabetic list of the combining forms used in Unit I.

- **Appendix D,** Prefixes, is a complete alphabetic list of the prefixes used in Unit I.

- **Appendix E,** Suffixes, is a complete alphabetic list of the suffixes used in Unit I.

- **Appendix F,** Abbreviations, is a complete list of the abbreviations referenced in Unit I.

- **Appendix G,** Further Text Resources, is a list of texts that you may want to obtain to supplement your study plan.

## DAY BEFORE THE EXAMINATION

- No cramming! Your study time is now over, and cramming the day before the test is not a good idea because it just increases your anxiety level. This day is your day to prepare yourself. Do some things you enjoy this day. Take your mind off the examination. Pamper yourself: you deserve it.

- Prepare pencils (no. 2), erasers, picture identification, CPT (AMA standard or professional version only), ICD-9-CM (Vols. 1 and 2), HCPCS code manuals, and examination admission card. For a paper/pencil examination, take a ruler so that if you skip a question and want to mark that question to return to later, you can use the ruler to make certain you return to the correct question.

- You cannot have excessive writing, sticky notes, labels, etc. in your code books. Check the AAPC examination information to ensure that your books meet the specifications identified by the testing organization.

- Review the certification packet information one last time to ensure that you have all the required material.

- Pack quiet snacks and bottled water sufficient for 5 hours and 40 minutes.

- Listen to the weather and traffic reports. Plan your route to the examination site. If it is in a new location, drive to the location before the big day.

- Eat a light supper and get to bed early. Set the alarm in plenty of time to arrive at the site early. It is a good idea to have a friend or family member give you an early wake-up call to ensure that you do not oversleep.

## DAY OF THE EXAMINATION

- Wear comfortable clothes and be prepared for any room temperature. A short-sleeved shirt with a sweater is a good plan. Dress in layers so you can ensure that you will be comfortable in any environment.

- Take a watch with you.

- Eat a good breakfast. Avoid caffeine because it initially stimulates you, but in the long run will decrease your concentration.

- Arrive early. The doors are locked to those who arrive late. This is a day to be early.

- Ensure that you have the correct room for your examination. Often there are several examinations being administered at one time, so be certain you are in the correct room for your examination.

## THE CERTIFICATION EXAMINATION

You are ready for this! You have planned your work and have worked your plan. Now it is time to reap the rewards for all that hard work.

- Choose a good location in which to sit. Choose a location that will not get a lot of traffic from those leaving the room.

- Place all your supplies on the table.

- Take several deep breaths before you begin to help relax you.

- Some prefer to take the parts of the examination out of order, taking those questions they are most confident of first. Others prefer to start at the beginning and work through all questions in order. The approach that you use will depend on your individual test-taking style.

- When you come to a question for which you are unsure of the answer, you may wish to skip over and come back to all those ones you were unsure of at the end of the examination, depending on the time available. Or you may want to attempt each question and note those you are unsure of to return to when you have finished the exam section. Again, the approach you will use depends on your individual style.

- Read the directions. This may sound too simple, but many persons do not completely read the directions, only to find that the directions gave specific directions about what or what not to code on a certain case (for example, "code only this certain portion of the procedure"). Yet the choices for answers included the full coding of the case as a selection; if you did not read all the directions, you would choose the response with codes for all the items listed in the report. For example, the question may have directed you to code the service only, not the diagnosis, and yet one of the choices would be the correct service and diagnosis codes, which of course would be an incorrect answer based on the directions. So read all of the directions.

- Your speed and accuracy are being tested. You do not have time to labor over each question for a long time if you intend to complete all the questions. Read the directions, read the question, put down your best assessment of the answer, and then move on to the next question.

- Words such as *always, every, never,* and *all* generally indicate broad terms that, with true/false questions, usually indicate a false question.

- If you do not know the answer to the question, try eliminating those that you know are incorrect first and then select that answer that seems more likely to be correct.

- Judge the time as you are moving through the examination. Keep assessing whether you are making sufficient progress or whether you can slow down or need to speed up.

- Answer all questions. Even if you have to guess quickly, at least fill in an answer. The best situation is that you answer all questions and have time left over to go back over the questions about which you are in doubt.

- Be certain to carefully complete the information sheet that accompanies the examination. This sheet will include your name, address, and other information that ensures that your test results are accurately recorded.

- Use every minute of the test time, but it is not a good idea to begin second-guessing yourself. Do not return to those questions for which you did not have serious doubts about the correct answer. Usually, your first answer is the best.

- When the time is finished, hand in your examination, and pat yourself on the back! You have done an excellent job. Now it is time to go get a good supper and a good night's sleep.

## DAYS AFTER THE EXAMINATION

- You will miss the preparation! Okay, maybe not miss it exactly, but your life will be different now without that constant preparation.

- Relax and await the results in confidence. You have done your best. That is always good enough!

- Be proud of yourself; this was no small undertaking, and you did it.

My personal best wishes to you as you prepare for your certification. You can do this!

Best regards,
**Carol J. Buck, MS, CPC, CPC-H, CCS-P**

*Our goals can only be reached through a vehicle of a plan, in which we must fervently believe, and upon which we must vigorously act. There is no other route to success.*

*Stephen A. Brennan*

# Course Syllabus and Student Calendar

The following documents are the syllabus and the course calendar that would be used in a classroom setting. It is suggested that these documents be used in development of your personal educational plan.

## COURSE SYLLABUS

### Course Description

The focus of this class is a review of terminology, anatomy, pathophysiology, and reimbursement as a preparation to take the coding certification examination. A review of CPT, ICD-9-CM, and HCPCS coding will be an integral part of this review course. Two practice certification review examinations will be taken under timed conditions. The course assists the learner in establishing a personal plan for continued development in preparation for a certification examination.

### Texts

*CPC® Coding Exam Review 2012: The Certification Step,* by Carol J. Buck, Elsevier

*The Practice Step: Physician-Based Coding Cases,* 2012 edition, by Carol J. Buck, Elsevier

*2012 ICD-9-CM, Volumes 1 & 2,* by Carol J. Buck, Elsevier

*2012 HCPCS Level II,* by Carol J. Buck, Elsevier

*2012 CPT,* American Medical Association

Medical dictionary

### Performance Objectives

1. Write a personal plan for preparation for a certification examination.

2. Review the structure, function, terminology, pathophysiology, and abbreviations of the integumentary system.

3. Review the structure, function, terminology, pathophysiology, and abbreviations of the musculoskeletal system.

4. Review the structure, function, terminology, pathophysiology, and abbreviations of the respiratory system.

5. Review the structure, function, terminology, pathophysiology, and abbreviations of the cardiovascular system.

6. Review the structure, function, terminology, pathophysiology, and abbreviations of the female genital system and pregnancy.

7. Review the structure, function, terminology, pathophysiology, and abbreviations of the male genital system.

8. Review the structure, function, terminology, pathophysiology, and abbreviations of the urinary system.

9. Review the structure, function, terminology, pathophysiology, and abbreviations of the digestive system.

10. Review the structure, function, terminology, pathophysiology, and abbreviations of the mediastinum and diaphragm.

11. Review the structure, function, terminology, pathophysiology, and abbreviations of the hemic and lymphatic systems.

12. Review the structure, function, terminology, pathophysiology, and abbreviations of the endocrine system.

13. Review the structure, function, terminology, pathophysiology, and abbreviations of the nervous system.

14. Review the structure, function, terminology, pathophysiology, and abbreviations of the senses of the body.

15. Demonstrate knowledge of organ system structure, function, terminology, pathophysiology, and abbreviations.

16. Review medical reimbursement issues.

17. Demonstrate knowledge of medical reimbursement issues.

18. Review CPT E/M section.

19. Review CPT Anesthesia section.

20. Review CPT Surgery section.

21. Review CPT Radiology section.

22. Review CPT Pathology and Laboratory section.

23. Review CPT Medicine section.

24. Review HCPCS.

25. Review format and conventions of ICD-9-CM.

26. Review assignment of ICD-9-CM codes.

27. Review *ICD-9-CM Official Guidelines for Coding and Reporting.*

28. Demonstrate coding ability by assigning CPT codes.

29. Demonstrate coding ability by assigning HCPCS codes.

30. Demonstrate coding ability by assigning ICD-9-CM codes.

## Personal Objectives

The student will:

- Attend class sessions.

- Prepare for class sessions.

- Complete assignments in a timely manner.

- Demonstrate a high level of responsibility.

- Display respect for other members of the class.

- Participate in class discussions.

## Evaluation and Grading

- Evaluation is directly related to the performance objectives.

- Performance is measured by examination, assignments, and/or quizzes.

- The letter grade is based on the percentage of the total points earned throughout the semester based on the following scale:

  - A = 93% to 100%

  - B = 85% to 92%

  - C = 79% to 84%

  - D = 70% to 78%

  - F = 69% and below

- Examinations are scheduled in advance. To qualify for the total points on the examinations, the student must take the examination at the scheduled time. Five points will be deducted from each examination if the examination is not taken at the scheduled time. This rule reinforces the need for on-time performance. Any make-up examination must be completed within 3 days of the scheduled examination or no points will be awarded for the examination.

- Assignments are scheduled in advance. To qualify for the total points on the assignment, the student must submit the completed assignment at the scheduled time. Five points are deducted from each assignment if the assignment is not submitted at the scheduled time. This rule reinforces the need for on-time performance. Any late assignment must be completed within 3 days from the date the assignment was due or no points will be awarded for the assignment.

- Quizzes are scheduled in advance. Quizzes cannot be made up, and no points are awarded for missed quizzes.

## Methods of Instruction

The instructional methods used include lecture, class discussion, and assignments.

# COURSE CALENDAR

## Lesson 1

Reading assignment(s):     Success Strategies, pages S1-S8

Assignment(s):     Complete the Pre-Examination located on the companion Evolve website, and at **Lesson 3** class period, hand in your summary sheet with your score for 75 points. The Pre-Examination is NOT graded if each question has been attempted. 1 point will be deducted for each question not attempted.
Download certification examination information at http://www.aapc.com/certification
Print one page to hand in at **Lesson 2** to demonstrate successful access to certification information from web (10 points—nongraded)
*The Practice Step: Physician-Based Coding Cases,* 2012 edition, Integumentary, Cases 1-4 (8 points)

## Lesson 2

Student hand in:     One printed page to demonstrate successful access to certifying organization's information from web (10 points—nongraded)
*The Practice Step: Physician-Based Coding Cases,* 2012 edition, Integumentary, Cases 1-4 (8 points)

Reading assignment(s):     Unit 1, pages 1-54 (through Musculoskeletal System)

Assignment(s):     Develop a personal plan for preparation for Certification Review (20 points—graded) to be submitted at **Lesson 6** class period
Integumentary Anatomy/Terminology (10 points) and Pathophysiology Quizzes (10 points)
Musculoskeletal Anatomy/Terminology (10 points) and Pathophysiology Quizzes (10 points)
*The Practice Step: Physician-Based Coding Cases,* 2012 edition, Orthopedics, Cases 1-4 (8 points)

## Lesson 3

Student hand in:     Integumentary System Quizzes (20 points)
Musculoskeletal Quizzes (20 points)
Pre-Examination (175 points, nongraded if each question attempted, deduct 1 point for each question not attempted)
*The Practice Step: Physician-Based Coding Cases,* 2012 edition, Orthopedics, Cases 1-4 (8 points)

Reading assignment(s):     Unit 1, pages 55-122 (through Female Genital System and Pregnancy)

Assignment(s):     Respiratory Anatomy/Terminology (10 points) and Pathophysiology Quizzes (10 points)
Cardiovascular Anatomy/Terminology (10 points) and Pathophysiology Quizzes (10 points)

Female Genital System and Pregnancy Anatomy/
Terminology (10 points) and Pathophysiology
Quizzes (10 points)
*The Practice Step: Physician-Based Coding Cases,*
2012 edition, Emergency Medicine, Cases 11-12
(4 points)
Cardiology, Cases 1-6 (12 points)
Obstetrics and Gynecology, Cases 1-4 (8 points)
Pediatrics, Neonatology, and Adolescent Medicine,
Cases 1-4 (8 points)

## Lesson 4

Student hand in:

Respiratory Quizzes (20 points)
Cardiovascular Quizzes (20 points)
Female Genital System and Pregnancy Quizzes
(20 points)
*The Practice Step: Physician-Based Coding Cases,*
2012 edition, Emergency Medicine, Cases 11-12
(4 points)
Cardiology, Cases 1-6 (12 points)
Obstetrics and Gynecology, Cases 1-4 (8 points)
Pediatrics, Neonatology, and Adolescent Medicine,
Cases 1-4 (8 points)

Reading assignment(s):

Unit 1, pages 123-194 (through Mediastinum and
Diaphragm)

Assignment(s):

Male Genital System Anatomy/Terminology
(10 points) and Pathophysiology Quizzes (10 points)
Urinary System Anatomy/Terminology (10 points) and
Pathophysiology Quizzes (10 points)
Digestive System Anatomy/Terminology (10 points)
and Pathophysiology Quizzes (10 points)
Mediastinum and Diaphragm Quiz (10 points) (There
is no pathophysiology quiz for Mediastinum and
Diaphragm.)
*The Practice Step: Physician-Based Coding Cases,* 2012
edition, Urology, Cases 1-4 (8 points)
Gastroenterology, Cases 1-4 (8 points)
Nephrology, Cases 1-4 (8 points)
Pediatrics, Neonatology, and Adolescent Medicine,
Cases 5-6 (4 points)

## Lesson 5

Student hand in:

Male Genital System Quizzes (20 points)
Urinary System Quizzes (20 points)
Digestive System Quizzes (20 points)
Mediastinum and Diaphragm Quiz (10 points) (There
is no pathophysiology quiz for Mediastinum and
Diaphragm.)
*The Practice Step: Physician-Based Coding Cases,* 2012
edition, Urology, Cases 1-4 (8 points)
Gastroenterology, Cases 1-4 (8 points)
Nephrology, Cases 1-4 (8 points)

Pediatrics, Neonatology, and Adolescent Medicine,
Cases 5-6 (4 points)

| | |
|---|---|
| Reading assignment(s): | Unit 1, pages 195-228 (through Endocrine System) |
| Assignment(s): | Hemic and Lymphatic Anatomy/Terminology (10 points) and Pathophysiology Quizzes (10 points) |
| | Endocrine Anatomy/Terminology (10 points) and Pathophysiology Quizzes (10 points) |
| | Prepare to submit Personal Plan for Preparation for Certification Examination (20 points—graded) |
| | *The Practice Step: Physician-Based Coding Cases,* 2012 edition, Nephrology, Cases 5-7 (6 points) |

## Lesson 6

| | |
|---|---|
| Student hand in: | Hemic and Lymphatic Quizzes (20 points) |
| | Endocrine Quizzes (20 points) |
| | Submit Personal Plan for Preparation for Certification Examination |
| | *The Practice Step: Physician-Based Coding Cases,* 2012 edition, Nephrology, Cases 5-7 (6 points) |
| Reading assignment(s): | Unit 1, pages 229-276 (through end of Unit 1) |
| Assignment(s): | Nervous System Anatomy/Terminology (10 points) and Pathophysiology Quizzes (10 points) |
| | Senses Anatomy/Terminology (10 points) and Pathophysiology Quizzes (10 points) |
| | Prepare for Unit 1, Anatomy, Terminology, and Pathophysiology, Test 1 (50 points, 25 questions, 15 minutes) |
| | *The Practice Step: Physician-Based Coding Cases,* 2012 edition, Neurology and Ophthalmology, Cases 1-4 (8 points) |

## Lesson 7

**UNIT 1: ANATOMY, TERMINOLOGY, AND PATHOPHYSIOLOGY, TEST 1**
**Timed Test: 15 Minutes**

| | |
|---|---|
| Student hand in: | Nervous System Quizzes (20 points) |
| | Senses Quizzes (20 points) |
| | *The Practice Step: Physician-Based Coding Cases,* 2012 edition, Neurology and Ophthalmology, Cases 1-4 (8 points) |
| Reading assignment(s): | Unit 2, pages 277-294 (through end of Unit 2) |
| Assignment(s): | None |

## Lesson 8

| | |
|---|---|
| Student hand in: | Reimbursement Quiz (10 points) |
| Reading assignment(s): | Unit 3, pages 295-301 (up to E/M section) |
| Assignment(s): | Prepare for Reimbursement, Test 2 (20 points, 10 questions, 10 minutes) |

## Lesson 9

**UNIT 2: REIMBURSEMENT, TEST 2**
**Timed Test: 10 Minutes**

Student hand in:     None

Reading assignment(s):     Unit 3, pages 302-311 (up to Contributory Factors)
Read E/M Guidelines

Assignment(s):     *The Practice Step: Physician-Based Coding Cases,*
2012 edition, Evaluation and Management,
Cases 1-8 (16 points)
Emergency Medicine, Cases 1-6 (12 points)

## Lesson 10

Student hand in:     *The Practice Step: Physician-Based Coding Cases,*
2012 edition, Evaluation and Management,
Cases 1-8 (16 points)
Emergency Medicine, Cases 1-6 (12 points)

Reading assignment(s):     Unit 3, pages 311-320 (up to Anesthesia section)

Assignment(s):     *The Practice Step: Physician-Based Coding Cases,*
2012 edition, Evaluation and Management,
Cases 9-19 (22 points)
Emergency Medicine, Cases 7-10 (8 points)

## Lesson 11

Student hand in:     *The Practice Step: Physician-Based Coding Cases,* 2012
edition, Evaluation and Management, Cases 9-19
(22 points)
Emergency Medicine, Cases 7-10 (8 points)

Reading assignment(s):     Unit 3, pages 321-323 (up to CPT/HCPCS Level I
Modifiers)

Read Anesthesia Guidelines

Assignment(s):     Prepare for E/M, Test 3 (25 points, 5 Guidelines
questions [10 points] and 3 cases [15 points],
15 minutes)
*The Practice Step: Physician-Based Coding Cases,* 2012
edition, Anesthesiology, Cases 1-6 (12 points)

## Lesson 12

**E/M, TEST 3**
**Timed Test: 15 Minutes**

Student hand in:     *The Practice Step: Physician-Based Coding Cases,* 2012
edition, Anesthesiology, Cases 1-16 (12 points)

Reading assignment(s):     Unit 3, pages 324-330 (up to Surgery section)

Assignment(s):     Prepare for Anesthesia, Test 4 (20 points, 5 Guidelines
questions [10 points], 2 cases [10 points], 15
minutes)
*The Practice Step: Physician-Based Coding Cases,* 2012
edition, Anesthesiology, Cases 7-11 (10 points)

## Lesson 13

**ANESTHESIA, TEST 4**
**Timed Test: 15 Minutes**

Student hand in:         *The Practice Step: Physician-Based Coding Cases*, 2012 edition, Anesthesiology, Cases 7-11 (10 points)

Reading assignment(s):     Unit 3, pages 330-332 (up to Integumentary System Subsection)
Read Surgery Guidelines

Assignment(s):         None

## Lesson 14

Student hand in:         None

Reading assignment(s):     Unit 3, pages 332-341 (up to Musculoskeletal System Subsection)

Assignment(s):         *The Practice Step: Physician-Based Coding Cases*, 2012 edition, Integumentary, Cases 5-9 (10 points)

## Lesson 15

Student hand in:         *The Practice Step: Physician-Based Coding Cases*, 2012 edition, Integumentary, Cases 5-9 (10 points)

Reading assignment(s):     Unit 3, pages 341-347 (up to Respiratory System Subsection)

Assignment(s):         *The Practice Step: Physician-Based Coding Cases*, 2012 edition, Orthopedics, Cases 5-13 (18 points)

## Lesson 16

Student hand in:         *The Practice Step: Physician-Based Coding Cases*, 2012 edition, Orthopedics, Cases 5-13 (18 points)

Reading assignment(s):     Unit 3, pages 347-351 (up to Cardiovascular System Subsection)

Assignment(s):         *The Practice Step: Physician-Based Coding Cases*, 2012 edition, Cardiology, Case 7 (Respiratory case) (2 points)
Otorhinolaryngology, Cases 2, 8, 11-13 (10 points)

## Lesson 17

Student hand in:         *The Practice Step: Physician-Based Coding Cases*, 2012 edition, Cardiology, Case 7 (Respiratory case) (2 points)
Otorhinolaryngology, Cases 2, 8, 11-13 (10 points)

Reading assignment(s):     Unit 3, pages 351-356 (up to Venous Reconstruction)

Assignment(s):         *The Practice Step: Physician-Based Coding Cases*, 2012 edition, Cardiology, Cases 8-10 (Cardiology cases) (6 points)

## Lesson 18

| | |
|---|---|
| Student hand in: | *The Practice Step: Physician-Based Coding Cases,* 2012 edition, Cardiology, Cases 8-10 (Cardiology cases) (6 points) |
| Reading assignment(s): | Unit 3, pages 356-363 (up to Hemic and Lymphatic System Subsection) |
| Assignment(s): | None |

## Lesson 19

| | |
|---|---|
| Student hand in: | None |
| Reading assignment(s): | Unit 3, pages 363-368 (up to Female Genital System Subsection) |
| Assignment(s): | *The Practice Step: Physician-Based Coding Cases,* 2012 edition, Gastroenterology, Cases 5-6 (4 points) Urology, Cases 5-10 (12 points) |

## Lesson 20

| | |
|---|---|
| Student hand in: | *The Practice Step: Physician-Based Coding Cases,* 2012 edition, Gastroenterology, Cases 5-6 (4 points) Urology, Cases 5-10 (12 points) |
| Reading assignment(s): | Unit 3, pages 368-378 (through Auditory System Subsection) |
| Assignment(s): | *The Practice Step: Physician-Based Coding Cases,* 2012 edition, Obstetrics and Gynecology, Cases 5-11 (14 points) General Surgery, Cases 1-11 (22 points) |

## Lesson 21

| | |
|---|---|
| Student hand in: | *The Practice Step: Physician-Based Coding Cases,* 2012 edition, Obstetrics and Gynecology, Cases 5-11 (14 points) General Surgery, Cases 1-11 (22 points) |
| Reading assignment(s): | None |
| Assignment(s): | *The Practice Step: Physician-Based Coding Cases,* 2012 edition, Neurology and Ophthalmology, Cases 5-10 (12 points) Otorhinolaryngology, Cases 1, 3-7, 9, and 10 (16 points) Diagnostic Radiology, Cases 1-13 (26 points) |

## Lesson 22

| | |
|---|---|
| Student hand in: | *The Practice Step: Physician-Based Coding Cases,* 2012 edition, Neurology and Ophthalmology, Cases 5-10 (12 points) Otorhinolaryngology, Cases 1, 3-7, 9, and 10 (16 points) Diagnostic Radiology, Cases 1-13 (26 points) |

| | |
|---|---|
| Reading assignment(s): | Unit 3, pages 378-385 (through Nuclear Medicine Subsection) |
| Assignment(s): | Prepare for Surgery, Test 5 (30 points, 9 questions, 5 Guidelines questions [10 points], 4 cases [20 points], 20 minutes) |
| | *The Practice Step: Physician-Based Coding Cases,* 2012 edition, Interventional Radiology and Radiation Oncology, Cases 1-7 (14 points) |

## Lesson 23

**SURGERY, TEST 5**
**Timed Test: 20 Minutes**

| | |
|---|---|
| Student hand in: | *The Practice Step: Physician-Based Coding Cases,* 2012 edition, Interventional Radiology and Radiation Oncology, Cases 1-7 (14 points) |
| Reading assignment(s): | Unit 3, pages 385-391 (up to Medicine Section) |
| Assignment(s): | Prepare for Radiology, Test 6 (22 points, 5 Guidelines questions, 1 non-Guidelines question [12 points], 2 cases [10 points], 15 minutes) |
| | *The Practice Step: Physician-Based Coding Cases,* 2012 edition, Interventional Radiology and Radiation Oncology, Cases 8-14 (14 points) |

## Lesson 24

**RADIOLOGY, TEST 6**
**Timed Test: 15 Minutes**

| | |
|---|---|
| Student hand in: | *The Practice Step: Physician-Based Coding Cases,* 2012 edition, Interventional Radiology and Radiation Oncology, Cases 8-14 (14 points) |
| Reading assignment(s): | Unit 3, pages 391-395 (up to Ophthalmology) |
| Assignment(s): | Prepare for Pathology and Laboratory, Test 7 (47 points, 5 Guidelines questions, 1 non-Guidelines question [12 points], 7 cases [35 points], 20 minutes) |
| | *The Practice Step: Physician-Based Coding Cases,* 2012 edition, Pathology, Cases 1-10 (20 points) |

## Lesson 25

**PATHOLOGY AND LABORATORY, TEST 7**
**Timed Test: 20 Minutes**

| | |
|---|---|
| Student hand in: | *The Practice Step: Physician-Based Coding Cases,* 2012 edition, Pathology, Cases 1-10 (20 points) |
| Reading assignment(s): | Unit 3, pages 395-403 (up to HCPCS Coding) |
| Assignment(s): | *The Practice Step: Physician-Based Coding Cases,* 2012 edition, Medicine, Cases 1-5 (10 points) |

## Lesson 26

Student hand in:  *The Practice Step: Physician-Based Coding Cases,* 2012 edition, Medicine, Cases 1-5 (10 points)

Reading assignment(s):  Unit 3, pages 403-410 (up to Using the ICD-9-CM)

Assignment(s):  Prepare for Medicine/HCPCS, Test 8 (36 points, 5 Guidelines questions, 3 non-Guidelines questions [16 points], 4 cases [20 points], 10 minutes)
*The Practice Step: Physician-Based Coding Cases,* 2012 edition, Medicine, Cases 6-10 (10 points)

## Lesson 27

**MEDICINE/HCPCS, TEST 8**
**Timed Test: 10 Minutes**

Student hand in:  *The Practice Step: Physician-Based Coding Cases,* 2012 edition, Medicine, Cases 6-10 (10 points)

Reading assignment(s):  Unit 3, pages 410-412 (up to Selection of Primary Diagnosis)

Assignment(s):  None

## Lesson 28

Student hand in:  None

Reading assignment(s):  Unit 3, pages 412-423 (up to Chapter 8, Diseases of Respiratory System)

Assignment(s):  Post-Examination (to hand in results at Lesson 30 class period)

## Lesson 29

Student hand in:  None

Reading assignment(s):  Unit 3, pages 423-430 (through end of Unit 3)

Assignment(s):  None

## Lesson 30

Student hand in:  Post-Examination results (75 points, nongraded if each question attempted, deduct 1 point for each question not attempted; hand in printed copy of summary of your score)

Reading assignment(s):  None

Assignment(s):  Prepare for ICD-9-CM, Test 9 (25 points, 5 cases, 20 minutes)
Bring ICD-9-CM, CPT, and HCPCS to class to begin Final Examination

## Lesson 31

**ICD-9-CM, TEST 9**
**Timed Test: 20 Minutes**

Final Examination beginning

| | |
|---|---|
| Student hand in: | None |
| Reading assignment(s): | None |
| Assignment(s): | Complete Final Examination (150 points) |

## Lesson 32

Final grade calculation
Course evaluation

# Anatomy, Terminology, and Pathophysiology

Make sure to check

evolve
learning system

for the latest
content updates

# ■ INTEGUMENTARY SYSTEM

## INTEGUMENTARY SYSTEM—ANATOMY AND TERMINOLOGY

The skin and accessory organs (nails, hair, and glands)

### Layers (Fig. 1–1)

### Two layers make up skin: epidermis and dermis

**Epidermis.** Outermost layer; containing keratin

Stratum corneum, most superficial layer of four layers called stratum

Basal layer, deepest region of epidermis (stratum germinativum or stratum basale), is growth layer

**Dermis.** The second layer of skin

Two layers are papillare and reticulare and contain:

    Fibrous connective tissue or skin appendages

    Blood vessels

    Nerves

    Hair

    Nails

    Glands

**Subcutaneous Tissue or Hypodermis.** Not considered a layer of skin

Contains fat tissue and fibrous connective tissue

AKA: superficial fascia

Connects skin to underlying muscle

### Nails

Keratin plates covering dorsal surface of each finger and toe

Lunula—semilunar or half-moon

    White area at base of nail plate is growth area

    Thickens and lengthens nail

Eponychium or cuticle: narrow band of epidermis at base and sides of nail

Paronychium: soft tissue around nail border

### Glands

**Sebaceous glands** located in dermal layer

Secrete sebum that lubricates skin/hair

Influenced by sex hormones so they hypertrophy in adolescence and atrophy in old age

**Sudoriferous glands** originate in dermis. See Fig. 1–1.

AKA: sweat glands

Extend up through epidermis opening as pores

Secrete mostly water and salts to cool body

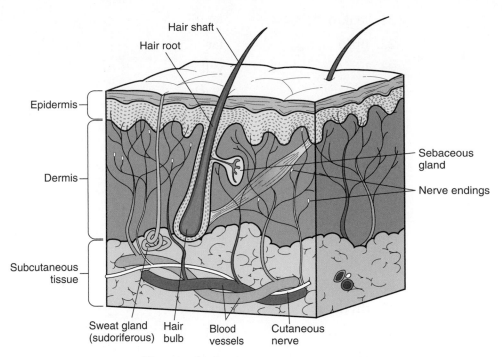

Figure **1-1** Integumentary system.

## COMBINING FORMS

| | | |
|---|---|---|
| 1. | aden/o | in relationship to a gland |
| 2. | adip/o | fat |
| 3. | albin/o | white |
| 4. | aut/o | self |
| 5. | bi/o | life |
| 6. | caus/o | burning sensation |
| 7. | cauter/o | burn |
| 8. | crypt/o | hidden |
| 9. | cutane/o | skin |
| 10. | cyan/o | blue |
| 11. | derm/o, dermat/o | skin |
| 12. | diaphor/o | profuse sweating |
| 13. | eosin/o | rosy |
| 14. | erythem/o | red |
| 15. | erythr/o | red |
| 16. | heter/o | different |
| 17. | hidr/o | sweat |
| 18. | ichthy/o | dry/scaly |
| 19. | jaund/o | yellow |
| 20. | kerat/o | hard |

| | | |
|---|---|---|
| 21. | leuk/o | white |
| 22. | lip/o | fat |
| 23. | lute/o | yellow |
| 24. | melan/o | black |
| 25. | myc/o | fungus |
| 26. | necr/o | death |
| 27. | onych/o | nail |
| 28. | pachy/o | thick |
| 29. | pht/o | plant |
| 30. | pil/o | hair |
| 31. | poli/o | gray matter |
| 32. | py/o | pus |
| 33. | rhytid/o | wrinkle |
| 34. | rube/o | red |
| 35. | seb/o | sebum/oil |
| 36. | staphyl/o | clusters |
| 37. | steat/o | fat |
| 38. | strept/o | twisted chain |
| 39. | steat/o | fat |
| 40. | squam/o | flat/scalelike |
| 41. | trich/o | hair |
| 42. | ungu/o | nail |
| 43. | xanth/o | yellow |
| 44. | xer/o | dry |

## PREFIXES

| | | |
|---|---|---|
| 1. | epi- | on/upon |
| 2. | hyper- | over |
| 3. | hypo- | under |
| 4. | intra- | within |
| 5. | para- | beside |
| 6. | per- | through |
| 7. | peri- | surrounding |
| 8. | sub- | under |

## SUFFIXES

1. -coccus        spherical bacterium
2. -ectomy        removal
3. -ia        condition
4. -malacia        softening
5. -opsy        view of
6. -plasty        surgical repair
7. -rrhea        discharge
8. -tome        an instrument to cut
9. -tomy        to cut

## MEDICAL ABBREVIATIONS

1. bx        biopsy
2. ca        cancer
3. derm        dermatology
4. I&D        incision and drainage
5. subcu, subq, SC, SQ        subcutaneous
6. PPD        tuberculin skin test

## MEDICAL TERMS

| | |
|---|---|
| Absence | Without |
| Adipose | Fatty |
| Albinism | Lack of color pigment |
| Allograft | Homograft, same species graft |
| Alopecia | Condition in which hair falls out |
| Anhidrosis | Deficiency of sweat |
| Autograft | From patient's own body |
| Avulsion | Ripping or tearing away of part either surgically or accidentally |
| Biopsy | Removal of a small piece of living tissue for diagnostic purposes |
| Causalgia | Burning pain |
| Collagen | Protein substance of skin |
| Debridement | Cleansing of or removal of dead tissue from a wound |
| Delayed flap | Pedicle of skin with blood supply that is separated from origin over time |
| Dermabrasion | Planing of skin by means of sander, brush, or sandpaper |
| Dermatologist | Physician who treats conditions of skin |
| Dermatoplasty | Surgical repair of skin |
| Electrocautery | Cauterization by means of heated instrument |
| Epidermolysis | Loosening of epidermis |

| | |
|---|---|
| Epidermomycosis | Superficial fungal infection |
| Epithelium | Surface covering of internal and external organs of body |
| Erythema | Redness of skin |
| Escharotomy | Surgical incision into necrotic (dead) tissue |
| Fissure | Cleft or groove |
| Free full-thickness graft | Graft of epidermis and dermis that is completely removed from donor area |
| Furuncle | Nodule in skin caused by *Staphylococcus* entering through hair follicle |
| Hematoma | A localized collection of blood, usually result of a break in a blood vessel |
| Hemograft | Allograft, same species graft |
| Ichthyosis | Skin disorder characterized by scaling |
| Incise | To cut into |
| Island pedicle flap | Contains a single artery and vein that remains attached to origin temporarily or permanently |
| Leukoderma | Depigmentation of skin |
| Leukoplakia | White patch on mucous membrane |
| Lipocyte | Fat cell |
| Lipoma | Fatty tumor |
| Melanin | Dark pigment of skin |
| Melanoma | Tumor of epidermis, malignant and black in color |
| Mohs surgery or Mohs micrographic surgery | Removal of skin cancer in layers by a surgeon who also acts as a pathologist during surgery |
| Muscle flap | Transfer of muscle from origin to recipient site |
| Neurovascular flap | Contains artery, vein, and nerve |
| Pedicle | Growth attached with a stem |
| Pilosebaceous | Pertains to hair follicles and sebaceous glands |
| Sebaceous gland | Secretes sebum |
| Seborrhea | Excess sebum secretion |
| Sebum | Oily substance |
| Split-thickness graft | All epidermis and some of dermis |
| Steatoma | Fat mass in sebaceous gland |
| Stratified | Layered |
| Stratum (strata) | Layer |
| Subungual | Beneath nail |
| Xanthoma | Tumor composed of cells containing lipid material, yellow in color |
| Xenograft | Different species graft |
| Xeroderma | Dry, discolored, scaly skin |

# INTEGUMENTARY SYSTEM ANATOMY AND TERMINOLOGY QUIZ

1. This is the outermost layer of skin:
   a. basal
   b. dermis
   c. epidermis
   d. subcutaneous

2. Which of the following is NOT a part of skin or accessory organs:
   a. sudoriferous glands
   b. sebaceous gland
   c. nail
   d. arterioles

3. This prefix means beside:
   a. para-
   b. intra-
   c. per-
   d. epi-

4. This combining form means hair:
   a. xanth/o
   b. trich/o
   c. ichthy/o
   d. kerat/o

5. Lunula is the:
   a. narrow band of epidermis at base of nail
   b. opening of pores
   c. outermost layer of epidermis
   d. white area at base of nail plate

6. Subcutaneous tissue is also known as:
   a. dermal
   b. adipose
   c. hypodermis
   d. stratum corneum

7. Which of the following combining forms does NOT refer to a color?
   a. cyan/o
   b. jaund/o
   c. eosin/o
   d. pachy/o

8. This medical term means surgical incision into dead tissue:
   a. onychomycosis
   b. escharotomy
   c. keratotomy
   d. curettage

9. This suffix means surgical repair:
   a. -opsy
   b. -rrhea
   c. -plasty
   d. -tome

10. Soft tissue around nail border is the:
   a. cuticle
   b. lunula
   c. paronychium
   d. corium

# INTEGUMENTARY SYSTEM—PATHOPHYSIOLOGY

## Lesions and Other Abnormalities (Fig. 1–2)

### Macule
Flat area of color change (mostly reddened)

No elevation or depression

*Example:* flat moles, freckles

### Papule
Solid elevation

Less than 1.0 cm in diameter

May run together and form plaques

*Example:* warts, lichen planus, elevated mole

### Nodule
Solid elevation 1-2 cm in diameter

Extends deeper into dermis than papule

*Example:* lipoma, erythema nodosum, enlarged lymph nodes

### Pustule
Elevated area

Filled with purulent fluid

*Example:* pimple, impetigo, abscess

### Tumor
Solid mass

Uncontrolled, progressive growth of cells

*Example:* hemangioma, neoplasm, lipoma

### Plaque
Flat, elevated surface

Equal or greater than 1.0 cm

*Example:* psoriasis, seborrheic keratosis

### Wheal
Temporary localized elevation of skin

Results in transient edema in dermis

*Example:* insect bite, allergic reaction

### Vesicle
Small blister

Less than 1 cm in diameter

Filled with serous fluid in epidermis

*Example:* herpes zoster (shingles), varicella (chickenpox)

### Bulla
Large blister

Greater than 1.0 cm in diameter

*Example:* blister

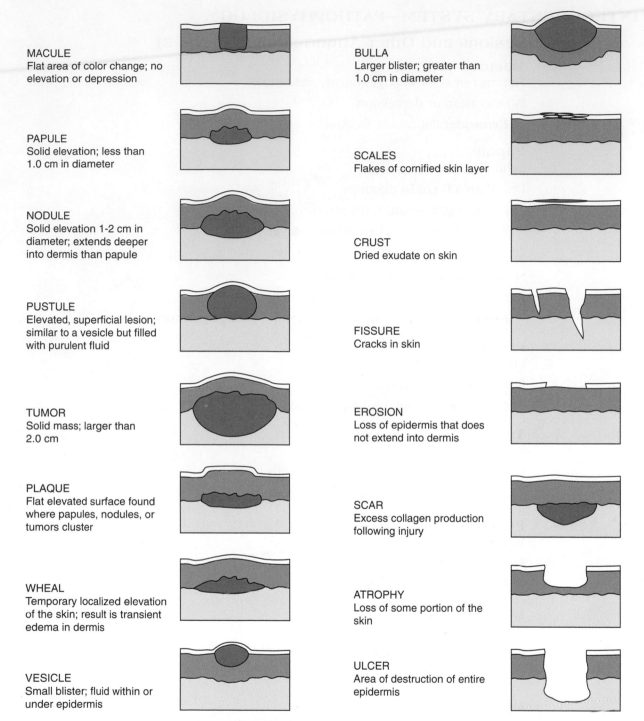

**MACULE**
Flat area of color change; no elevation or depression

**PAPULE**
Solid elevation; less than 1.0 cm in diameter

**NODULE**
Solid elevation 1-2 cm in diameter; extends deeper into dermis than papule

**PUSTULE**
Elevated, superficial lesion; similar to a vesicle but filled with purulent fluid

**TUMOR**
Solid mass; larger than 2.0 cm

**PLAQUE**
Flat elevated surface found where papules, nodules, or tumors cluster

**WHEAL**
Temporary localized elevation of the skin; result is transient edema in dermis

**VESICLE**
Small blister; fluid within or under epidermis

**BULLA**
Larger blister; greater than 1.0 cm in diameter

**SCALES**
Flakes of cornified skin layer

**CRUST**
Dried exudate on skin

**FISSURE**
Cracks in skin

**EROSION**
Loss of epidermis that does not extend into dermis

**SCAR**
Excess collagen production following injury

**ATROPHY**
Loss of some portion of the skin

**ULCER**
Area of destruction of entire epidermis

Figure **1-2** Lesions of skin.

## Scales
Flakes of cornified skin layer

**Example:** dry skin

## Crust
Dried exudate on skin

**Example:** scab

## Fissure
Cracks in skin

**Example:** athlete's foot, openings in corners of mouth

## Erosion
Loss of epidermis

Does not extend into dermis

**Example:** blisters

## Scar
Excess collagen production following surgery or trauma

**Example:** healed surgical wound

## Atrophy
Loss of some portion of skin and appears translucent

**Example:** aged skin

- Not a lesion, but a physiologic response in aging process

## Ulcer
Area of destruction of entire epidermis

**Example:** missing tissue on heel, decubitus bedsore (pressure sore)

## Pressure Ulcer (Decubitis Ulcer) (Fig. 1–3)
**Result of pressure or force**
Occludes blood flow, causing ischemia and tissue death

Develops over bony prominence

**Locations**
- Coccygeal (end of spine)
- Sacral (between hips)
- Heel
- Elbow
- Ischial (lower hip)
- Trochanteric (outer hip)

**Staging or classification system**
- Stage I: erythema (redness) of skin
- Stage II: partial loss of skin (epidermis or dermis)

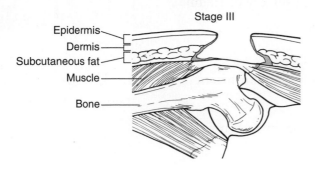

Figure **1-3** Stages I, II, III, and IV of pressure ulcers.

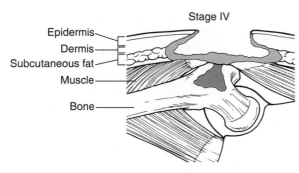

- Stage III: full thickness loss of skin (up to but not through fascia)
- Stage IV: full thickness loss (extensive destruction and necrosis)

  Deep ulcers may require surgical debridement

### Keloids

Sharply elevated, irregularly shaped scars that progressively enlarge

Due to excessive collagen in corneum during connective tissue repair

Result of tissue repair or trauma

Familial tendency for formation

**Cicatrix**
Normal scar left after wound healing

## Inflammatory Disorders

### Atopic Dermatitis
Unknown etiology

**Exogenous (external) causes include**
   Irritant dermatitis

   Allergic contact dermatitis

**Endogenous (internal) cause includes**
   Seborrheic dermatitis

**Results in activation of**
- Mast cells

- Eosinophils

- T lymphocytes

- Monocytes

**Greater in those with family history of**
- Asthma

- Dry skin

- Eczema

- Allergic rhinitis

**Common in**
- Children

- Infants

**Results in**
- Chronic inflammation

- Scratching

- Erythema

- Thickened, leathery skin (lichenification)

- Secondary *Staphylococcus aureus* infection

**Treatment**
- Topical steroid

- Antibiotic for secondary infection

- Antihistamines

### Allergic Contact Dermatitis
Most common in infants and children

**Potential causes**
- Hypersensitivity to allergens

  - Microorganisms

  - Drugs

- Foreign proteins
- Chemicals
- Latex
- Metals
- Plants

**Manifestations**
- Scaling
- Lichenification (leathery, thickened skin)
- Erythema
- Itching (pruritus)
- Vesicular lesions
- Edema

**Diagnosis and treatment**
- Check medical history
- Patch test
- Avoidance of irritant
- Skin lubrication and hydration
- Steroids
  - Topical
  - Systemic
- Topical tacrolimus (immunosuppressive agent)

## Irritant Contact Dermatitis
**Response to**
- Chemical
- Exposure to irritant

**Treatment**
- Removal of irritant
- Topical agents

## Stasis Dermatitis
Usually on the legs from venous stasis

**Associated with**
- Phlebitis
- Vascular trauma
- Varicosities

**Progress**
- Begins with erythema and pruritus
- Progresses to scaling, hyperpigmentation, petechia (small hemorrhagic areas)
- Lesion becomes ulcerated

**Treatment**
- Elevate legs
- Reduce standing
- No constricting clothes
- Eliminate external compression
- Antibiotics for acute lesions
- Silver nitrate or Burow's solution dressings for chronic lesions

## Seborrheic Dermatitis
Common chronic inflammation of sebaceous glands—cause unknown

Periods of remission and exacerbation

**Commonly occurs on**
- Scalp (cradle cap in infants)
- Ear canals
- Eyelids
- Eyebrow
- Nose
- Axillae
- Chest
- Groin

**Lesions are**
- Scaly (dry or greasy)
- White or yellowish
- Mildly pruritic

**Treatment of mild cases**
- Soap/shampoo of
  - Coal tar
  - Sulfur
  - Salicylic acid

**Treatment of more severe cases**
- Corticosteroid

## Papulosquamous Disorders
**Conditions associated with**
- Scales
- Papules
- Plaque
- Erythema

**Three types**
- Psoriasis

- Pityriasis

- Lichen planus

## Psoriasis
Chronic, relapsing, proliferating skin disorder

Usually begins by age 20

**Cause unknown, suggested to be**
- Exacerbated by anxiety; appears to run in families

- Immunologic

- Biochemical alterations

- Triggering agent

**Commonly occurs on**
- Face

- Scalp

- Forearms and elbows

- Knees and legs

**Results in**
- Thickened dermis and epidermis

- Well-demarcated plaque

- Cell hyperproliferation/scaly

- Inflammation (pruritus)

- Lesions that are deep red color

**Treatment**
- Only palliative (treatment of symptoms)

Mild cases

- Keratolytic agents

- Corticosteroids

- Emollients

Moderate cases

- Interleukin-2 inhibitors

- Psoralens and ultraviolet A (PUVA) light therapy

- Coal tar

- Cyclosporin

- Vitamin D analogs

Severe cases

- Topical agents

- Systemic corticosteroids

- Antimetabolic
- Hospitalization

## Pityriasis Rosea

Unknown cause

Self-limiting inflammatory disorder

Occurs most often in young adults

**Primary lesion**
- Begins with herald patch 3 to 4 cm
- Salmon-pink colored
- Circular and well-defined lesions

**Secondary lesions**
- 14 to 21 days

Trunk and upper extremities
- Oval lesions
- Severe pruritus

**Diagnosis**
May be confused with
- Secondary syphilis
- Seborrheic dermatitis
- Psoriasis

**Treatment**
- Antipruritics
- Antihistamines
- Corticosteroids
- Ultraviolet light
- Sunlight

## Lichen Planus

Occurs on skin and mucous membranes

Unknown cause (idiopathic)

Autoimmune inflammatory disorder

Onset ages 30 to 70

**Lesions**
- Begin as pink lesions that turn into violet-colored pruritic papules
- Results in hyperpigmentation
- 2- to 10-mm flat lesions with central depression
- Last 12 to 18 months
- Tend to reoccur

**Treatment**
- Antihistamines
- Corticosteroids

  Topical

  Systemic

## Acne Vulgaris

Site of lesion is sebaceous (pilosebaceous) follicles

Primarily on face and upper trunk

Occurs in 85% of the population between the ages of 12 and 25

Exact cause: unknown

Causative factor: sebum accumulation/inflammation in pores of skin

**Types**

Noninflammatory acne
- Whiteheads
- Blackheads

Inflammatory acne
- Follicle walls rupture
- Sebum expels into dermis
- Inflammation begins
  - Pustules, cysts, and papules result

**Cause**

Unknown

**Treatment**

Topical
- Antibiotics
- Salicylic acid
- Benzoyl peroxide
- Tretinoin

Systemic
- Antibiotic
- Hormones
- Corticosteroids
- Isotretinoin

## Diaper Dermatitis

Variety of disorders

**Causes**

Urine

Feces

Plastic diaper cover

Allergic reaction

Secondary *Candida albicans* infection

**Treatment**
Clean, dry area

Expose to air

Topical antifungal medications

Topical steroids

## Pruritus (Itching)
Symptom of skin disorder/dermatitis

Can be localized or generalized and is a condition not an inflammation

Results from stimulation of nerves of skin reacting to an allergen or irritation from substances in blood or foreign bodies

**Causes**
Primary skin disorder

    ***Example:*** eczema or lice

Systemic disease

    ***Example:*** chronic renal failure

Opiates

Allergic reaction

**Treatment is for underlying condition**
Antihistamines

Minor tranquilizers

Application of emollients (lotions)

Topical steroids

# Skin Infections

## ■ Bacterial
## Impetigo
Most common in infants and children

Usually on face and begins as small vesicles

Caused primarily by *Staphylococcus*

• Sometimes by group A beta-hemolytic *Streptococcus*

It is a highly contagious pyoderma

**Treatment in mild cases**
Topical antibiotics

Topical antiseptics

**Treatment in moderate cases**
Systemic antibiotics

Local compresses

Analgesics

## Cellulitis

Caused primarily by *Staphylococcus*

Often secondary to an injury

**Results in**

Erythema, usually of lower trunk and legs

Fever

Localized pain

Lymphangitis

**Treatment**

Systemic antibiotics

Burow's soaks for pain relief

## Furuncles (Boils)

Infected hair follicle

Usually caused by *Staphylococcus*

Developed boil drains pus and necrotic tissue

Squeezing spreads infection

Collection of furuncles that have merged is a carbuncle

## Folliculitis

Infection of hair follicles

**Results in**

Erythema

Pustules

**Causes**

Skin trauma, such as irritation or friction

Poor hygiene

Excessive skin moisture

**Treatment**

Cleansing of area

Topical antibiotics

## Erysipelas

Infection of skin

**Cause**

Group A beta-hemolytic *Streptococcus*

Common occurrence: face, ears, lower legs

Prior to outbreak, presents with

- Fever
- Malaise
- Chills

**Lesions appear as**
Bright red and hot

- Develops raised borders

- Itching

- Burning

- Tenderness

## Acute Necrotizing Fasciitis
**Flesh-eating disease**
Virulent strain of gram-positive, group A beta-hemolytic *Streptococcus*

Mortality rate of over 40%

**Causes**
　Skin trauma

　Skin infection

**Areas secrete tissue-destroying enzyme, proteases**
Extreme inflammation and pain

Rapidly increasing

Dermal gangrene develops

**Systemic toxicity may develop with**
　Fever

　Disorientation

　Hypotension

　Tachycardia (fast heart rate)

May lead to organ failure

**Treatment**
　Antimicrobial therapy

　Fluid replacement

　Removal of areas of infection

## ■ Viral
## Herpes Simplex (Cold Sores)
**Causes**
Herpes simplex virus type 1 (HSV-1)

- Most common type

- Results in fever blisters or cold sores on or near lips or canker sores of the mouth

Herpes simplex virus type 2 (HSV-2)

- Genital and oral type

- Prominent sexually transmitted disease

Primary infections may show no symptoms (asymptomatic)

Virus remains in nerve tissue to later reactivate

**Reactivation may be triggered by**
   Stress

   Common cold

   Exposure to sun

**Presents with**
   Burning or tingling

**Develops painful vesicles that rupture**
Causes spreading

May cause secondary infection of eye

- Episode lasts several weeks

- Treatment may include antiviral medication

   • No permanent cure exists

## Herpes Zoster (Shingles)
Usually older adult

**Caused by varicella-zoster virus (VZV)**
Virus was dormant and then reactivates

Result of varicella or chickenpox, usually in childhood

**Affects**
   One cranial nerve or one dermatome (an area of skin supplied with afferent nerve fibers by a posterior spinal root)

**Results in**
   Pain

   Rash (unilateral)

   Paresthesia (abnormal touch sensation, such as burning)

**Course**
   Several weeks

   Pain may continue even after lesion disappears

**Treatment**
   Clears spontaneously

   Antiviral medications provide symptomatic relief

   Sedatives

   Analgesic

   Antipruritics

## Warts (Verrucae)
Verruca vulgaris (common wart)

Caused by human papillomavirus (HPV)

- Numerous types of HPV

Spread by contact

Appear anywhere on body

Present with a grayish appearance

Variety of shapes and sizes

Transmitted by touch

Plantar warts (verrucae) are located on pressure points of body (such as feet; *plantar* means the bottom surface of foot)

Painful when pressure is applied

Juvenile warts occur on feet and hands of children

Venereal warts occur on genitals/anus

**Treatment**
> Liquid nitrogen
>
> Topical keratolytics
>
> Laser
>
> Electrocautery
>
> Often persist even with treatment

## Fungal (Mycoses)
Usually superficial dermatophytes (fungus)

Fungus lives off dead cells

**Tinea**
Superficial skin infections

Tinea capitis

- Infection of scalp
- Common in children
- Treatment with oral antifungal medication

Tinea corporis (ringworm)

- Infection of body
- Presents as a red ring
- Produces burning sensation and pruritus
- Treatment with topical antifungal medication

Tinea pedis (athlete's foot)

- Involves feet and toes
- Produces pain, inflammation, fissures, and foul odor
- Treatment with topical antifungal medication

Tinea unguium (onychomycosis)

- Nail infection
  - Usually toenails
- Nail turns white then brown, thickens and cracks
- Spreads to other nails

**Candidiasis**
Caused by *Candida albicans*

Normally on mucous membranes of gastrointestinal tract and vagina

Poor health and certain conditions predispose individuals to overarching infection by *Candida*

- Antibiotic therapy, which changes the balance of the normal flora in the body

Treatment is topical or oral antifungal medications

## Tumors of Skin

### ■ Benign Tumors
### Keratosis(es)
**Seborrheic keratosis**

Proliferation of basal cells

Dark colored lesion

Found on trunk and face

**Actinic keratosis**

Pigmented, scaly patch

Often caused by exposure to sun

Often in fair-skinned individuals

Premalignant lesion

May develop into squamous cell carcinoma

Treatment with cryosurgery (freezing area) or excision

**Keratoacanthoma**

Occurs in hair follicles

Usually in those over 60

Often on face, neck, back of hands, and other locations exposed to the sun

Resolve spontaneously or are excised

**Moles (Nevi)**

Located on any body part

Various shapes and sizes

May become malignant

- Especially if located in area of continual irritation

### ■ Malignant Tumors
### Squamous Cell Carcinoma
Similar to basal cell carcinoma

Grows wherever squamous epithelium is located (mouth, pharynx, esophagus, lungs, bladder)

Most often appears in areas exposed to sun (actinic keratosis—precancerous)

Scaly appearance

Rarely metastatic (spreading)

Easily treated with good prognosis

Surgical excision

Cryotherapy

Curettage

Electrodesiccation

Radiotherapy

## Basal Cell Carcinoma
Common type of skin cancer

Developed in deeper skin layers (basal cells) than squamous cell carcinoma

Often occurs with sun exposure in fair-skinned individuals

Shiny appearance and slow growing

Easily treated with good prognosis

## Malignant Melanoma
Originates in cells that produce pigment (melanocytes) or nevi

**Increased incidence with**
Sun exposure

Fair hair and skin, freckles

Genetic predisposition

Skin nevus (mole) often brown and evenly colored with irregular borders

Grow downward into tissues

- Metastasize quickly

Treatment is removal with extensive border excision

- Depending on extent, chemotherapy or radiation therapy may be used

## Kaposi's Sarcoma
Rare form of vascular skin cancer

**Associated with**
Human immunodeficiency virus (HIV)

Acquired immunodeficiency syndrome (AIDS)

Herpes virus may be found in lesions

Cells originate from endothelium in small blood vessels

Painful lesions develop rapidly, appearing as purple papules; spreads quickly to lymph nodes and internal organs

Treatment

Radiation

Chemotherapy

# INTEGUMENTARY SYSTEM PATHOPHYSIOLOGY QUIZ

1. A pimple is an example of a:
   a. papule
   b. vesicle
   c. pustule
   d. nodule

2. A Stage III pressure ulcer involves:
   a. erythema of skin
   b. partial loss of epidermis and dermis
   c. full thickness loss of skin up to but not through fascia
   d. full thickness loss of skin with extensive destruction and necrosis

3. This type of dermatitis may be exogenous or endogenous and is common in children and infants:
   a. atopic
   b. irritant contact
   c. stasis
   d. seborrheic

4. Psoriasis, pityriasis, and lichen planus are three types of this disorder:
   a. dermatitis
   b. inflammatory
   c. acne
   d. papulosquamous

5. This condition begins with a herald spot:
   a. psoriasis
   b. pityriasis
   c. lichen planus
   d. dermatitis

6. This skin infection is caused by group A beta-hemolytic *Streptococcus*, and the lesions appear as firm red spots with itching, burning, and tenderness:
   a. furuncles
   b. folliculitis
   c. erysipelas
   d. fasciitis

7. This type of herpes produces cold sores:
   a. herpes zoster
   b. shingles
   c. VZV
   d. herpes simplex

8. This condition is caused by human papillomavirus:
   a. mycoses
   b. verrucae
   c. shingles
   d. folliculitis

9. This type of tumor occurs in hair follicles:
   a. keratoses
   b. nevi
   c. Kaposi's sarcoma
   d. keratoacanthoma

10. This type of superficial carcinoma is rarely metastatic:
   a. squamous cell
   b. basal cell
   c. melanoma
   d. Kaposi's sarcoma

# ■ MUSCULOSKELETAL SYSTEM
## MUSCULOSKELETAL SYSTEM—ANATOMY AND TERMINOLOGY

### Skeletal System

Comprises 206 bones, cartilage, and ligaments

Provides organ protection, movement, framework, stores calcium, hematopoiesis (formation of blood cells)

### Classification of Bones
#### Long bones (tubular)
Length exceeds width of bone

Broad at ends, such as thigh, lower leg, upper arm, and lower arm

#### Short bones (cuboidal)
Cubelike bones, such as carpals (wrist) and tarsals (ankle)

#### *Flat*
Thin—flattened with curved surfaces

Cover body parts, such as skull, scapula, sternum, ribs

#### *Irregular*
Varied shapes, such as zygoma of face or vertebrae

#### *Sesamoid*
Rounded

Found near joint, such as patella (kneecap)

Patella is largest sesamoid bone in body

### Structure

#### Long Bones (Fig. 1–4)
Diaphysis: shaft

Epiphysis: both ends of long bones—bulbular shape with muscle attachments

• Articular cartilage covers epiphyses and serves as a cushion

Epiphyseal line or plate: growth plate that disappears when fully grown

Metaphysis: flared portion of bone near epiphyseal plate

Periosteum: dense, white outer covering (fibrous)

Cortical or compact bone: hard bone beneath periosteum mainly found in shaft

• Medullary cavity contains yellow marrow (fatty bone marrow)

Cancellous bones: spongy or trabecular

• Contains red bone marrow (blood cell development)

Endosteum is thin epithelial membrane lining medullary cavity of long bone

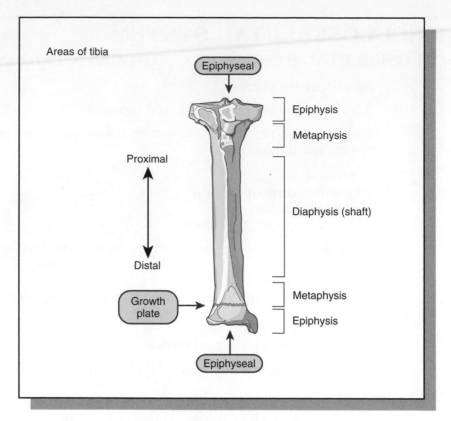

Figure **1-4** Structure of bones.

## Two Skeletal Divisions
Axial (trunk)

Appendicular (appendages)

## Axial Skeleton, comprised of 80 bones
Skull, hyoid bone, vertebral column, sacrum, ribs, and sternum

### Skull (Fig. 1–5)
*Cranial*
Frontal (forehead)

Parietal (sides and top)

Temporal (lower sides)

Occipital (posterior of cranium)

Sphenoid (floor of cranium)

Ethmoid (area between orbits and nasal cavity)

Styloid process (below ear)

Zygomatic process (cheek)

*Middle ear bones (Fig. 1–6)*
Malleus (hammer)

Incus (anvil)

Stapes (stirrup)

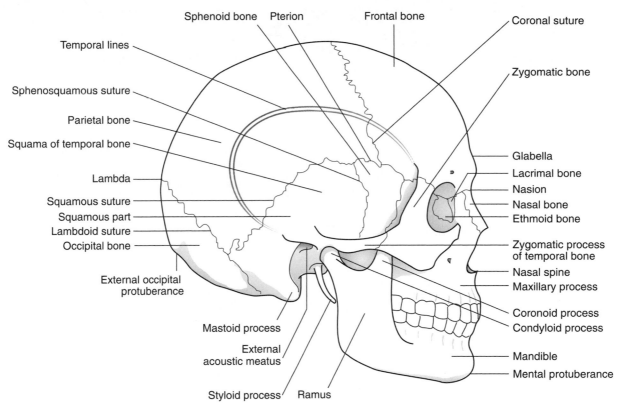

Temporal lines
Sphenosquamous suture
Parietal bone
Squama of temporal bone
Lambda
Squamous suture
Squamous part
Lambdoid suture
Occipital bone
External occipital protuberance
Mastoid process
External acoustic meatus
Styloid process
Ramus

Sphenoid bone
Pterion
Frontal bone
Coronal suture
Zygomatic bone
Glabella
Lacrimal bone
Nasion
Nasal bone
Ethmoid bone
Zygomatic process of temporal bone
Nasal spine
Maxillary process
Coronoid process
Condyloid process
Mandible
Mental protuberance

Figure **1-5** Lateral view of skull.

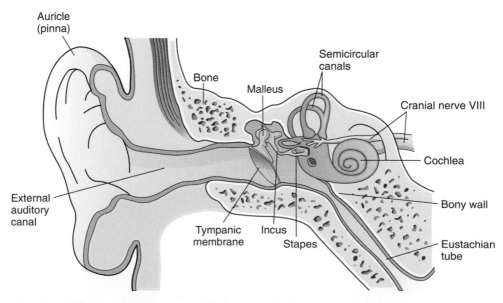

Auricle (pinna)
Bone
Malleus
Semicircular canals
Cranial nerve VIII
Cochlea
External auditory canal
Tympanic membrane
Incus
Stapes
Bony wall
Eustachian tube

Figure **1-6** Structure of ear and three divisions of external, middle, and inner ear.

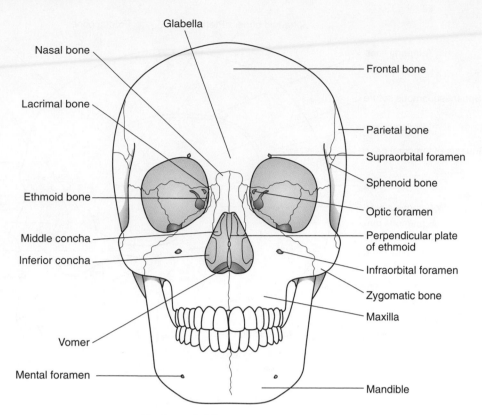

Figure **1-7** Frontal view of skull.

*Face (Fig. 1–7)*

Nasal (bridge of nose)

Maxilla (upper jaw)

Zygomatic (arch of cheekbone)

Mandible (lower jawbone)

Lacrimal (near orbits)

Palate (separates oral and nasal cavities)

Vomer (base, nasal septum)

Nasal conchae (turbinates)

    Interior

    Middle

    Superior

*Hyoid*

Supports tongue

U shaped

Attached by ligaments and muscles to larynx and skull

**Spine (33 vertebrae) (Fig. 1–8)**

Cervical vertebrae (7)

- C1-7

- (C1)-atlas

- (C2)-axis

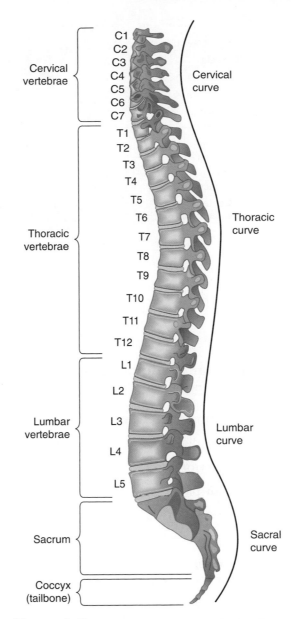

Figure **1-8** Anterior view of vertebral column.

Thoracic vertebrae (12) (T1-12)

Lumbar vertebrae (5) (L1-5)

Sacrum (5)—fused in adults

Coccyx (4)—fused in adults

**Thorax (Fig. 1–9)**
Ribs, 12 pairs

- True ribs, 1-7

- False ribs, 8-10

- Floating ribs, 11 and 12

Sternum

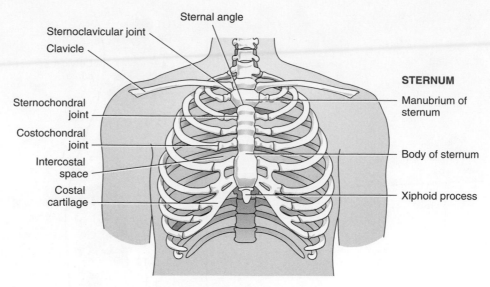

Figure **1-9** The thoracic cage.

## Appendicular Skeleton, comprised of 126 bones (Fig. 1-10)
Shoulder, girdle, pelvic girdle, and extremities
*Pelvis*
Ilium (uppermost part) wing shaped

• Acetabulum, depression on lateral hip surface into which head of femur fits

Ischium (posterior part)

Pubis (anterior part)

Pubis symphysis (cartilage between pubic bones)

**Lower extremities**
*Femur (thighbone)*
Trochanter (processes at neck of femur)

Head fits into acetabulum

Patella (kneecap)

Tibia (shinbone)

Fibula (smaller lateral bone in lower leg)

Talus (ankle bone)

Calcaneus (heel bone)

Metatarsals (foot instep)

Phalanges (toes)

Lateral malleolus (lower part of fibula)

Medial malleolus (lower part of tibia)

**Upper extremities**
Clavicle (collarbone)

Scapula (shoulder blade)

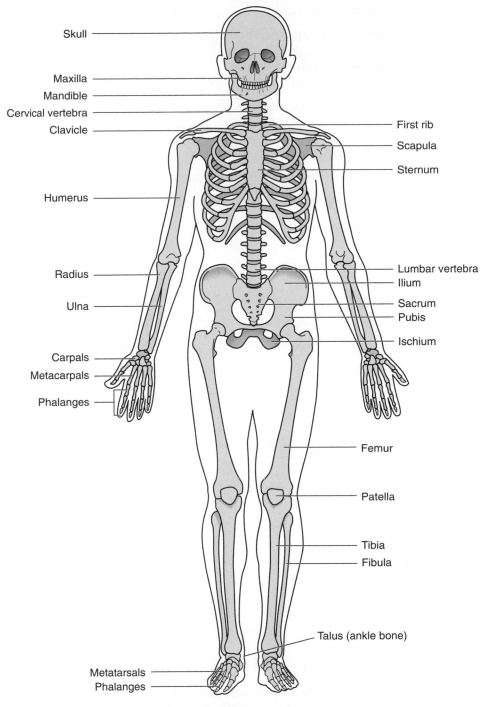

Skull

Maxilla
Mandible
Cervical vertebra
Clavicle

First rib
Scapula
Sternum

Humerus

Radius

Lumbar vertebra
Ilium

Ulna

Sacrum
Pubis

Ischium

Carpals
Metacarpals

Phalanges

Femur

Patella

Tibia
Fibula

Talus (ankle bone)

Metatarsals
Phalanges

Figure **1-10** Skeletal system.

Humerus (upper arm)

Radius (forearm, thumb side)

Ulna (forearm, little finger side)

Olecranon (projection of ulna at elbow)

Carpals (wrist)—eight bones bound by ligaments in two rows with 4 bones in each

Metacarpals (hand)—framework or palm of hand (5 bones)

Phalanges (finger)

Olecranon (tip of elbow)

### Joints (Articulations)
Condyle, rounded end of bone

Classified by degree of movement

- Synarthrosis (immovable and fibrous)

   ***Example:*** joint between cranial bones

- Amphiarthrosis (slightly movable and cartilaginous)

   ***Example:*** intervertebral (joint between bodies of vertebra)

- Diarthrosis (considerably movable and synovial)

Types

- Uniaxial—hinge and pivot joints

   Example—elbow (hinge and pivot) and cervical 2 (axis) (pivot)

- Biaxial—saddle and condyloid joints

   Example—thumb and joints between radius and carpal bones

- Multiaxial—ball and socket and gliding

   Example—shoulder and hip/joints between articular surfaces of vertebrae

***Example:*** elbow, hip

- Bursa, sac of synovial fluid located in the tissues to prevent friction

## Muscular System

### Functions
Heat production

Movement

Posture

Protection

Shape

## Muscle Tissue Types

### Skeletal—600 muscles constituting 40% to 50% of body weight
Striated (cross stripes) (Figs. 1–11 and 1–12)

Move body

Voluntary

Attaches to bones

- Most attach to two bones with a joint in between

- Origin, point where muscle attaches to stationary bone

- Insertion, where muscle attaches to movable bone

- Body of muscle, main part of muscle

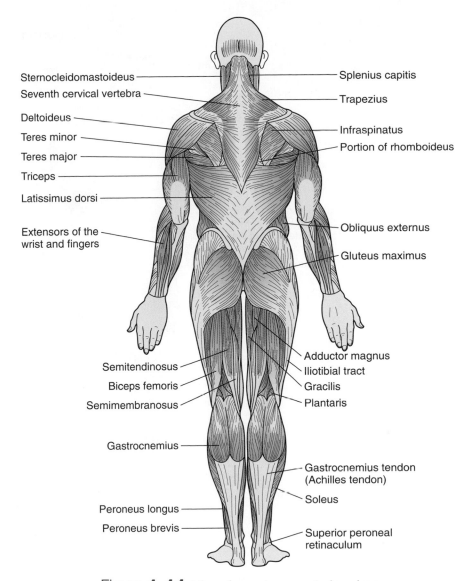

Sternocleidomastoideus
Seventh cervical vertebra
Deltoideus
Teres minor
Teres major
Triceps
Latissimus dorsi
Extensors of the wrist and fingers

Splenius capitis
Trapezius
Infraspinatus
Portion of rhomboideus
Obliquus externus
Gluteus maximus

Semitendinosus
Biceps femoris
Semimembranosus

Adductor magnus
Iliotibial tract
Gracilis
Plantaris

Gastrocnemius

Gastrocnemius tendon (Achilles tendon)
Soleus

Peroneus longus
Peroneus brevis

Superior peroneal retinaculum

Figure **1-11** Muscular system, posterior view.

### Cardiac/Heart Muscle
Striated and smooth muscle

   Specialized cells that interlock so that muscle cells contract together

Involuntary

Moves blood by means of contractions

### Smooth/Visceral
Linings such as bowel, urethra, blood vessels

Nonstriated

Involuntary

### Tendons Anchor Muscle to Bone

### Ligaments Anchor Bones to Bones

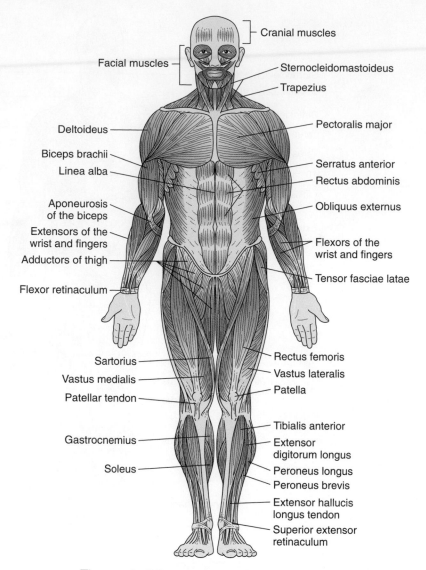

**Cranial muscles**

Facial muscles —

Sternocleidomastoideus

Trapezius

Deltoideus —

Pectoralis major

Biceps brachii —

Linea alba —

Serratus anterior

Rectus abdominis

Aponeurosis
of the biceps —

Obliquus externus

Extensors of the
wrist and fingers —

Flexors of the
wrist and fingers

Adductors of thigh —

Flexor retinaculum —

Tensor fasciae latae

Sartorius —

Rectus femoris

Vastus medialis —

Vastus lateralis

Patellar tendon —

Patella

Tibialis anterior

Gastrocnemius —

Extensor
digitorum longus

Soleus —

Peroneus longus

Peroneus brevis

Extensor hallucis
longus tendon

Superior extensor
retinaculum

Figure **1-12** Muscular system, anterior view.

## Muscle Action

### Muscle Capabilities
Stretches

Contracts

Receives and responds to stimulus

Returns to original shape and length

### Muscle Movement
Prime mover, responsible for movement (agonist)

Synergist, assists prime mover

Antagonist, relaxes as prime mover and synergists contract, resulting in movement

Fixator, acts as joint stabilizer

## Terms of Movement—from midline of body

Flexion (bend)

Extension (straighten)

Abduction (away)

Adduction (toward)

Rotation (turn on axis)

Circumduction (circular)

Supination (turning palm upward or forward [anteriorly] or lying down with face upward)

Pronation (turning palm downward or backward or act of lying face down)

Hyperextension (overextension)

Inversion (inward)

Eversion (outward)

## Names of Muscles

### Head and neck
Facial expression

- Occipitofrontalis (raises eyebrows and wrinkles forehead horizontally)

- Corrugator supercilii (wrinkles forehead vertically)

- Orbicularis oris (opens mouth)

- Zygomaticus (elevates corners of mouth)

- Orbicularis oculi (opens and closes eyelid)

- Buccinator (smiling and blowing)

Mastication (chewing)

- Masseter (used to chew closing jaw)

- Temporalis (closes jaw)

- Pterygoids (grates teeth)

Muscles moving head

- Sternocleidomastoid (flexes head)

- Semispinalis capitis (complexus) (extends head)

- Splenius capitis (extends head, bends and rotates head to side where muscle is contracting)

- Longissimus capitis (trachelomastoid muscle) (extends head, bends and rotates to contracting side)

- Trapezius (extends head)

### Upper extremities
Biceps brachii (flexes elbow)

Triceps brachii and anconeus (extends elbow)

Brachialis (flexes prone forearm)

Brachioradialis (flexes semi-prone/supinated forearm)

Deltoid (abducts upper arm)

Latissimus dorsi (extends upper arm)

Pectoralis major (flexes upper arm)

Trapezius (raises/lowers shoulder)

**Trunk**
External oblique (compresses abdomen)

Internal oblique (compresses abdomen)

Transversus abdominis (compresses abdomen)

Rectus abdominis (flexes trunk)

Quadratus lumborum (flexes vertebral column laterally)

**Respiratory**
Diaphragm (enlarges thorax/inspiration)

External intercostals (raise ribs)

Internal intercostal (depress ribs)

**Lower extremities**
Thigh

* Gluteus group, maximus, medius, minimus (abducts thigh)

* Tensor fasciae latae (abducts thigh)

* Abductor group, brevis, longus, magnus (adducts thigh)

* Gracilis (adducts thigh)

* Iliopsoas (flexes thigh)

* Rectus femoris (flexes thigh)

Hamstring group, biceps femoris, semitendinosus, semimembranosus (extends thigh)

Quadriceps group, rectus femoris, vastus lateralis, vastus medialis, vastus intermedius (extends lower leg)

Sartorius (flexes, abducts, and rotates leg)

Lower leg

Tibialis anterior (dorsiflexes foot)

Peroneus group, longus, brevis, tertius (everts foot)

Gastrocnemius (calf, with soleus extends foot, also flexes knee)

Soleus (calf, extends foot)

Extensor digitorum longus (extends toes, flexes foot)

Achilles tendon (largest tendon, extending from gastrocnemius to calcaneus)

## COMBINING FORMS

1. acetabul/o          hip socket

2. ankyl/o            bent, fused

| | | |
|---|---|---|
| 3. | aponeur/o | tendon type |
| 4. | arthr/o | joint |
| 5. | articul/o | joint |
| 6. | burs/o | fluid-filled sac in a joint |
| 7. | calc/o, calci/o | calcium |
| 8. | calcane/o | calcaneus (heel) |
| 9. | carp/o | carpals (wrist bones) |
| 10. | chondr/o | cartilage |
| 11. | clavic/o, clavicul/o | clavicle (collar bone) |
| 12. | cost/o | rib |
| 13. | crani/o | cranium (skull) |
| 14. | disc/o | intervertebral disc |
| 15. | femor/o | thighbone |
| 16. | fibul/o | fibula |
| 17. | humer/o | humerus (upper arm bone) |
| 18. | ili/o | ilium (upper pelvic bone) |
| 19. | ischi/o | ischium (posterior pelvic bone) |
| 20. | kinesi/o | movement |
| 21. | kyph/o | hump |
| 22. | lamin/o | lamina |
| 23. | lord/o | curve |
| 24. | lumb/o | lower back |
| 25. | malleol/o | malleolus (process on lateral ankle) |
| 26. | mandibul/o | mandible (lower jawbone) |
| 27. | maxill/o | maxilla (upper jawbone) |
| 28. | menisc/o | meniscus |
| 29. | menisci/o | meniscus |
| 30. | metacarp/o | metacarpals (hand) |
| 31. | metatars/o | metatarsals (foot) |
| 32. | myel/o | bone marrow |
| 33. | my/o, muscul/o | muscle |
| 34. | olecran/o | olecranon (elbow) |
| 35. | orth/o | straight |
| 36. | oste/o | bone |
| 37. | patell/o | patella (kneecap) |
| 38. | pelv/i | pelvis (hip) |
| 39. | perone/o | fibula |

| | | |
|---|---|---|
| 40. | petr/o | stone |
| 41. | phalang/o | phalanges (finger or toe) |
| 42. | plant/o | sole of foot |
| 43. | pub/o | pubis |
| 44. | rachi/o | spine |
| 45. | radi/o | radius (lower arm) |
| 46. | rhabdomy/o | skeletal (striated muscle) |
| 47. | rheumat/o | watery flow (collection of fluids in joints) |
| 48. | sacr/o | sacrum |
| 49. | scapul/o | scapula (shoulder) |
| 50. | scoli/o | bent |
| 51. | spondyl/o | vertebra |
| 52. | stern/o | sternum (breast bone) |
| 53. | synovi/o | synovial joint membrane |
| 54. | tars/o | tarsal (ankle/foot) |
| 55. | ten/o | tendon |
| 56. | tend/o | tendon (connective tissue) |
| 57. | tendin/o | tendon (connective tissue) |
| 58. | tibi/o | shin bone |
| 59. | uln/o | ulna (lower arm bone) |
| 60. | vertebr/o | vertebra |

## PREFIXES

| | | |
|---|---|---|
| 1. | inter- | between |
| 2. | supra- | above |
| 3. | sym- | together |
| 4. | syn- | together |

## SUFFIXES

| | | |
|---|---|---|
| 1. | -asthenia | weakness |
| 2. | -blast | embryonic |
| 3. | -clast, -clasia, -clasis | break |
| 4. | -desis | bind together |
| 5. | -listhesia | slipping |
| 6. | -malacia | softening |
| 7. | -physis | to grow |
| 8. | -porosis | passage, cavity formation |
| 9. | -schisis | split |
| 10. | -stenosis | narrowing |

| | | |
|---|---|---|
| 11. | -tome | instrument that cuts |
| 12. | -tomy | incision |

## MEDICAL ABBREVIATIONS

| | | |
|---|---|---|
| 1. | ACL | anterior cruciate ligament |
| 2. | AKA | above-knee amputation |
| 3. | BKA | below-knee amputation |
| 4. | C1-C7 | cervical vertebrae |
| 5. | CTS | carpal tunnel syndrome |
| 6. | fx | fracture |
| 7. | L1-L5 | lumbar vertebrae |
| 8. | OA | osteoarthritis |
| 9. | RA | rheumatoid arthritis |
| 10. | T1-T12 | thoracic vertebrae |
| 11. | TMJ | temporomandibular joint |

## MEDICAL TERMS

| | |
|---|---|
| Arthrocentesis | Injection and/or aspiration of joint |
| Arthrodesis | Surgical immobilization of a joint |
| Arthrography | Radiography of joint |
| Arthroplasty | Reshaping or reconstruction of a joint |
| Arthroscopy | Use of scope to view inside joint |
| Arthrotomy | Incision into a joint |
| Articular | Pertains to a joint |
| Aspiration | Use of a needle and a syringe to withdraw fluid |
| Atrophy | Wasting away |
| Bunion | Hallux valgus, abnormal increase in size of metatarsal head that results in displacement of great toe |
| Bursitis | Inflammation of bursa (joint sac) |
| Chondral | Referring to the cartilage |
| Carpal tunnel syndrome | Compression of medial nerve |
| Closed fracture repair | Not surgically opened with/without manipulation and with/without traction |
| Closed treatment | Fracture site that is not surgically opened and visualized |
| Colles' fracture | Fracture at lower end of radius that displaces bone posteriorly |
| Dislocation | Placement in a location other than original location |
| Endoscopy | Inspection of body organs or cavities using a lighted scope that may be inserted through an existing opening or through a small incision |

| | |
|---|---|
| Fasciectomy | Removal of band of fibrous tissue |
| Fissure | Groove |
| Fracture | Break in a bone |
| Ganglion | Knot or knotlike mass |
| Internal/External fixation | Application of pins, wires, screws, placed externally or internally to immobilize a body part |
| Kyphosis | Humpback |
| Lamina | Flat plate |
| Ligament | Fibrous band of tissue that connects cartilage or bone |
| Lordosis | Anterior curve of spine |
| Lumbodynia | Pain in lumbar area |
| Lysis | Releasing |
| Manipulation or reduction | Alignment of a fracture or joint dislocation to normal position |
| Open fracture repair | Surgical opening (incision) over or remote opening as access to a fracture site |
| Osteoarthritis | Degenerative condition of articular cartilage |
| Osteoclast | Absorbs or removes bone |
| Osteotomy | Cutting into bone |
| Percutaneous | Through skin |
| Percutaneous fracture repair | Repair of a fracture by means of pins and wires inserted through the fracture site |
| Percutaneous skeletal fixation | Considered neither open nor closed; fracture is not visualized, but fixation is placed across fracture site under x-ray imaging |
| Reduction | Replacement to normal position |
| Scoliosis | Lateral curve of spine |
| Skeletal traction | Application of pressure to bone by means of pins and/or wires inserted into bone |
| Skin traction | Application of pressure to bone by means of tape applied to the skin |
| Spondylitis | Inflammation of vertebrae |
| Subluxation | Partial dislocation |
| Supination | Supine position—lying on back, face upward |
| Synchondrosis | Union between two bones (connected by cartilage) |
| Tendon | Attaches a muscle to a bone |
| Tenodesis | Suturing of a tendon to a bone |
| Tenorrhaphy | Suture repair of tendon |
| Traction | Application of pressure to maintain normal alignment |
| Trocar needle | Needle with a cannula that can be removed; used to puncture and withdraw fluid from a cavity |

# MUSCULOSKELETAL SYSTEM ANATOMY AND TERMINOLOGY QUIZ

1. Tubular is another name for these bones:
   a. short
   b. long
   c. flat
   d. irregular

2. These bones are found near joints:
   a. irregular
   b. flat
   c. sesamoid
   d. broad

3. Zygoma is an example of this type of bone:
   a. irregular
   b. flat
   c. sesamoid
   d. broad

4. Diaphysis is this part of bone:
   a. end
   b. surface
   c. shaft
   d. marrow

5. Which is NOT a part of cranium?
   a. condyle
   b. sphenoid
   c. ethmoid
   d. parietal

6. This is NOT an ear bone:
   a. malleus
   b. stapes
   c. incus
   d. styloid

7. This term describes growth plate:
   a. endosteum
   b. epiphyseal
   c. metaphysis
   d. periosteum

8. This is a depression on lateral hip surface into which head of femur fits:
   a. ilium
   b. ischium
   c. patella
   d. acetabulum

9. Tip of elbow is the:
   a. olecranon
   b. trapezium
   c. humerus
   d. tarsal

10. This term describes an immovable joint:
    a. amphiarthrosis
    b. diarthrosis
    c. synarthrosis
    d. ischium

# MUSCULOSKELETAL SYSTEM—PATHOPHYSIOLOGY

## Injuries

### ■ Fractures

### Classification of fractures

**Open/closed**

Open (compound): broken bone penetrates skin

Closed (simple): broken bone does not penetrate skin

**Complete/incomplete**

Complete: bone is broken all way through

    ***Example:*** oblique, linear, spiral, and transverse

Incomplete: bone is not broken all way through

    ***Example:*** greenstick, bowing, torus, stress, and transchondral

**Treatment**

Closed reduction (realignment of bone fragments by manipulation)

Reduction (the returning of the bone to normal alignment)

Immobilization (returns to normal alignment and holds in place)

Traction (application of pulling force to hold bone in alignment)

- Skeletal traction uses internal devices (pins, screws, wires, etc.) inserted into bone with ends sticking out through skin for attachment of traction device (Fig. 1–13)

- Skin traction is use of strapping, elastic wrap, or tape attached to skin to which weights are attached (Fig. 1–14)

Figure **1-13** Skeletal traction uses patient's bones to secure internal devices to which traction is attached.

Figure **1-14** Skin traction utilizes strapping, wraps, or tape to which traction is attached.

**Improper union**

Nonunion: failure of bone ends to grow together

Malunion: incorrect alignment of bone ends

Delayed union: delay of bone union 8 or 9 months

**Dislocations**

Bone and soft tissue damage usually caused by trauma

Any part of bone is displaced

Can result in nerve and tissue damage

**Treatment**

Reduction

Immobilization

**Sprains and strains**

Soft tissue damage usually caused by trauma to tendons and ligaments

Strain: partial tear of a tendon

Sprain results from overuse or overextension/tearing or rupture of some part of musculature

## Bone Disorders

### Osteomyelitis

Bone infection

Usually caused by bacteria

- Exogenous osteomyelitis is caused by bacteria that enter from outside body
- Hematogenous osteomyelitis (endogenous) is caused by a bacterial infection within body

### Osteoporosis

Common disorder in postmenopausal women and elderly and most common metabolic disease

- Malabsorption of calcium and magnesium; certain trace elements and vitamins C and D contribute to bone loss

Decreased bone mass and density

- Fractures more common due to decrease in strength of bone

**Treatment**

Increased intake of calcium, magnesium, and vitamin D

Increased weight-bearing activity

## Osteomalacia and Rickets

Osteomalacia is softened adult bones, while rickets is softened growing bones in children

Caused by vitamin D and phosphate deficiency

## Osteitis Deformans (Paget's Disease)

Abnormal bone remodeling and resorption resulting in enlarged, soft bones

Unknown cause but strong genetic considerations

**Treatment**

Calcitonin and biophosphates

## Spinal Curvatures

Lordosis: swayback

- Inward curvature of spine

Kyphosis: humpback

- Outward curvature of spine

Scoliosis

- Lateral curvature of spine

## Spina Bifida

Congenital abnormality in which vertebrae do not close correctly around the spinal cord

# Joint Disorders

Bursitis: inflammation of bursa (joint sac)

Arthritis: inflammation of joints

## Osteoarthritis (OA)

This is degenerative or wear/tear arthritis

- DJD, degenerative joint disease

Chronic inflammation of joint

Increased pain on weightbearing or movement

Affects weight-bearing joints

- Loss of articular cartilage
- Sclerosis of bone—eburnation

  Turning bone into ivorylike mass—polished

- Osteophytes (bone spurs)

**Symptoms**

Pain and stiffness

Crepitation (bone on bone creates characteristic grinding sound)

**Classifications**

Primary (idiopathic)

- No known cause

Secondary

- Associated with joint instability, joint stress, or congenital abnormalities

**Treatment**

Symptomatic

Arthroplasty

## Rheumatoid Arthritis (RA)

Progressive inflammatory connective tissue disease of the joints

Systemic autoimmune disease

- Can invade arteries, lung, skin, and other organs with nodules

Affects small joints

- Destroys synovial membrane, articular cartilage, and surrounding tissues

Leads to loss of function due to fixation and deformity

**Treatment**

Pharmaceuticals to modify autoimmune and inflammatory processes

Gene therapy and stem cell transplantation are being researched

Symptomatic

Arthroplasty

## Infectious and Septic Arthritis

Infectious process

Usually affects single joint

Without antimicrobial intervention, permanent joint damage results

*Example:* Lyme disease

**Treatment**

Antibiotics—early intervention

## Gout (Gouty Arthritis)

Inflammatory arthritis

Often affects the joint of the great toe

Caused by excessive amounts of uric acid that crystallizes in connective tissue of joints

Leads to inflammation and destruction of joint

**Treatment**

Pharmaceuticals—nonsteroidal antiinflammatory drugs

## Ankylosing Spondylitis (AS)

Inflammatory disease that is progressive

Affects vertebral joints and insertion points of ligaments, tendons, and joint capsules

Leads to rigid spinal column and sacroiliac joints

**Treatment**
Nonsteroidal anti-inflammatory drugs relieve symptoms

Analgesics for pain

# Tendon, Muscle, and Ligament Disorders

## Muscular Dystrophy—Familial Disorder
Progressive degenerative muscle disorder

Multiple types of muscular dystrophy

Most often affects boys

- Genetic predisposition—Duchenne muscular dystrophy

## Primary Fibromyalgia Syndrome
**Symptoms**
Generalized aching and pain

Tender points

Fatigue

Depression

**Usually appears in**
Middle-aged women

## Polymyositis
General muscle inflammation causing weakness

- With skin rash = dermatomyositis

# Tumors

## Bone Tumors
**Origin of bone tumors**
Osteogenic (bone cells)

Chondrogenic (cartilage cell)

Collagenic (fibrous tissue cell)

Myelogenic (marrow cell)

**Osteoma**
Benign

Abnormal outgrowth of bone

**Chondroblastoma**
Rare

Usually benign

**Osteosarcoma**
Malignant tumor of long bones

Usually in young adults

Typically causes bone pain

**Multiple myeloma**

Malignant plasma cells in skeletal system and soft tissue

Progressive and generally fatal

Usually in those over 40

**Chondrosarcoma**

Malignant cartilage tumor

Usually in middle-aged and older individuals

In late stages, symptoms include local swelling and pain

- Worsens with time

Surgical excision is usually treatment of choice

If diagnosed in early stages, it is treatable with long-term survival possible

## Muscle Tumors

Rare

Rhabdomyosarcoma

Aggressive, invasive carcinoma with widespread metastasis

# MUSCULOSKELETAL SYSTEM PATHOPHYSIOLOGY QUIZ

1. A compound fracture is also known as:
   a. complete
   b. incomplete
   c. closed
   d. open

2. This is a common bone disorder in postmenopausal women resulting from lower levels of calcium and potassium:
   a. Paget's disease
   b. lordosis
   c. osteoporosis
   d. rheumatoid arthritis

3. This inflammatory disease is progressive and leads to a rigid spinal column:
   a. polymyositis
   b. ankylosing spondylitis
   c. primary fibromyalgia syndrome
   d. septic arthritis of spine

4. This type of tumor arises from bone cells:
   a. osteogenic
   b. chondrogenic
   c. collagenic
   d. myelogenic

5. This type of tumor is the most common type of malignant bone tumor that occurs in those over 40 and is progressive and generally fatal:
   a. rhabdomyosarcoma
   b. chondrosarcoma
   c. osteosarcoma
   d. multiple myeloma

6. A general muscle inflammation with an accompanying skin rash is:
   a. muscular dystrophy
   b. dermatologic arthritis
   c. ankylosing spondylitis
   d. dermatomyositis

7. A cartilage tumor that usually occurs in middle-aged and older individuals:
   a. chondrosarcoma
   b. osteosarcoma
   c. chondroblastoma
   d. rhabdomyosarcoma

8. Returning of bone to normal alignment is:
   a. immobilization
   b. traction
   c. reduction
   d. manipulation

9. Result of overuse or overextension of a ligament is:
   a. strain
   b. sprain
   c. fracture
   d. displacement

10. Primary osteoarthritis is also known as:
    a. secondary
    b. functional
    c. congenital
    d. idiopathic

# ■ RESPIRATORY SYSTEM
## RESPIRATORY SYSTEM—ANATOMY AND TERMINOLOGY

Supplies oxygen to body and helps clean body of waste (carbon dioxide)

Two tracts (Fig. 1–15A)

- Upper respiratory tract (nose, pharynx, and larynx)

- Lower respiratory tract (trachea, bronchial tree, and lungs)

Lined with ciliated mucosa

- Purifies air by trapping irritants

Warms and humidifies air

### Upper Respiratory Tract (URT)

### Nose
Sense of smell (olfactory)

Moistens and warms air

Nasal septum divides interior

### Sinuses (Paranasal or Accessory Sinuses) (4 pair)
Frontal

Ethmoid

Maxillary

Sphenoid

### Turbinates (Conchae)
Bones on inside of nose

Divided into inferior, middle, and superior (Fig. 1–15B)

Warms and humidifies air

### Pharynx (Throat)
Passageway for both food and air

Nasopharynx contains adenoids

Oropharynx contains tonsils

Laryngopharynx leads to larynx

### Larynx (Voice Box) (opening to trachea)
Contains vocal cords

- Cartilages of larynx, thyroid, epiglottis, and arytenoid

### Lower Respiratory Tract (LRT)

### Trachea (Windpipe)—Air-Conducting Structure
Mucus-lined tube with C-shaped cartilage rings to hold windpipe open

### Segmental Bronchi
Trachea divides into right and left main bronchus which further divide into lobar bronchii—3 on right, 2 on left

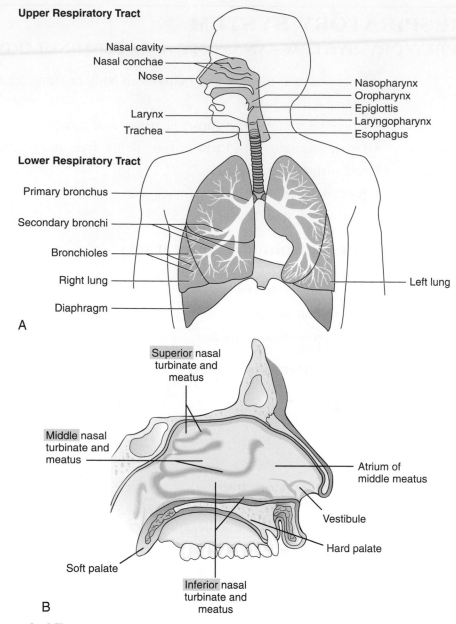

**Upper Respiratory Tract**

Nasal cavity
Nasal conchae
Nose

Nasopharynx
Oropharynx
Epiglottis
Larynx
Laryngopharynx
Trachea
Esophagus

**Lower Respiratory Tract**

Primary bronchus

Secondary bronchi

Bronchioles

Right lung

Diaphragm

Left lung

A

Superior nasal turbinate and meatus

Middle nasal turbinate and meatus

Atrium of middle meatus

Vestibule

Hard palate

Soft palate

Inferior nasal turbinate and meatus

B

Figure **1-15 A,** Upper and lower respiratory system. **B,** Superior, inferior, and middle nasal turbinates.

## Bronchioles
Branches divide into secondary bronchi, then smaller bronchioles

## Alveolar Ducts (minute branches of bronchial tree)
End in alveoli (sacs) of simple squamous cells

- Primary gas-exchange units

  Surrounded by capillaries and where exchange of oxygen and carbon dioxide takes place

## Lungs

Covered by pleura

Cone-shaped organs filling thoracic cavity

Base rests on diaphragm and apex (top of lungs) extends to above clavicles

Hilum is medial surface of lung where pulmonary artery, pulmonary veins, nerves, lymphatics, and bronchial tubes enter and exit

Left lung contains two lobes divided by fissures

Right lung contains three lobes

## Respiration

Inspiration—oxygen moves in, downward movement of lungs enlarging thoracic cavity

Expiration—carbon dioxide moves out, upward movement of diaphragm decreasing lung space

## COMBINING FORMS

| | | |
|---|---|---|
| 1. | adenoid/o | adenoid |
| 2. | alveol/o | alveolus |
| 3. | atel/o | incomplete |
| 4. | bronch/o | bronchus |
| 5. | bronchi/o | bronchus |
| 6. | bronchiol/o | bronchiole |
| 7. | capn/o | carbon dioxide |
| 8. | coni/o | dust |
| 9. | cyan/o | blue |
| 10. | diaphragmat/o | diaphragm |
| 11. | epiglott/o | epiglottis |
| 12. | laryng/o | larynx |
| 13. | lob/o | lobe |
| 14. | mediastin/o | mediastinum |
| 15. | muc/o | mucus |
| 16. | nas/o | nose |
| 17. | orth/o | straight |
| 18. | ox/o | oxygen |
| 19. | oxy/o | oxygen |
| 20. | pector/o | chest |
| 21. | pharyng/o | pharynx |
| 22. | phon/o | voice |

| | | |
|---|---|---|
| 23. | phren/o | diaphragm |
| 24. | pleur/o | pleura |
| 25. | pneum/o | lung/air |
| 26. | pneumat/o | air |
| 27. | pneumon/o | lung/air |
| 28. | pulmon/o | lung |
| 29. | py/o | pus |
| 30. | rhin/o | nose |
| 31. | sept/o | septum |
| 32. | sinus/o | sinus |
| 33. | spir/o | breath |
| 34. | tel/o | complete |
| 35. | thorac/o | thorax |
| 36. | tonsill/o | tonsil |
| 37. | trache/o | trachea |

## PREFIXES

| | | |
|---|---|---|
| 1. | a- | not |
| 2. | an- | not |
| 3. | endo- | within |
| 4. | eu- | good |
| 5. | dys- | difficult |
| 6. | pan- | all |
| 7. | poly- | many |

## SUFFIXES

| | | |
|---|---|---|
| 1. | -algia | pain |
| 2. | -ar | pertaining to |
| 3. | -ary | pertaining to |
| 4. | -capnia | carbon dioxide |
| 5. | -centesis | puncture to remove (drain) |
| 6. | -dynia | pain |
| 7. | -eal | pertaining to |
| 8. | -ectasis | stretching |
| 9. | -emia | blood |
| 10. | -gram | record |

11. -graph            recording instrument

12. -graphy         recording process

13. -itis              inflammation

14. -meter          measurement or instrument that measures

15. -metry          measurement of

16. -osmia          smell

17. -oxia            oxygen

18. -pexy           fixation

19. -phonia         sound

20. -pnea           breathing

21. -ptysis          spitting

22. -rrhage, -rrhagia   abnormal, excessive flow

23. -scopy          to examine

24. -spasm          contraction of muscle

25. -sphyxia        pulse

26. -stenosis       blockage, narrowing

27. -stomy          opening

28. -thorax          chest

29. -tomy           cutting, incision

## MEDICAL ABBREVIATIONS

1. ABG           arterial blood gas

2. AFB            acid-fast bacillus

3. ARDS          adult respiratory distress syndrome

4. BiPAP         bi-level positive airway pressure

5. COPD         chronic obstructive pulmonary disease

6. CPAP         continuous positive airway pressure

7. DLCO         diffuse capacity of lungs for carbon monoxide

8. FEF            forced expiratory flow

9. $FEV_1$          forced expiratory volume in 1 second

10. $FEV_1{:}FVC$    maximum amount of forced expiratory volume in 1 second

11. FRC            functional residual capacity

12. FVC            forced vital capacity

13. HHN           hand-held nebulizer

14. IPAP          inspiratory positive airway pressure

15. IRDS          infant respiratory distress syndrome

| 16. MDI | metered-dose inhaler |
| 17. MVV | maximum voluntary ventilation |
| 18. PAWP | pulmonary artery wedge pressure |
| 19. PCWP | pulmonary capillary wedge pressure |
| 20. PEAP | positive end-airway pressure |
| 21. PEEP | positive end-expiratory pressure |
| 22. PFT | pulmonary function test |
| 23. PND | paroxysmal nocturnal dyspnea |
| 24. RDS | respiratory distress syndrome |
| 25. RSV | respiratory syncytial virus |
| 26. RV | respiratory volume |
| 27. RV:TLC | ratio of respiratory volume to total lung capacity |
| 28. TLC | total lung capacity |
| 29. TLV | total lung volume |
| 30. URI | upper respiratory infection |
| 31. V/Q | ventilation/perfusion scan |

## MEDICAL TERMS

| Ablation | Removal or destruction by cutting, chemicals, or electrocautery |
| Adenoidectomy | Removal of adenoids |
| Apnea | Cessation of breathing |
| Asphyxia | Lack of oxygen |
| Asthma | Shortage of breath caused by contraction of bronchi |
| Atelectasis | Incomplete expansion of lung, collapse |
| Auscultation | Listening to sounds, such as to lung sounds |
| Bacilli | Plural of bacillus, a rod-shaped bacteria |
| Bilobectomy | Surgical removal of two lobes of a lung |
| Bronchiole | Smaller division of bronchial tree |
| Bronchoplasty | Surgical repair of bronchi |
| Bronchoscopy | Inspection of bronchial tree using a bronchoscope |
| Catheter | Tube placed into body to put fluid in or take fluid out |
| Cauterization | Destruction of tissue by use of cautery |
| Cordectomy | Surgical removal of vocal cord(s) |
| Crackle | Abnormal sound when breathing (heard on auscultation) |
| Croup | Acute viral infection (obstruction of larynx), stridor |
| Cyanosis | Bluish discoloration |

| | |
|---|---|
| Drainage | Free flow or withdrawal of fluids from a wound or cavity |
| Dysphonia | Speech impairment |
| Dyspnea | Shortage of breath, difficult breathing |
| Emphysema | Air accumulated in organ or tissue |
| Epiglottidectomy | Excision of covering of larynx |
| Epistaxis | Nose bleed |
| Glottis | True vocal cords |
| Hemoptysis | Bloody sputum |
| Intramural | Within organ wall |
| Intubation | Insertion of a tube |
| Laryngeal web | Congenital abnormality of connective tissue between vocal cords |
| Laryngectomy | Surgical removal of larynx |
| Laryngoplasty | Surgical repair of larynx |
| Laryngoscope | Fiberoptic scope used to view inside of larynx |
| Laryngoscopy | Direct visualization and examination of interior of larynx with a laryngoscope |
| Laryngotomy | Incision into larynx |
| Lavage | Washing out |
| Lobectomy | Surgical excision of a lobe of lung |
| Nasal button | Synthetic circular disc used to cover a hole in the nasal septum |
| Orthopnea | Difficulty in breathing, relieved by assuming upright position |
| Percussion | Tapping with sharp blows as a diagnostic technique |
| Pertussis | Whooping cough—highly contagious bacterial infection of pharynx, larynx, and trachea |
| Pharyngolaryngectomy | Surgical removal of pharynx and larynx |
| Pleura | Covers lungs and lines thoracic cavity |
| Pleurectomy | Surgical excision of pleura |
| Pleuritis | Inflammation of pleura |
| Pneumocentesis/ pneumonocentesis | Surgical puncturing of a lung to withdraw fluid |
| Pneumonia | Inflammation of lungs with consolidation |
| Pneumonolysis/ pneumolysis | Surgical separation of lung from chest wall to allow lung to collapse |
| Pneumonotomy/ pneumotomy | Incision of lung |
| Pulmonary edema | Accumulation of fluid in pulmonary tissues and air spaces |
| Pulmonary embolism | Thrombus or other foreign material lodged in pulmonary artery or one of its branches |
| Rales | An abnormal respiratory sound heard in auscultation, indicating some pathologic condition |

| | |
|---|---|
| Rhinoplasty | Surgical repair of nose |
| Rhinorrhea | Free discharge of a thin nasal mucus |
| Sarcoidosis | Chronic inflammatory disease with nodules developing in lungs, lymph nodes, other organs |
| Segmentectomy | Surgical removal of the smaller subdivisions (segment) of lobes of a lung |
| Septoplasty | Surgical repair of nasal septum |
| Sinusotomy | Surgical incision into a sinus |
| Spirometry | Measuring breathing capacity |
| Tachypnea | Quick, shallow breathing |
| Thoracentesis/ thoracocentesis (pleuracentesis/ pleurocentesis) | Surgical puncture of thoracic cavity, usually using a needle, to remove fluids |
| Thoracoplasty | Surgical procedure that removes rib(s) and thereby allows collapse of a lung |
| Thoracoscopy | Use of a lighted endoscope to view pleural spaces and thoracic cavity or to perform surgical procedures |
| Thoracostomy | Surgical incision into chest wall and insertion of a chest tube |
| Thoracotomy | Surgical incision into chest wall |
| Total pneumonectomy | Surgical removal of an entire lung |
| Tracheostomy | Creation of an opening into trachea |
| Tracheotomy | Incision into trachea |
| Transtracheal | Across trachea |
| Tuberculosis | Infection of the lungs caused by bacteria (tubercle bacillus) |

# RESPIRATORY SYSTEM ANATOMY AND TERMINOLOGY QUIZ

1. This is NOT a part of lower respiratory tract:
   a. trachea
   b. larynx
   c. bronchi
   d. lungs

2. Another name for voice box is:
   a. oropharynx
   b. pharynx
   c. laryngopharynx
   d. larynx

3. This is the windpipe:
   a. pharynx
   b. larynx
   c. trachea
   d. sphenoid

4. Interior of nose is divided by the:
   a. septum
   b. sphenoid
   c. oropharynx
   d. apical

5. This combining form means "incomplete":
   a. atel/o
   b. alveol/o
   c. ox/i
   d. pneumat/o

6. This combining form means "breath":
   a. py/o
   b. lob/o
   c. spir/o
   d. pleur/o

7. This prefix means "all":
   a. a-
   b. an-
   c. pan-
   d. poly-

8. This abbreviation refers to a syndrome that involves difficulty in breathing:
   a. ABG
   b. ARDS
   c. BiPAP
   d. FEF

9. This abbreviation refers to amount of air patient can expel from the lungs in 1 second:
   a. PFT
   b. PND
   c. RDS
   d. $FEV_1$

10. This suffix means "breathing":
    a. -stenosis
    b. -spasm
    c. -pexy
    d. -pnea

# RESPIRATORY SYSTEM—PATHOPHYSIOLOGY

## Signs and Symptoms of Pulmonary Disorders

### Dyspnea
Difficult breathing (sense of air hunger)

Increased respiratory effort

### Hypoventilation
Decreased alveolar ventilation

### Hyperventilation
Increased alveolar ventilation

### Hemoptysis
Bloody sputum

### Hypoxia
Reduced oxygenation of tissue cells

### Cough
Caused by irritant

Protective reflex

Acute cough is up to 3 weeks

Chronic cough is over 3 weeks

### Tachypnea
Rapid breathing

### Apnea
Lack of breathing

### Orthopnea
Requiring sitting upright to facilitate breathing

## Pulmonary Diseases and Disorders

### Hypercapnia
Increased carbon dioxide in arterial blood

Caused by inadequate ventilation of alveoli

Can result in respiratory acidosis

### Hypoxemia
Reduced oxygenation of arterial blood

### Acute Respiratory Failure
Inadequate gas exchange

Hypoxemia

Can result from trauma or disease

### Adult Respiratory Distress Syndrome (ARDS)

Acute injury to alveolocapillary membrane

Results in edema and atelectasis

In infants, infant respiratory distress syndrome (IRDS)

### Pulmonary Edema

Accumulation of fluid in lung tissue

Most common cause is left ventricular failure

### Aspiration

Passage of fluid and solid particles into lung

Can cause severe pneumonitis

- Localized inflammation of lung

### Atelectasis

Collapse of lung

Three most common types are:

- Adhesive
- Compression
- Obstruction

May be chronic or acute

- Acute, such as compression as a result of an automobile accident
- Chronic from structural defect

### Absorption Atelectasis

Results from absence of air in alveoli

Caused by

> Foreign body
>
> Tumor
>
> Abnormal external pressure

### Bronchiectasis

Chronic, irreversible dilation of bronchi

**Common types that describe severity of condition**
- Cylindrical
- Varicose
- Sacular or cystic

### Respiratory Acidosis

Decreased level of pH

> Due to excess retention of carbon dioxide

### Bronchiolitis

Inflammation and obstruction of bronchioles

Usually in children less than 2—preceded by URI

Viral infection (respiratory syncytial virus, or RSV)

**Common types**
- Constrictive
- Proliferative
- Obliterative

## Pneumothorax
Air collected in pleural cavity

Leads to lung collapse

Communicating pneumothorax is barometric air pressure in pleural space

Spontaneous pneumothorax is spontaneous rupture of visceral pleura

Secondary pneumothorax is a result of trauma to chest

## Pneumoconiosis
Dust particles or other particulate matter in lung

**Common types**
- Coal
- Asbestos
- Fiberglass

## Pleural Effusion-Fluid in Pleural Space
**Common types**
- Hemothorax—hemorrhage into pleural cavity
- Empyema—Infectious materials in pleural space
- Exudate—Fluid remaining after infection, inflammation, malignancy

## Empyema
**Infectious pleural effusion**
Pus in pleural space

Complication of respiratory infection

Commonly follows pneumonia and is treated like pneumonia

## Pulmonary Embolism
Air, tissue, or clot occlusion

Lodges in pulmonary artery or branch of artery

Risk with congestive heart failure

Most clots originate in leg veins

## Cor Pulmonale
Hypertrophy or failure of right ventricle

Result of lung, pulmonary vessels, or chest wall disorders

Acute is secondary to pulmonary embolus

Chronic is secondary to obstructive lung disease

## Pleurisy (Pleuritis)
Inflammation of pleura

Often preceded by an upper respiratory infection

### Infectious Disease
**Upper respiratory infection (URI)**
Acute inflammatory process of mucous membranes in trachea and above

**Common types**
- Common cold
- Croup
- Sinusitis
- Laryngitis

## Lower Respiratory Infection (LRI)

### Pneumonia
Inflammation of lungs with consolidation

Categorized according to causative organism

Can be caused by

Aspiration

Bacteria

Protozoa

Fungi

Chlamydia

Virus

**Common types**

Aspiration pneumonia

Bacterial

Chlamydial

Drug resistant

Eosinophil

Fungal

Hospital acquired (nosocomial)

Legionnaires' disease

Mycoplasma

Pneumococcal

Viral

### Tuberculosis
Communicable lung disease—airborne droplet

Caused by *Mycobacterium tuberculosis* (bacilli)

### Chronic Obstructive Pulmonary Disease (COPD)
Irreversible airway obstruction that decreases expiration

**Includes**

Chronic bronchitis

- Bronchial spasms

- Dyspnea

- Wheezing

- Productive cough

- Cyanosis

- Chronic hypoventilation

- Polycythemia

- Cor pulmonale

- Prolonged expiration

Emphysema

- Loss of elasticity and enlargement of alveoli

- Mimics symptoms of chronic bronchitis but more exaggerated

# RESPIRATORY SYSTEM PATHOPHYSIOLOGY QUIZ

1. Acute injury to alveolocapillary membrane that results in edema and atelectasis:
   a. hypoxemia
   b. adult respiratory distress syndrome
   c. bronchiolitis
   d. pneumoconiosis

2. Condition in which pus is in pleural space and is often a complication of pneumonia:
   a. empyema
   b. cor pulmonale
   c. pneumothorax
   d. atelectasis

3. Which of the following is NOT one of the most common types of atelectasis?
   a. adhesive
   b. compression
   c. obstruction
   d. expansion

4. This condition is a result of accumulation of dust particles in lung:
   a. pleurisy
   b. tuberculosis
   c. chronic obstructive pulmonary disease
   d. pneumoconiosis

5. An irreversible airway obstructive disease in which symptoms are bronchial spasm, dyspnea, and wheezing:
   a. pleurisy
   b. empyema
   c. bronchiolitis
   d. COPD

6. Cylindrical, varicose, and secular/cystic are examples of:
   a. bronchiectasis
   b. cor pulmonale
   c. pneumothorax
   d. atelectasis

7. Condition in which there is a loss of elasticity and enlargement of alveoli:
   a. chronic bronchitis
   b. asthma
   c. emphysema
   d. empyema

8. Definition of a chronic cough is one that lasts for more than this number of weeks:
   a. 2
   b. 3
   c. 4
   d. 5

9. A condition marked by an increase in carbon dioxide in arterial blood and decreased ability to breathe that can result in respiratory acidosis:
   a. hypercapnia
   b. hypoxemia
   c. acute respiratory failure
   d. pulmonary edema

10. This condition often follows a viral infection and occurs in children under 2 years of age. Examples of various types of this condition are constrictive, proliferating, and obliterative.
    a. pneumoconiosis
    b. pulmonary edema
    c. bronchiolitis
    d. bronchiectasis

# ■ CARDIOVASCULAR SYSTEM
## CARDIOVASCULAR SYSTEM—ANATOMY AND TERMINOLOGY

Consists of blood, blood vessels, and heart

### Blood (function is to maintain a constant environment)

Composed of cells suspended in plasma (clear, straw-colored liquid)

### Carries

Oxygen and nutrients to cells

Waste and carbon dioxide to kidneys, liver, and lungs

Hormones from endocrine system

### Regulates

Temperature by circulating blood

### Protection

White cells (leukocytes) produce antibodies

### Composed of Two Parts

Liquid part (extracellular) is plasma

Water 91%

Protein 1%, albumin, globulins, fibrinogen, ferritin, transferrin

2% ions, nutrients, waste products, gases, regulating substances

Cellular structures

Leukocytes (WBCs)—granular and agranular—fight infections

- Neutrophils
- Lymphocytes
- Monocytes
- Eosinophils
- Basophils

Erythrocytes (red blood cells)—hemoglobin carries oxygen

Thrombocytes (platelets)—important for hemostasis

Blood types: A, B, AB, and O are genetically endowed

- Blood type O negative is known as universal donor (no Rh and no red cell antigens present)

### Vessels—Circulatory System

### Function

To carry blood delivering nutrients and oxygen (arterial system) and carry away cell waste and carbon dioxide (venous system)

### Types

Arteries (Fig. 1–16) carrying oxygenated blood

Inner layer, endothelium

Lead away from heart

Branches are arterioles

Figure **1-16** Arteries of circulatory system.

### Capillaries
Connection between arterioles and venules

Exchange structure (oxygen and carbon dioxide, nutrients, and waste)

### Veins (Fig. 1–17) carrying deoxygenated blood
Carry blood to heart

Venules are small branches

## Heart
Circulates blood

## Four Chambers (Fig. 1–18)
### Two upper
Right and left atria (singular: atrium) receive blood

### Two lower
Right and left ventricles discharge blood (pump)

Figure **1-17** Veins of circulatory system.

## Chamber Walls

Composed of three layers

- Endocardium: smooth inner layer

- Myocardium: middle muscular layer

- Epicardium: outer layer

## Septa (singular: septum)

Divide chambers

- Interatrial septum

  Separates two upper chambers

- Interventricular septum

  Separates two lower chambers

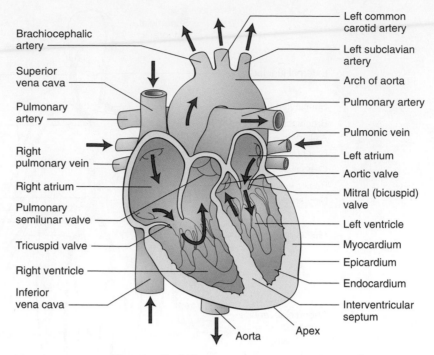

Figure **1-18** Internal view of heart.

## Major Blood Vessels

Inferior vena cava—carries deoxygenated blood from lower extremities, pelvic and abdominal viscera to right atrium

Superior vena cava—drains deoxygenated blood from head, neck, upper extremities, and chest to right atrium

Pulmonary artery bifurcates and becomes right and left pulmonary artery—carries deoxygenated blood from right ventricle to lungs

Right and left pulmonary veins (4)—carry oxygenated blood from lungs to left atrium

Aorta—carries oxygenated blood from left side of heart to body

## Pericardium

Sac comprised of two layers that covers heart

• Parietal pericardium: outermost covering

• Visceral pericardium: innermost (epicardium)

• Pericardial cavity: contains about 30 cc of fluid

## Valves (4 in heart)

Tricuspid: between right atrium and right ventricle

Pulmonary: at entrance of pulmonary artery leading from right ventricle

Aortic: at entrance of aorta leading from left ventricle

Bicuspid (mitral): between left atrium and left ventricle

## Conduction System (Fig. 1-19)

Sinoatrial node: SAN, nature's pacemaker, sends impulses to atrioventricular node

Figure **1-19** Electrical system of heart.

Atrioventricular node (AVN): located on interatrial septum and sends impulses to bundle of His

Bundle of His: divides into right bundle branch (RBB) and left bundle branch (LBB) in septum

Purkinje fibers: merge from bundle branches into specialized cells of myocardium, located at base of heart

## Heartbeat

### Two Phases—Correspond to Blood Pressure Readouts
Systole: contraction—top number reading

Diastole: relaxation—lower number reading

Trace a drop of blood from trunk of body (deoxygenated) to trunk of body (oxygenated)

Inferior vena cava to right atrium

Through tricuspid valve to right ventricle

From right ventricle to pulmonary artery to lung capillaries

From lung capillaries to pulmonary veins

To left atrium through mitral (bicuspid) valve to left ventricle

Though aortic valve to aorta

## COMBINING FORMS

| | | |
|---|---|---|
| 1. | angi/o | vessel |
| 2. | aort/o | aorta |
| 3. | ather/o | yellow plaque (fat) |
| 4. | arter/o | artery |
| 5. | arteri/o | artery |
| 6. | atri/o | atrium |
| 7. | brachi/o | arm |

8. cardi/o      heart

9. cholesterol/o      cholesterol

10. coron/o      heart

11. cyan/o      blue

12. my/o, muscul/o      muscle

13. myx/o      mucous

14. ox/o      oxygen

15. pericardi/o      pericardium

16. phleb/o      vein

17. sphygm/o      pulse

18. steth/o      chest

19. thromb/o      clot

20. valv/o      valve

21. valvul/o      valve

22. vascul/o      vessel

23. vas/o      vessel

24. ven/o      vein

25. ventricul/o      ventricle

## PREFIXES

1. a-      not

2. an-      not

3. bi-      two

4. brady-      slow

5. de-      lack of

6. dys-      bad, difficult, painful

7. endo-      in

8. hyper-      over

9. hypo-      under

10. inter-      between

11. intra-      within

12. meta-      change, after

13. peri-      surrounding

14. tachy-      fast

15. tetra-      four

16. tri-      three

## SUFFIXES

| | | |
|---|---|---|
| 1. | -dilation | widening, expanding |
| 2. | -emia | blood |
| 3. | -graphy | recording process |
| 4. | -lysis | separation |
| 5. | -megaly | enlargement |
| 6. | -oma | tumor |
| 7. | -osis | condition |
| 8. | -plasty | repair |
| 9. | -sclerosis | hardening |
| 10. | -stenosis | blockage, narrowing |
| 11. | -tomy | cutting, incision |

## MEDICAL ABBREVIATIONS

| | | |
|---|---|---|
| 1. | ASCVD | arteriosclerotic cardiovascular disease |
| 2. | ASD | atrial septal defect |
| 3. | ASHD | arteriosclerotic heart disease |
| 4. | AV | atrioventricular |
| 5. | CABG | coronary artery bypass graft |
| 6. | CHF | congestive heart failure |
| 7. | CK | creatine kinase |
| 8. | CPK | creatine phosphokinase |
| 9. | CVI | cerebrovascular insufficiency |
| 10. | DSE | dobutamine stress echocardiography |
| 11. | HCVD | hypertensive cardiovascular disease |
| 12. | LBBB | left bundle branch block |
| 13. | LVH | left ventricular hypertrophy |
| 14. | MAT | multifocal atrial tachycardia |
| 15. | MI | myocardial infarction |
| 16. | NSR | normal sinus rhythm |
| 17. | PAC | premature atrial contraction |
| 18. | PAT | paroxysmal atrial tachycardia |
| 19. | PST/PSVT | paroxysmal supraventricular tachycardia |
| 20. | PTCA | percutaneous transluminal coronary angioplasty |
| 21. | PVC | premature ventricular contraction |
| 22. | RBBB | right bundle branch block |
| 23. | RSR | regular sinus rhythm |

| 24. | RVH | right ventricular hypertrophy |
| 25. | SVT | supraventricular tachycardia |
| 26. | TEE | transesophageal echocardiography |
| 27. | TST | treadmill stress test |

## MEDICAL TERMS

| Acute coronary syndrome (ACS) | An umbrella term used to cover clinical symptoms compatible with acute myocardial ischemia |
|---|---|
| Anastomosis | Surgical connection of two tubular structures, such as two pieces of the intestine |
| Aneurysm | Abnormal dilation of vessels, usually an artery |
| Angina | Spasmotic, choking, or suffocative pain |
| Angiography | Radiography of blood vessels |
| Angioplasty | Procedure in a vessel to dilate vessel opening |
| Atherectomy | Removal of plaque from an artery (can be done by a percutaneous or open procedure) |
| Auscultation | Listening for sounds within body |
| Bundle of His | Muscular cardiac fibers that provide heart rhythm to ventricles |
| Bypass | To go around |
| Cardiopulmonary | Refers to heart and lungs |
| Cardiopulmonary bypass | Blood bypasses heart through a heart-lung machine |
| Cardioverter-defibrillator | Surgically placed or wearable device that directs an electric shock to the heart to restore rhythm |
| Circumflex | A coronary artery that circles heart |
| Cutdown | Incision into a vessel for placement of a catheter |
| Edema | Swelling due to abnormal fluid collection in tissue spaces |
| Electrode | Lead attached to a generator that carries electric current from the generator to atria or ventricles |
| Electrophysiology | Study of electrical system of heart, including study of arrhythmias |
| Embolectomy | Removal of blockage (embolism) from vessel |
| Endarterectomy | Incision into an artery to remove inner lining |
| Epicardial | Over heart |
| False aneurysm | Sac of clotted blood that has completely destroyed vessel and is being contained by tissue that surrounds vessel |
| Fistula | Abnormal opening from one area to another area or to outside of the body |
| Hematoma | Mass of blood that forms outside vessel |
| Hemolysis | Breakdown of red blood cells |
| Hypoxemia | Low level of oxygen in blood |

| | |
|---|---|
| Hypoxia | Low level of oxygen in tissue |
| Intracardiac | Inside heart |
| Invasive | Entering body, breaking skin |
| Noninvasive | Not entering body, not breaking skin |
| Nuclear cardiology | Diagnostic specialty that uses radiologic procedures to aid in diagnosis of cardiologic conditions |
| Order | Shows subordination of one thing to another; family or class |
| Pericardiocentesis | Procedure in which a surgeon withdraws fluid from pericardial space by means of a needle inserted percutaneously |
| Pericardium | Membranous sac enclosing heart and ends of great vessels |
| Swan-Ganz catheter | A catheter that measures pressure in right side of heart and in pulmonary artery |
| Thoracostomy | Incision into chest wall and insertion of a chest tube |
| Thromboendarterectomy | Removal of thrombus and atherosclerotic lining from an artery (percutaneous or open procedure) |
| Transvenous | Through a vein |

# CARDIOVASCULAR SYSTEM ANATOMY AND TERMINOLOGY QUIZ

1. These carry blood to the heart:
   a. capillaries
   b. arteries
   c. arterioles
   d. veins

2. Relaxation phase of heartbeat:
   a. diastole
   b. systole

3. Nature's pacemaker is this node:
   a. atrioventricular
   b. Bundle of His
   c. sinoatrial
   d. mitral

4. Node located on interatrial septum:
   a. atrioventricular
   b. Bundle of His
   c. sinoatrial
   d. Purkinje

5. Which of the following is NOT one of the three layers of chamber walls of the heart?
   a. endocardium
   b. myocardium
   c. epicardium
   d. parietal

6. Septum that divides upper two chambers of heart:
   a. intraventricular
   b. interatrial
   c. tricuspid
   d. myocardium

7. Valve between right atrium and right ventricle:
   a. pulmonary
   b. aortic
   c. bicuspid
   d. tricuspid

8. Outer two-layer covering of heart:
   a. pericardium
   b. mitral
   c. myocardium
   d. epicardium

9. These are chambers that receive blood:
   a. right and left ventricle
   b. left ventricle and right atrium
   c. right atrium and right ventricle
   d. right and left atria

10. This combining form means "plaque":
    a. atri/o
    b. brachi/o
    c. cyan/o
    d. ather/o

# CARDIOVASCULAR SYSTEM—PATHOPHYSIOLOGY

## Vascular Disorders

### Coronary Artery Disease (CAD)/Ischemic Heart Disease (IHD)

Thickening and hardening of arterial intima (innermost layer) with lipid and fibrous plaque (atherosclerosis)

- Produces narrowing and stiffening of vessel

Location of lesions leads to various vascular diseases

- Femoral and popliteal arteries = peripheral vascular disease
- Carotid arteries = stroke
- Aorta = aneurysms (dilation/weakening of vessel walls)
- Coronary arteries = ischemic heart disease or myocardial infarction

Resulting in decreased oxygen supply

Risk factors increased by:

- Age
- Family history of CAD
- Hyperlipidemia
- Low HDL-C (good cholesterol)
- Hypertension
- Cigarette smoking
- Diabetes mellitus
- Obesity, particularly abdominal

### Ischemia

Deficiency of oxygenated blood

- Often due to constriction or obstruction of blood vessel

**Localized myocardial ischemia—most common cause: atherosclerosis of vessels**
Oxygen demand of tissues greater than supply

Presenting symptoms

- Chest pain (angina pectoris)
- Hypotension
- Changes in ECG

**Transient ischemia**
Heart muscle begins to perform at a low level due to lack of oxygen (reversible ischemia)

**Irreversible ischemia—is cause of an MI (myocardial infarction)**
Heart muscle dies—necrosis (myocardial infarction)

- Prolonged ischemia of 30 minutes or more
- Reestablishment of blood flow reduces residual necrosis
  - Thrombolytic agents to dissolve or split up thrombus
  - Primary percutaneous transluminal coronary angioplasty (PTCA)

Cardiac enzymes are released from damaged cells

- Blood test reveals elevation of enzymes, confirming myocardial infarction

**Hypertension (HTN)**
Normal is less than 120/80 for adults

- Fig. 1–20 illustrates new hypertension classifications

Leading cause of death in United States, due to damage to brain, heart, kidneys, eyes, and arteries of the lower extremities

Cause is unknown in 95% of cases

- Known as
  - Primary hypertension
  - Essential hypertension

5% of cases are secondary to underlying disease

Increased resistance damages heart and blood vessels

- Retinal vascular changes are monitored to assess therapy and disease progression

Chronic hypertension often leads to end-stage renal disease

- Result of progressive sclerosis of renal vessels

**Treatment**
Medications

- ACE (angiotensin-converting enzyme) inhibitor
- Alpha-adrenergic or beta-adrenergic receptor blocker
- Diuretic
- Calcium channel blocker

Lifestyle changes

Classification of blood pressure for
adults aged 18 years or older[1]

| Category | Systolic (mm Hg) | Diastolic (mm Hg) |
|---|---|---|
| Normal | <120 | <80 |
| Prehypertension (stays between) | 120–139 | 80–89 |
| Hypertension[2] | | |
| Stage 1 (mild) | 140–159 | 90–99 |
| Stage 2 (moderate) | 160–179 | 100–109 |
| Stage 3 (severe) | ≥180 | ≥110 |

[1] Not taking antihypertensive drugs and not acutely ill. When systolic and diastolic pressures fall into different categories, the higher category should be selected.

[2] Based on the average of two or more readings taken at each of two or more visits after an initial screening.

Figure **1-20** Classification of blood pressure.

## Hypotension
**Abnormally low blood pressure**
*Types*
Orthostatic (postural) hypotension

- Fall in both systolic and diastolic arterial blood pressure on standing

- Associated with

  - Dizziness

  - Blurred vision

  - Fainting (syncope)

- Caused by insufficient oxygenated blood flow through brain

- Can be acute (temporary) or chronic

Chronic orthostatic hypotension—types

- Primary of unknown cause

- Secondary to certain disease processes

- Such as:

  - Endocrine

  - Metabolic

  - Central nervous system disorders

- Treatment for secondary hypotension is correction of underlying disease

## Aneurysm
Dilation of an arterial blood vessel wall or cardiac chamber

- Danger is rupture of aneurysm

Atherosclerosis is common cause

Arteriosclerosis and hypertension also common in persons with aneurysms

**True aneurysm**
Involves all three layers of arterial wall

Causes weakening and ballooning of arterial wall

**False or psuedoaneurysm**
Usually result of trauma

Also known as saccular

Separation of arterial wall layers (dissecting) in artery wall (crisis situation—a medical emergency)

Bleeds into dissected space and is contained by arterial connective tissue wall

## Thrombus
Blood clot that remains attached to vessel wall and occludes vessel

Dislodged thrombus is a thromboembolus

**Causes**
Trauma

Interior wall lining irritation/roughening

Infection

Inflammation

Low blood pressure/blood stagnation

Obstruction

Atherosclerosis

**Risks related to thrombus**
Dislodges and moves to lungs, brain, heart

Grows to occlude blood flow

**Treatment**
Pharmacologic, anticoagulants

Heparin

Warfarin derivatives

**Non-invasive intervention**
Balloon-tipped catheter to remove or compress thrombus

## Thrombophlebitis Caused by Inflammation (Phlebitis)
**Causes**
Trauma

Infection

Immobility

**Commonly associated with**
Endocarditis

Rheumatic heart disease

## Embolism
Mass that is present and circulating in blood

**Common types**
Air bubble

Fat

Bacterial mass

Cancer cells

Foreign substances

Dislodged thrombus

Amniotic fluid

**Obstructs vessel**
Pulmonary emboli travel through venous side or right side of the heart to the pulmonary artery

Systemic or arterial emboli originate in left side of the heart

Associated with

- Myocardial infarction
- Left-sided heart failure

- Endocarditis
- Valvular conditions
- Dysrhythmias

## Peripheral Arterial Disease

### Thromboangiitis obliterans (Buerger's disease)
Occurs most often in young men who are heavy smokers

Inflammatory disease of peripheral arteries creating thombi and vasospasms

Involves small or medium arteries of feet and often hands

- May necessitate amputation

### Raynaud's disease
Vasospasms and constriction of small arterioles of fingers and toes

Affects young women as a secodary condition

Triggered by cold temperatures, emotional stress, cigarette smoking

Fingertips thicken and nails become brittle

Raynaud's phenomenon is secondary to primary disease, such as

- Scleroderma
- Pulmonary hypertension

### Treatment of underlying condition
No known origin or treatment

## Varicose Veins
Blood pools in veins, distending them

Tends to be progressive/vein valve failure

Occurs most commonly in saphenous veins

Hemorroids are varicose veins of anus

### Leads to
Swelling and discomfort

Fatigue when in legs

Possible ulcerations

## Heart Disorders

### Congestive Heart Failure (CHF)—heart cannot pump required amounts of blood
Can be left-sided or right-sided heart failure

Left-sided heart failure (systolic); cannot generate adequate output, causing pulmonary edema

Common causes:

Myocardial infarction

Myocarditis

Cardiomyopathies leading to ischemia

Symptoms of left-sided congestive heart failure include:

Shortness of breath

Fatigue

Exercise intolerance

Right-sided heart failure (diastolic) results in right ventricle stasis, inadequate pulmonary circulation, and peripheral edema/hepatosplenomegaly

## Abnormal Heart Rhythms (Conduction Irregularities)

Bradycardia and heart block (atrioventricular block)

Inadequate conduction impulses from SA node though AV node to AV bundle

Treatment

Cardiac pacemaker to maintain proper heart rate

Flutter—rapid regular contractions (most commonly of atria)

Symptoms—palpitations

Treatment

Cardioversion (electronic shock to heart)

Ablation (radiofrequency catheter destroying tissue causing arrhythmia)

Fibrillation—rapid, erratic, inefficient contractions of atria and ventricles

Atrial fibrillation—most common (electrical impulses move randomly in atria)

Symptoms—palpitation, risk of stroke due to clot formations from poor atrial outputs

Treatment

Cardioversion

Ablation

Ventricular fibrillation—life-threatening, random electrical impulses throughout ventricles

Symptoms

Cardiac death or arrest without immediate treatment

Treatment

Cardioversion

Digoxin—drug used to slow heart rate

Implantable cardioverter-defibrillator (ICD)

Emergency treatment—automatic external defibrillators (AEDs)

Radiofrequency catheter ablation (RFA) is a minimally invasive technique used to treat cardiac arrhythmias

## Infective Endocarditis

Inflammation of interior-most lining of heart

Leads to destruction and permanent damage to heart valves

Caused by

> Bacteria (most common streptococci and staphylococci)
>
> Virus
>
> Fungi
>
> Parasites

Patients with heart defects or damage usually take antibiotics prior to invasive procedures

## Pericarditis
Inflammation of pericardium of heart

**Common types**
- Acute

- Pericardial effusion

- Constrictive

## Rheumatic Fever/Rheumatic Heart Disease
Results in formation of scar tissue of the endocardium and heart valves

In 10% of cases leads to rheumatic heart disease

Family tendency to develop

Begins as carditis (inflammation of all layers of heart wall)

Long-term effects:

Mitral and/or aortic valve disease

> Stenosis
>
> Regurgitation
>
> Insufficiency

Tricuspid valve

> Affected in about 10% of cases

Pulmonary valve

> Rarely affected

## Valvular Heart Disease

Valves are extensions of endocardial tissue

Endocardial damage can be congenital or acquired

Damage leads to stenosis and/or incompetent valve

Includes

- Valvular stenosis is narrowing, stiffness, thickening, fusion, or blockage of valve, creating resistance, resulting in increased pressure in cardiac chamber behind valve

- Valvular regurgitation is failure of valve leaflet to close tightly, allowing backflow of blood

  - Result of lesions causing valve leaflets to shrink

  - Functional valvular regurgitation results in increased chamber size (cardiomegaly)

## Stenosis

### Aortic valve stenosis

Caused by

Congenital malformation

Degeneration

Infection

Results in slowing blood circulatory rate

Symptoms

Bradycardia

Faint pulse

May lead to heart murmur and hypertrophy

### Mitral valve stenosis

Impaired flow from left atrium to left ventricle

Caused by

Rheumatic fever

Bacterial infections

Symptom

Decreased cardiac output

May lead to

- Pulmonary hypertension
- Right ventricular heart failure
- And/or edema

## Valvular Regurgitation

Flow in opposite direction from normal

Mitral regurgitation (MR)

Backflow of blood from left ventricle into left atrium

Aortic regurgitation (AR)

Backflow of blood from aorta into left ventricle

Pulmonic regurgitation (PR)

Backflow of blood from pulmonary artery into right ventricle

Tricuspid regurgitation (TR)

Backflow of blood from right ventricle into right atrium

## Heart Wall Disorders

### Acute Pericarditis

Roughening and inflammation of pericardium (sac around heart)

Treatment

Anti-inflammatory drugs and pain medication

### Constrictive Pericarditis (Restrictive Pericarditis)

**Forms fibrous lesions that encase heart**

Compresses heart—thickened pericardial sac prevents heart from expanding when blood enters it

> Tamponade occurs when fluid builds up in pericardial space

> Pressure stops heart from beating—pericardial effusion or bleeding after heart surgery

Reduces output

### Pericardial Effusion

Accumulation of fluid in pericardial cavity

Results in pressure on heart

- Sudden development of pressure on heart is tamponade

## Cardiomyopathies

Myocardium: muscular wall (middle layer) of heart musculature

Group of diseases that affect myocardium

Cause

> Idiopathic (most common)

> Underlying condition

### Types of Cardiomyopathy

Dilated cardiomyopathy (congestive cardiomyopathy)

- Ventricular distention and impaired systolic function

Hypertrophic cardiomyopathy

- Cause is often hypertensive or valvular heart disease
- Results in thickened interventricular septum (septum between the ventricle chambers)

Restrictive cardiomyopathy

- Myocardium becomes stiffened
- Heart enlarges (cardiomegaly)
- Dysrhythmias common
- Caused by infiltrative diseases such as amyloidosis

### Congenital Heart Defects

Coarctation of aorta (CoA)—narrowing of the aorta

- Treatment

> Surgical removal of narrow segment/end-to-end anastomosis

Patent ductus arteriosus (PDA)—opening between aorta and pulmonary artery

- Treatment

> Drugs to close/embolize or plug ductus or tying off surgically

Tetralogy of Fallot—malformation of heart includes four defects

Pulmonary artery stenosis—narrowing/obstruction

Ventricular septal defect

Hole between two bottom chambers (ventricles) of heart

Overriding aorta

Shift of aorta to right—aorta overrides the interventricular septum

Hypertrophy of right ventricle

Myocardium enlarges to pump blood through narrowed pulmonary artery

• Treatment

Open-heart technique with heart-lung machine support to relieve right ventricular outflow tract stenosis and repair of ventriculoseptal defect

# CARDIOVASCULAR SYSTEM PATHOPHYSIOLOGY QUIZ

1. Lesion of carotid artery may lead to:
   a. heart attack
   b. stroke
   c. peripheral vascular disease
   d. ischemic heart disease

2. This blood pressure is hypertension:
   a. 120/80
   b. 130/70
   c. 140/90
   d. 110/70

3. Infective endocarditis is inflammation of the interior of the lining of the heart, and when caused by streptococci or staphylococci, the infection is:
   a. viral
   b. fungal
   c. bacterial
   d. parasitic

4. Angina pectoris is:
   a. heart block
   b. heart murmur
   c. chest pain
   d. barrel chest

5. In this type of regurgitation there is a backflow of blood from left ventricle into left atrium:
   a. aortic
   b. pulmonic
   c. tricuspid
   d. mitral

6. In this type of heart wall disorder, fibrous lesions form and encase the heart:
   a. constrictive pericarditis
   b. acute pericarditis
   c. pericardial effusion
   d. cardiomyopathy

7. Which of the following terms means "of unknown cause"?
   a. etiology
   b. manifestation
   c. idiopathic
   d. late effect

8. This condition is also known as congestive cardiomyopathy:
   a. hypertrophic
   b. valvular
   c. dilated
   d. restrictive

9. This peripheral arterial disease most often occurs in young men who are heavy smokers:
   a. Buerger's
   b. Pick's
   c. Addison's
   d. Glasser's

10. This cardiomyopathy results in a thickened interventricular septum:
    a. restrictive
    b. congestive
    c. dilated
    d. hypertrophic

# ■ FEMALE GENITAL SYSTEM AND PREGNANCY

## FEMALE GENITAL SYSTEM AND PREGNANCY—ANATOMY AND TERMINOLOGY

### Terminology

#### Ovaries (Pair)
Produce ova (single female gamete) and hormones; ova: plural; ovum: singular (Fig. 1–21). Each ovum/gamete contains 23 chromosomes.

#### Fallopian Tubes (Uterine Tubes or Oviducts)
Ducts from ovary to uterus

#### Uterus (Womb)
Muscular organ that holds embryo

Three layers
- Endometrium: inner mucosa
- Myometrium: middle layer/muscle
- Perimetrium/Uterine serosa: outer layer
  - Cervix: lower narrow portion of uterus
  - Fundus: the upper rounded part of the uterus

#### Vagina
Tube from uterus to outside of body

#### Vulva
External genitalia
- Clitoris: erectile tissue
- Labia majora: outer lips of vagina
- Labia minora: inner lips of vagina
- Urinary meatus: opening to urethra
- Bartholin's gland: glands on either side of vagina
- Hymen: membrane partially or wholly occludes entrance to vagina

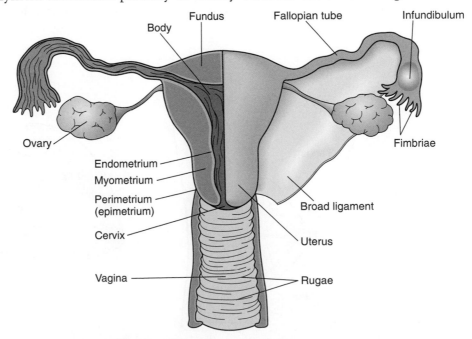

Figure **1-21** Female reproductive system.

### Perineum

Area between anus and vaginal orifice

## Accessory Organs (Fig. 1–22)

### Breasts

Mammary glands

Composed of glandular tissue containing milk glands/lactiferous ducts

In response to hormones from pituitary gland, milk is produced in acini (also known as alveolua) (lactation)

Lactiferous ducts transfer milk to nipple

Nipple, surrounded by areola

## Menstruation and Pregnancy

### Proliferation Phase

**Menstruation (Days 1-5):** discharge of blood fluid containing endometrial cells, blood cells, and glandular secretions from endometrium

**Endometrium repair (Days 6-12):** maturing follicle in ovary produces estrogen (hormone) which causes endometrium to thicken and ovum (egg) to mature in graafian follicle

### Secretory Phase

**Ovulation (Days 13-14):** occurs when graafian follicle ruptures and ovum travels down fallopian tube

Usually only one graffian follicle develops each month

**Premenstruation (Days 15-28):** a period of time in which graafian follicle converts to corpus luteum secreting progesterone to stimulate build-up of uterine lining. If after 5 days no fertilization occurs, cycle repeats.

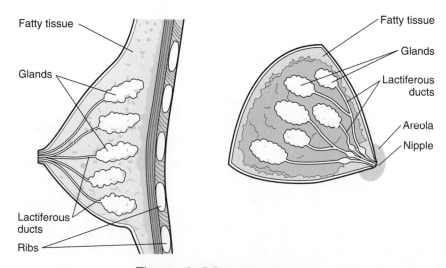

Figure **1-22** Breast structure.

## Pregnancy

Prenatal stage of development from fertilization to birth (39 weeks)

Fertilized ovum or zygote develops in a double cavity: yolk sac (produces blood cells) and amniotic cavity (contains amniotic fluid)

Embryo, stage of development from 4th to 8th week

Fetus, unborn offspring, 9 weeks until birth

## Placenta Forms Within Uterine Wall and Produces Hormone—Human Chorionic Gonadotropin (HCG)

HCG is horomone tested in urine pregnancy tests

HCG stimulates corpus luteum to produce estrogen and progesterone until the third month of pregnancy

Placenta then produces hormones

Expelled after delivery (afterbirth)

## Gestation, Approximately 266 Days

280 days used when calculating estimated date of delivery (EDD) or time from last menstrual period (LMP)

Three trimesters

- First    LMP-12 weeks
- Second   13-27 weeks
- Third    28 weeks-EDD

## COMBINING FORMS

1. amni/o — amnion
2. arche/o — first
3. cephal/o — head
4. cervic/o — cervix
5. chori/o — chorion
6. colp/o — vagina
7. crypt/o — hidden
8. culd/o — cul-de-sac
9. episi/o — vulva
10. fet/o — fetus
11. galact/o — milk
12. gynec/o — female
13. gyn/o — female
14. hymen/o — hymen
15. hyster/o — uterus
16. lact/o — milk

| 17. lapar/o | abdominal wall |
| 18. mamm/o | breast |
| 19. mast/o | breast |
| 20. men/o | menstruation, month |
| 21. metr/o | uterus, measure |
| 22. metr/i | uterus |
| 23. my/o, muscul/o | muscle |
| 24. nat/a | birth |
| 25. nat/i | birth |
| 26. obstetr/o | pregnancy/childbirth |
| 27. olig/o | few |
| 28. oo/o | egg |
| 29. oophor/o | ovary |
| 30. ov/o | egg |
| 31. ovari/o | ovary |
| 32. ovul/o | ovulation |
| 33. perine/o | perineum |
| 34. peritone/o | peritoneum |
| 35. phor/o | to bear |
| 36. salping/o | uterine tube, fallopian tube |
| 37. top/o | place |
| 38. uter/o | uterus |
| 39. vagin/o | vagina |
| 40. vulv/o | vulva |

## PREFIXES

| 1. ante- | before |
| 2. dys- | painful |
| 3. ecto- | outside |
| 4. endo- | in |
| 5. extra- | outside |
| 6. in- | into |
| 7. intra- | within |
| 8. multi- | many |
| 9. neo- | new |
| 10. nulli- | none |
| 11. nulti- | none |

12. post-         after

13. primi-        first

14. pseudo-       false

15. retro-        backwards

16. uni-          one

## SUFFIXES

1. -arche         beginning

2. -cyesis        pregnancy

3. -gravida       pregnancy

4. -rrhexis       rupture

5. -para          woman who has given birth

6. -parous        to bear

7. -rrhea         discharge

8. -salpinx       uterine tube

9. -tocia         labor

10. -version      turning

## MEDICAL ABBREVIATIONS

1. AFI            amniotic fluid index

2. AGA            appropriate for gestational age

3. ARM            artificial rupture of membrane

4. BPD            biparietal diameter

5. BPP            biophysical profile

6. BV             bacterial vaginosis

7. CHL            crown-to-heel length

8. CNM            certified nurse midwife

9. CPD            cephalopelvic disproportion

10. CPP           chronic pelvic pain

11. D&C           dilation and curettage

12. D&E           dilation and evacuation

13. DUB           dysfunctional uterine bleeding

14. ECC           endocervical curettage

15. EDC           estimated date of confinement

16. EDD           estimated date of delivery

17. EFM           electronic fetal monitoring

18. EFW           estimated fetal weight

| | | |
|---|---|---|
| 19. | EGA | estimated gestational age |
| 20. | EMC | endometrial curettage |
| 21. | ERT | estrogen replacement therapy |
| 22. | FAS | fetal alcohol syndrome |
| 23. | FHR | fetal heart rate |
| 24. | FSH | follicle-stimulating hormone |
| 25. | HPV | human papillomavirus |
| 26. | HSG | hysterosalpingogram |
| 27. | HSV | herpes simplex virus |
| 28. | IVF | in vitro fertilization |
| 29. | LEEP | loop electrosurgical excision procedure |
| 30. | LGA | large for gestational age |
| 31. | PID | pelvic inflammatory disease |
| 32. | PROM | premature rupture of membranes |
| 33. | SHG | sonohysterogram |
| 34. | SROM | spontaneous rupture of membranes |
| 35. | SUI | stress urinary incontinence |
| 36. | TAH | total abdominal hysterectomy |
| 37. | VBAC | vaginal birth after cesarean |

## MEDICAL TERMS

| | |
|---|---|
| Abortion | Termination of pregnancy |
| Amniocentesis | Percutaneous aspiration of amniotic fluid |
| Amniotic sac | Sac containing fetus and amniotic fluid |
| Antepartum | Before childbirth |
| Cesarean | Surgical opening through abdominal wall for delivery |
| Chorionic villus sampling | CVS, biopsy of outermost part of placenta |
| Cordocentesis | Procedure to obtain a fetal blood sample; also called a percutaneous umbilical blood sampling |
| Curettage | Scraping of a cavity using a spoon-shaped instrument |
| Cystocele | Herniation of bladder into vagina |
| Delivery | Childbirth |
| Dilation | Expansion (of cervix) |
| Ectopic | Pregnancy outside uterus (i.e., in fallopian tube) |
| Hysterectomy | Surgical removal of uterus |
| Hysterorrhaphy | Suturing of uterus |
| Hysteroscopy | Visualization of canal and cavity of uterus using a scope placed through vagina |

Introitus                 Opening or entrance to vagina

Ligation                  Binding or tying off, as in constricting blood flow of a vessel or
                          binding fallopian tubes for sterilization

Multipara                 More than one pregnancy

Oophorectomy              Surgical removal of ovary(ies)

Perineum                  Area between vulva and anus; also known as pelvic floor

Placenta                  A structure that connects fetus and mother during pregnancy

Postpartum                After childbirth

Primigravida              First pregnancy

Primipara                 First delivered infant/given birth to only one child

Salpingectomy             Surgical removal of uterine tube

Salpingostomy             Creation of a fistula into uterine tube

Tocolysis                 Repression of uterine contractions

Vesicovaginal fistula     Abnormal opening/channel between vagina and bladder

## FEMALE GENITAL SYSTEM AND PREGNANCY ANATOMY AND TERMINOLOGY QUIZ

1. This is NOT one of three layers of uterus:
   a. perimetrium
   b. endometrium
   c. myometrium
   d. barametrium

2. Located at the lower end of uterus is the:
   a. cervix
   b. vagina
   c. perineum
   d. labia majora

3. Approximate gestation of a human fetus is:
   a. 266 days
   b. 276 days
   c. 290 days
   d. 292 days

4. LMP is the:
   a. later maternity phase
   b. last menstrual period
   c. low metabolic pregnancy
   d. late menstruation phase

5. Name of stage that describes development of fetus from fertilization to birth is:
   a. postpartum
   b. antepartum
   c. prenatal
   d. natal

6. Which of the following correctly identifies three trimesters of gestation?
   a. LMP-12 weeks, 13-27 weeks, 28 weeks-EDD
   b. LMP-14 weeks, 15-27 weeks, 28 weeks-EDD
   c. LMP-14 weeks, 15-28 weeks, 29 weeks-EDD
   d. LMP-11 weeks, 12-26 weeks, 27 weeks-EDD

7. Combining form meaning "few":
   a. oopho/o
   b. olig/o
   c. nati/i
   d. top/o

8. Combining form meaning "hidden":
   a. amni/o
   b. crypt/o
   c. chori/o
   d. fet/o

9. Suffix meaning "beginning":
   a. -cyesis
   b. -rrhea
   c. -arche
   d. -orrhexis

10. Prefix meaning "within":
   a. ante-
   b. dys-
   c. ecto-
   d. endo-

# FEMALE GENITAL SYSTEM AND PREGNANCY—PATHOPHYSIOLOGY

## Menstrual and Hormonal Disorders

### Dysmenorrhea

Painful menstruation

**Common types**
- Primary and secondary

**Primary dysmenorrhea**

No underlying condition but begins with commencement of ovulation

Cramping is caused by excess of prostaglandin

- Causes contractions and uterine ischemia
- Develops 24 to 48 hours prior to menstruation

*Treatment*
- Nonsteroidal antiinflammatory agents
- Progesterone

**Secondary dysmenorrhea**

Caused by an underlying disorder, such as

- Polyps
- Tumors
- Endometriosis
- Pelvic inflammatory disease

*Treatment*

Directed at underlying disorder

### Amenorrhea

Amenorrhea is absence of menstruation

**Common types**
- Primary and secondary

**Primary amenorrhea**

Menstruation has never occurred

May be genetic disorder

- Turner's syndrome (ovaries do not function)

**Secondary amenorrhea**

Cessation of menstruation for 3 cycles or 6 months

- Individual has previously menstruated

Various causes of annovulation/amenorrhea

> ***Examples:***
> - Tumors
> - Stress
> - Eating disorders
> - Competitive sports participation

### Dysfunctional Uterine Bleeding (DUB)
Abnormal bleeding patterns

Occurs when no organic cause can be identified

### Abnormal Menstruation Types
Oligomenorrhea: in excess of 6 weeks between periods

Polymenorrhea: less than 3 weeks between periods

Metrorrhagia: bleeding between cycles

Menorrhagia: increase in amount and duration of flow

Hypomenorrhea: light or spotty flow

Menometrorrhagia: irregular cycle with varying amounts and duration of flow

Menorrhea: lengthy menstrual flow

Dysmenorrhea: painful menstruation

### Premenstrual Syndrome (PMS)
Also known as premenstrual tension (PMT)

Occurs before onset of menses (luteal phase) and ends at onset of menses

#### Cluster of common symptoms
Weight gain

Breast tenderness

Sleep disturbances

Headache

Irritability

Cause is unknown

#### Treatment
- Varies depending on individual symptoms

### Endometriosis
Endometrial tissue (uterine lining) develops outside the uterus (on ovaries, fallopian tubes, small intestine, etc.)

#### Responses to hormone cycle
Ectopic (out of place) endometrial tissue degenerates, sheds, and bleeds

#### Causes
- Irritation

- Inflammation

- Pain

Continued cycles produce fibrous tissue

- Adhesions and obstructions can then form

- Interferes with normal bodily function

- For example, fallopian tube endometriosis may lead to obstructed tubes

Primary symptom is dysmenorrhea

- May also cause painful intercourse (dyspareunia)

**Risks**

Increased risk for cancers

- Breast

- Ovaries

- Non-Hodgkin lymphoma

**Treatment Includes**

Hormonal suppression

Surgical removal of endometrial tissue

- May require hysterectomy and BSO (bilateral salpingo-oophorectomy)

# Infection, Inflammation, and Sexually Transmitted Diseases

## Pelvic Inflammatory Disease (PID)

Infection and inflammation of reproductive tract

- Primarily ovaries and fallopian tubes

- Usually originates in cervix or vagina

  - Migrates up through reproductive tract

**Types**

Acute

Chronic

Commonly forms adhesions and strictures

- May lead to infertility

## Candidiasis

Yeast infection

- *Candida albicans (Monilia)*

Not sexually transmitted

Opportunistic infection may follow

- Infection treated with antibiotics

- Period of reduced resistance

- Increased glucose or glycogen levels (often associated with diabetes mellitus)

Affects mucous membranes

Produces a white, thick, curdlike discharge

Result may be dyspareunia and dysuria

**Treatment**

Antifungal substances such as nystatin

Identification and treatment of underlying condition

## Chlamydia

Most common sexually transmitted disease (STD)

**Cause**
Bacteria, *Chlamydia trachomatis*

**Symptoms**
Asymptomatic or mild discharge and dysuria

**Treatment**
Antimicrobial

## Genital Herpes
**Cause**
Virus, herpes simplex 2 (HSV-2)

**Symptoms**
Ulcers and vesicles

**Treatment**
Antiviral, manage outbreaks

There is no cure for genital herpes

## Genital Warts
**Cause**
Virus, human papillomavirus

**Symptoms**
Polyps or grey lesions

**Treatment**
Excision

**Prevention**
Vaccine

There is no cure for genital warts

## Gonorrhea
**Cause**
Bacteria, *Neisseria gonorrhoeae*

Some strains are drug-resistant

**Symptoms**
Dysuria

Discharge

**Treatment**
Antibacterial drugs

## Syphilis
**Cause**
Bacteria, *Treponema pallidum*

**Symptoms**
Primary syphilis

- Ulcer or chancre at site of entry

Secondary syphilis

- Headache

- Fever

- Rash

- Tertiary

  - Affects cardiovascular and nervous systems

**Treatment**
Penicillin

## Trichomoniasis

**Cause**
Protozoan, *Trichomonas vaginalis*

**Symptoms**
Usually asymptomatic

**Treatment**
Antimicrobial drugs

## Benign Lesions

### Leiomyomas—Uterine Fibroids
Well-defined, solid uterine tumor

Also known as

- Uterine fibroids

- Fibromyoma

- Fibroma

- Myoma

- Fibroid

Classification is based on location of tumor within uterine wall

Submucous: beneath endometrium

Subserous: beneath serosa

Intramural: in muscle wall

**Symptoms**
May be asymptomatic

Abnormal uterine bleeding

Pressure on nearby structures, such as bladder and rectum

Constipation

Pain

Sensation of heaviness

**Treatment**
Surgical excision of lesions

Hysterectomy may be necessary

### Adenomyosis
Within uterine myometrium

**Symptoms**
Usually asymptomatic

Abnormal menstrual bleeding

Enlarged uterus

Commonly develops in late reproductive years

Common in those taking Tamoxifen

**Treatment**
Symptomatic in mild cases

Surgical in severe cases

- Excision of adenomyosis or hysterectomy

## Malignant Lesions

### Carcinoma of Breast
Accessory of reproductive system

Most often develops in upper outer quadrant

- Due to location, often spreads to lymph nodes

- May metastasize to lungs, brain, bone, liver, etc.

Majority arise from epithelial cells of ducts and lobules

Second most common cancer of women

Most are adenocarcinoma

- Invasive ductal carcinoma most common type

- Invasive lobular carcinoma second most common type

- Lymph node spread is determined by biopsying sentinel node (SNB)

- Small primary tumors are excised in a lumpectomy (tumor and immediate surrounding tissue only)

- Mastectomy is alternative surgical procedure removing entire breast

- Chemotherapy and radiation may be indicated to prevent reoccurrence

If neoplasm is responsive to hormone, hormone-blocking agents are administered

**Increased risks**
- Heredity

  - Especially history of mother or sister who developed breast cancer

  - Mutated breast cancer gene (BRCA-1)

  - Familial breast cancer syndrome associated with BRCA-2

- Lower socioeconomic status

- Radiation exposure

## Carcinoma of Uterus (Endometrial Cancer)

Most frequent pelvic cancer

Usually postmenopausal

Associated with higher levels of estrogen

**Increases risk**
  Obesity (estrogen produced by fat tissue)

  Early menarche

  Delayed menopause

  Hypertension

  Diabetes mellitus

  Nulliparity (no viable births)

  Some types of colorectal cancer

  Oral contraceptives (estrogen)

  Estrogen-producing tumors

**Symptoms**
  Abnormal, excessive uterine bleeding

  Postmenopausal bleeding

No simple screening test available

• Uterine cells may be aspirated for evaluation

**Staging of endometrial, cervical, and ovarian malignancies**
  I—Confined to corpus

  II—Involves corpus and cervix

  III—Extends outside uterus but not outside true pelvis

  IV—Extends outside true pelvis or involves rectum or bladder

**Treatment**
  Pharmaceutical

  Surgical

  Irradiation

  Chemotherapy

  Combination of above

## Carcinoma of Cervix

Routinely found on Papanicolaou (Pap) smear

Dysplasia is an early change in cervical epithelium

**Increases risks**
  Herpes simplex virus type 2 (HSV-2)

  Human papillomavirus (HPV)

  Young age of sexual activity

Smoking

Lower socioeconomic status

Stages of cervical cancer

Stage 1—Carcinoma of cervix

Stage 2—Carcinoma spread from cervix to upper vagina

Stage 3—Carcinoma spread to lower portion of vagina/pelvic wall

Stage 4—Most invasive stage spreading to other body parts

### Symptoms

Early stages asymptomatic

Later stages

- Bleeding

- Discharge

Biopsy is used to confirm

### Treatment

Pharmaceutical

Surgical

Irradiation

Chemotherapy

Combination of above

## Carcinoma of Ovary

Cause is unknown—considered silent killer

### Increased risks

Genetic factors (BRCA-1)

Endocrine

- Nulliparous

- Early menarche

- Late menopause

- Non–breast feeding

- Late first pregnancy

- Postmenopausal estrogen replacement therapy (ERT)

### Tumor categories

*Germ cell tumors*

Arise from primitive germ cells, usually the testis and ovum

### Types

- Germinoma

- Yolk sac

- Endodermal sinus tumor
- Teratoma
- Embryonal carcinoma
- Polyembryoma
- Gonadoblastoma
- Some types of choriocarcinoma

**Categories**

- Dermoid cysts (benign)
- Malignant tumors
- Primitive malignant
  - Embryonic
  - Extraembryonic cells

*Epithelial tumors*
Most common gynecologic cancer

*Gonadal stromal tumors*
**Symptoms**
    Pelvic heaviness

    Dysuria

    Increased urinary frequency

    Sometimes vaginal bleeding

**Treatment**
    Excision

        Hysterectomy, including bilateral salpingo-oophorectomy with omentectomy (fold of peritoneum)

    Chemotherapy

    Radiation therapy

    Combination of above

## Carcinoma of Fallopian Tubes
*Primary fallopian tube tumors*
Rare

Must be located within tube to be considered primary

- Adenocarcinoma most common primary tumor

Most tumors are secondary

**Symptoms**
    Often asymptomatic

    Bleeding or discharge

    Irregular menstruation

    Pain

**Treatment**
Hysterectomy, including bilateral salpingo-oophorectomy with any necessary omentectomy (fold of peritoneum)

Chemotherapy

Radiation therapy

Combination of above

## Carcinoma of Vulva
Usually squamous cell carcinoma (90%)

Increased risk with STDs

**Symptoms**
Can be asymptomatic

Pruritic vulvular lesion

**Treatment**
Radical vulvectomy with node dissection

Wide local excision

## Carcinoma of Vagina
Usually squamous cell carcinoma

**Increased risk**
Human papillomavirus (HPV)

Postmenopausal hysterectomy

History of abnormal Pap

History of other carcinomas

**Symptoms**
Often asymptomatic

Vaginal pain, discharge, or bleeding

**Treatment**
Squamous cell—radiation

Early tumors may be excised

Vaginectomy

Hysterectomy

Lymph node dissection

# Pregnancy

## Placenta Previa
Opening of cervix is obstructed by displaced placenta

**Types (Fig. 1–23)**
Marginal

Partial

Total

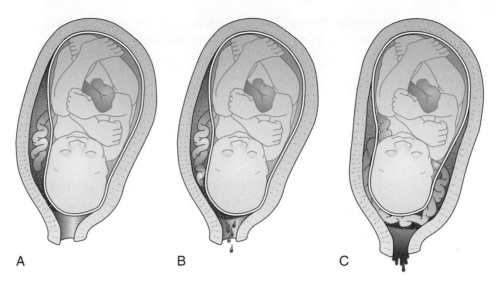

Figure **1-23** **A,** Marginal placenta previa. **B,** Partial placenta previa. **C,** Total placenta previa.

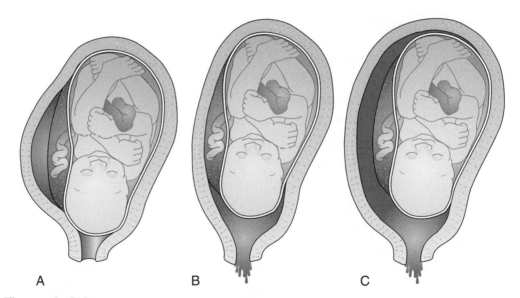

Figure **1-24** Abruptio placentae is classified according to the grade of separation of the placenta from uterine wall. **A,** Mild separation in which hemorrhage is internal. **B,** Moderate separation in which there is external hemorrhage. **C,** Severe separation in which there is external hemorrhage and extreme separation.

## Abruptio Placentae (Fig. 1–24)
Premature separation of placenta from uterine wall

### Eclampsia
Serious condition of pregnancy characterized by

• Hypertension

• Edema

• Proteinuria

### Ectopic Pregnancy (Extrauterine) (Fig. 1–25)
Implantation of fertilized ovum outside uterus

- Often fallopian tubes (tubal pregnancy)

### Hydatidiform Mole
Benign tumor of placenta

Secretes hormone (chorionic gonadotropic hormone, CGH)

Indicates positive pregnancy test

### Malpositions and Malpresentations (Fig. 1–26)

### Vaginal Delivery

Breech

Vertex

Face

Brow

Shoulder

### Abortion
**Types**

Spontaneous

- Miscarriage
- Happens naturally
- Uterus completely empties

Incomplete

- Uterus does not completely empty
- Requires intervention to remove remaining fetal material

Missed

- Fetus dies naturally
- Requires intervention to remove fetal material

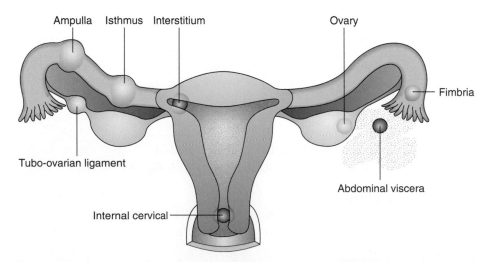

Figure **1-25** Ectopic pregnancy most often occurs in fallopian tube. Pregnancy outside the uterus may end in life-threatening rupture.

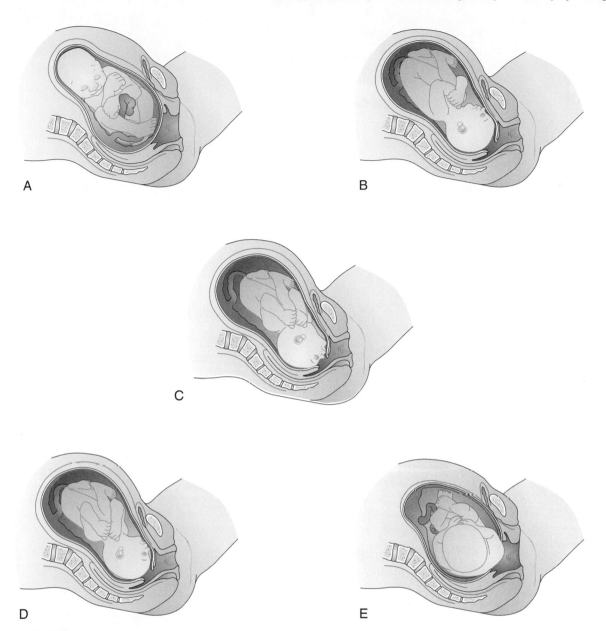

Figure **1-26** Five types of malposition and malpresentation of fetus: **A,** Breech. **B,** Vertex. **C,** Face. **D,** Brow. **E,** Shoulder.

Septic

- Similar to missed
- Has added complication of infection
- Requires intervention to remove fetal material
- Vigorous treatment of infection

**Methods**
D&C

- Dilation and curettage (scraping)

Evacuation (suction)

Intra-amniotic injections

- Saline (salt) solution

Vaginal suppositories

- Such as prostaglandin

# FEMALE GENITAL SYSTEM AND PREGNANCY PATHOPHYSIOLOGY QUIZ

1. Most common solution used for intra-amniotic injections is:
   a. prostaglandin
   b. saline
   c. estrogen
   d. chorionic gonadotropic hormone

2. This type of dysmenorrhea is treated with nonsteroidal antiinflammatory agents and progesterone:
   a. secondary
   b. constrictive
   c. periodic
   d. primary

3. In this type of amenorrhea there is a cessation of menstruation:
   a. secondary
   b. constrictive
   c. periodic
   d. primary

Match the abnormal menstruation type with correct definition.

4. oligomenorrhea _____    a. increased amount and duration of flow

5. metrorrhagia _____    b. bleeding between cycles

6. menorrhagia _____    c. in excess of 6 weeks

7. Increased risks of breast cancer, ovarian cancer, and non-Hodgkin lymphoma exist with this condition:
   a. endometriosis
   b. pelvic inflammatory disease
   c. sexually transmitted disease
   d. dysfunctional uterine bleeding

8. This benign lesion is also known as uterine fibroids:
   a. adenomyosis
   b. squamous cell
   c. leiomyoma
   d. extraembryonic cell primitive

9. Marginal, partial, and total are types of this condition:
   a. abruptio placentae
   b. placenta previa
   c. ectopic pregnancy
   d. hydatidiform mole

10. Which of the following is NOT a malposition of fetus?
    a. breech
    b. shoulder
    c. back
    d. brow

# ■ MALE GENITAL SYSTEM
## MALE GENITAL SYSTEM—ANATOMY AND TERMINOLOGY

Function, reproduction

Structure, essential organs, and accessory organs (Fig. 1–27)

### Essential Organs

#### Testes (Gonads)
Produce sperm (male gamete with 23 chromosomes) in seminiferous tubules

Covered by tunica albuginea, located in scrotum

Produce testosterone in Leydig cells

#### Vas Deferens
Is a tube

End of epididymis

### Accessory Organs

Ducts (carry sperm from testes to exterior), sex glands (produce solutions that mix with sperm), and external genitalia

Seminal vesicles produce most seminal fluid

Prostate gland produces some seminal fluid and activates sperm

Bulbourethral gland (Cowper's glands) secretes a very small amount of seminal fluid

**External genitalia:** penis and scrotum

- Penis contains three columns of erectile tissue: two corpora cavernosa and one spongiosum

- Urethra passes through corpora spongiosum

- Scrotum encloses testes

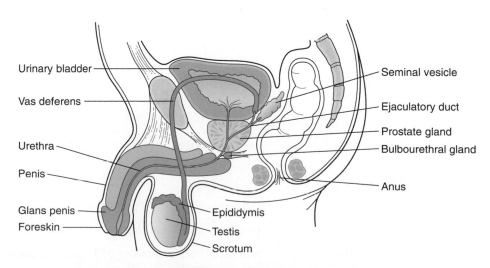

Figure **1-27** Male reproductive system.

Passage of sperm from production to exterior

Sperm are produced in seminiferous tubules (testes) and pass into

Epididymis then to vas deferens (within seminal vesicles) to

Ejaculatory duct then through urethra (prostate gland and Cowper's [bulbourethral] gland)

Pass though penis to outside of body

## COMBINING FORMS

| | | |
|---|---|---|
| 1. | andr/o | male |
| 2. | balan/o | glans penis |
| 3. | cry/o | cold |
| 4. | crypt/o | hidden |
| 5. | epididym/o | epididymis |
| 6. | gon/o | seed |
| 7. | hydr/o | water, fluid |
| 8. | orch/i | testicle |
| 9. | orch/o | testicle |
| 10. | orchi/o | testicle |
| 11. | orchid/o | testicle |
| 12. | prostat/o | prostate gland |
| 13. | semin/i | semen |
| 14. | sperm/o | sperm |
| 15. | spermat/o | sperm |
| 16. | test/o | testicle |
| 17. | varic/o | varicose veins |
| 18. | vas/o | vessel, vas deferens |
| 19. | vesicul/o | seminal vesicles |

## SUFFIXES

| | | |
|---|---|---|
| 1. | -one | hormone |
| 2. | -pexy | fixation |
| 3. | -ectomy | removal |
| 4. | -stomy | new opening |

## MEDICAL ABBREVIATIONS

| | | |
|---|---|---|
| 1. | BPH | benign prostatic hypertrophy |
| 2. | PSA | prostate-specific antigen |
| 3. | TURBT | transurethral resection of bladder tumor |
| 4. | TURP | transurethral resection of prostate |

## MEDICAL TERMS

| | |
|---|---|
| Cavernosa | Connection between cavity of penis and a vein |
| Cavernosography | Radiographic recording of a cavity, e.g., pulmonary cavity or main part of penis |
| Cavernosometry | Measurement of pressure in a cavity, e.g., penis |
| Chordee | Condition resulting in penis being bent downward |
| Corpora cavernosa | The two cavities of penis |
| Epididymectomy | Surgical removal of epididymis |
| Epididymis | Tube located at the top of testes that stores sperm |
| Epididymovasostomy | Creation of a new connection between vas deferens and epididymis |
| Meatotomy | Surgical enlargement of opening of urinary meatus |
| Orchiectomy | Castration, removal of testes |
| Orchiopexy | Surgical procedure to release undescended testis and fixate within scrotum |
| Penoscrotal | Referring to penis and scrotum |
| Plethysmography | Determining changes in volume of an organ part or body |
| Priapism | Painful condition in which penis is constantly erect |
| Prostatotomy | Incision into prostate |
| Transurethral resection, prostate | Procedure performed through urethra by means of a cystoscopy to remove part or all of prostate |
| Tumescence | State of being swollen |
| Tunica vaginalis | Covering of testes |
| Varicocele | Swelling of a scrotal vein |
| Vas deferens | Tube that carries sperm from epididymis to ejaculatory duct and seminal vesicles |
| Vasectomy | Removal of segment of vas deferens |
| Vasogram | Recording of the flow in vas deferens |
| Vasotomy | Incision in vas deferens |
| Vasorrhaphy | Suturing of vas deferens |
| Vasovasostomy | Reversal of a vasectomy |
| Vesiculectomy | Excision of seminal vesicle |
| Vesiculotomy | Incision into seminal vesicle |

# MALE GENITAL SYSTEM ANATOMY AND TERMINOLOGY QUIZ

1. This gland activates sperm and produces some seminal fluid:
   a. seminal vesicle
   b. bulbourethral gland
   c. prostate gland
   d. scrotum

2. Carries sperm from testes to ejaculatory duct:
   a. vas deferens
   b. sex gland
   c. tunica
   d. seminal

3. Penis contains these erectile tissues:
   a. one corpora cavernosa and two spongiosa
   b. two corpora cavernosa and two spongiosa
   c. one corpora cavernosa and one spongiosum
   d. two corpora cavernosa and one spongiosum

4. Also known as Cowper's gland:
   a. seminal vesicles
   b. bulbourethral gland
   c. prostate gland
   d. scrotum

5. Which of the following is NOT an accessory organ?
   a. gonads
   b. seminal vesicles
   c. prostate
   d. penis

6. Combining form meaning "male":
   a. andr/o
   b. balan/o
   c. orchi/o
   d. test/o

7. Combining form meaning "glans penis":
   a. balan/o
   b. vas/o
   c. vesicul/o
   d. orch/o

8. Testes are covered by the:
   a. seminal vesicles
   b. androgen
   c. chancre
   d. tunica albuginea

9. This abbreviation describes a surgical resection of prostate that is accomplished by means of an endoscope inserted into the urethra:
   a. TURBT
   b. BPH
   c. UPJ
   d. TURP

10. This abbreviation describes a condition of prostate in which there is an enlargement that is benign:
    a. TURBT
    b. BPH
    c. UPJ
    d. TURP

# MALE GENITAL SYSTEM—PATHOPHYSIOLOGY

## Male Genital System Disorders

### Disorders of Scrotum, Testes, and Epididymis

#### Cryptorchidism

Undescended testes—condition at birth

- Unilateral or bilateral
- Primarily result from obstruction
- Risk neoplastic processes
- May descend spontaneously

Treatment

- Administration of hormone to stimulate testosterone production
- Surgical intervention (orchiopexy) near age 1 to avoid risk of infertility

#### Orchitis

Inflammation of testes

Most common cause is virus

- Such as mumps orchitis
- Atrophy with irreversible loss of sperm production at risk

May be associated with

- Mumps or epidemic parotitis
- Gonorrhea
- Syphilis
- Tuberculosis

Symptoms

- Mild to severe pain in testes
- Mild to severe edema
- Feeling of weight in testicular area

Treatment

- Depends upon presence of underlying condition

#### Epididymitis

Inflammation of epididymis

Inflammatory response to trauma or infection

Abscess may form

#### Types

Sexually transmitted epididymitis

- Gonorrhea
- *T. pallidum*
- *T. vaginalis*

Nonspecific bacterial epididymitis

- *E. coli*
- Streptococci
- Staphylococci
- Associated with underlying urological disorder

*Symptoms*
Scrotal pain

Swelling

Erythema

Perhaps hydrocele formation

*Treatment*
Antibiotic

Bed rest

Ice packs

Scrotal support

Analgesics

**Hydrocele (Fig. 1–28)**
Collection of fluid in membranes of tunica vaginalis

May be congenital or acquired (response to infection or tumors)

Congenital hydrocele may reabsorb due to a communication between the scrotal sac and peritoneal cavity and require no intervention

*Symptoms*
Scrotal enlargement

Usually painless

- Unless infection is present

**Varicocele**
Abnormal dilation of plexus of veins

Decreases sperm production and motility

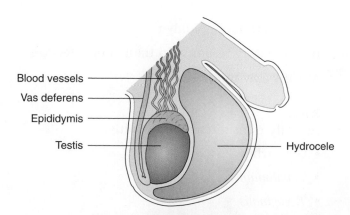

Figure **1-28** Hydrocele.

*Symptoms*
Usually painless

In elderly, may signal renal tumor

*Treatment*
Surgical intervention

**Torsion of testes (Fig. 1–29)**
Twisting of testes

Congenital abnormal development of tunica vaginalis and spermatic cord

Trauma may precipitate

*Symptoms*
Sudden onset of severe pain

Nausea

Vomiting

Scrotal edema and tenderness

Fever

*Treatment*
Immediate surgical intervention

**Cancer of testes**
Rare form of cancer

Cure rate high (95%)

Cause unknown

Usually occurs in younger men

Two main groups

- Germ cell tumors (GCT)—90% of testicular tumors

- Sex cord-stromal tumors

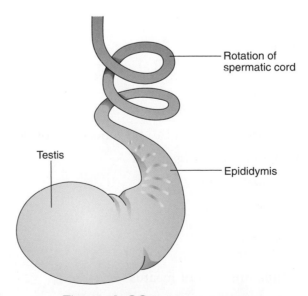

Figure **1-29** Torsion of testis.

**Cancer of scrotum**
Rare form of cancer

- Squamous cell carcinoma

*Symptoms*
Asymptomatic in early stages

Ulcerations in later stages

*Treatment*
Wide local excision

Mohs micrographic surgery

- Precise removal of tumor

- Layers are removed until no further microscopic evidence of abnormal cells is seen

Laser therapy

Lymph nodes are examined for metastasis

## Disorders of Urethra

**Epispadias**
Congenital anomaly

Urethral meatus is located on dorsal side of penis

Usually occurs in conjunction with other abnormalities

*Treatment*
Surgical reconstruction

**Hypospadias**
Most common abnormality of penis

Urethral opening on ventral side of penis

Results in curvature of penis

- Due to chordee

*Treatment*
Surgical reconstruction

**Urethritis**
Inflammation of urethra

Infectious urethritis can be gonococcal or nongonococcal

Nongonococcal organisms

- *C. trachomatis*

- *U. urealyticum*

*Symptoms*
Discharge

Inflammation of meatus

Burning

Itching

Urgent and frequent urination

In nongonococcal, symptoms are fewer

### Treatment
Antibiotics based on organism

## Disorders of Penis
### Balanitis
Inflammation of glans

### Causes
Syphilis

Trichomoniasis

Gonorrhea

*Candida albicans*

Tinea

Underlying disease—diabetes mellitus and candidiasis

No circumcision

### Symptoms
Irritation

Tenderness

Discharge

Edema

Ulceration

Swelling of lymph nodes

### Treatment
Culture of discharge

Saline irrigation

Antibiotics

### Phimosis and paraphimosis
### Phimosis
Condition in which prepuce (foreskin) is constricted

• Prepuce cannot be retracted over glans penis

Can occur at any age

Associated with poor hygiene and chronic infection in uncircumcised males

### Symptoms
Erythema

Edema

Tenderness

Purulent discharge

*Treatment*
Surgical circumcision

*Paraphimosis*
Condition in which prepuce (foreskin) is constricted

Prepuce is retracted over glans penis and cannot be moved forward

*Symptom*
Edema

*Treatment*
Surgical

### Peyronie's disease
Also known as bent nail syndrome

Fibrotic condition

- Results in lateral curvature of penis during erection

Occurs most often in middle-aged men

Cause is unknown but associated with

- Diabetes
- Keloid development
- Dupuytren's contracture (flexion deformity of toes and fingers)

*Treatment*
Sometimes spontaneous remission

Pharmacologic oxygenation increasing therapies

Surgical resection of fibrous bands

### Cancer of penis
Rare form of cancer

Occurs most often in men over age 60

Squamous cell carcinoma

Increased risks

- More common in uncircumcised men
- Sexual partner with cervical carcinoma
- Human papillomavirus

Usually begins with small lesion beneath prepuce

Intraepithelial neoplasia is also known as

- Bowen's disease
- Erythroplasia of Queyrat
- Begins as noninvasive

Progresses to invasive if untreated

Metastasis to lymph nodes

*Treatment*

Excision

Mohs micrographic surgery

Radiation therapy

Laser therapy

Cryosurgery

Advanced tumors are treated with partial or total penectomy and chemotherapy

## Disorders of Prostate Gland

**Benign prostatic hyperplasia/hypertrophy (BPH)**

Multiple fibroadenomatous nodules; usually located on outside of gland, so easily palpable on digital exam

- Related to aging; common in men over 60 years of age

- Enlarging prostate obstructs bladder neck and urethra

- Decreases urine flow

It is thought that increased levels of estrogen/androgen cause BPH

*Symptoms*

Increased frequency and urgency of urination

Nocturia

Incontinence

Hesitancy

Diminished force

Postvoiding dribble

*Screening*

Prostate-specific antigen (PSA)

Digital rectal examination (DRE)

*Treatment*

Partial prostatectomy

Transurethral resection of prostate (TURP)

Excision of nodules

Hormone therapy

Placement of urethral stents

Pharmaceuticals—those that inhibit production of testosterone and those that relax smooth muscle of gland and neck of bladder

**Prostatitis**

Inflammation of prostate

- Acute or chronic bacterial prostatitis

*Causes*

*Escherichia coli*

Enterococci

Staphylococci

Streptococci

*Chlamydia trachomatis*

*Ureaplasma urealyticum*

*Neisseria gonorrhea*

### Nonbacterial
Spontaneous

Prostatodynia

### Symptoms
#### Acute prostatitis
Fever and chills

Lower back pain

Perineal pain

Dysuria

Tenderness, suprapubic

Urinary tract infection

#### Chronic prostatitis
Recurring

Same as acute only with no infection in urinary tract

### Treatment
#### Acute
Antibiotic based on culture

#### Chronic
No treatment available

### Cancer of prostate
Most common diagnosed malignancy in men, occurring in men over age 60

Indications are that the cause is related to androgens

Predominately adenocarcinoma (95%)

No relationship between BPH and cancer of prostate

### Symptoms
Asymptomatic in early stages

Later symptoms include

- Dysuria
- Back pain
- Hematuria
- Frequent urination

- Urinary retention

- Increased incidence of uremia

### Stages
Two systems used to stage prostate cancer

- Whitmore-Jewett stages as indicated in Fig. 1–30

- Tumor node metastasis (TNM) as indicated in Fig. 1–31

### Treatment
Dependent upon stage

**WHITMORE-JEWETT STAGES:**

Stage A is clinically undetectable tumor confined to the gland and is an incidental finding at prostate surgery.
A1: well-differentiated with focal involvement
A2: moderately or poorly differentiated or involves multiple foci in the gland
Stage B is tumor confined to the prostate gland.
B0: nonpalpable, PSA-detected
B1: single nodule in one lobe of the prostate
B2: more extensive involvement of one lobe or involvement of both lobes
Stage C is a tumor clinically localized to the periprostatic area but extending through the prostatic capsule; seminal vesicles may be involved.
C1: clinical extracapsular extension
C2: extracapsular tumor producing bladder outlet or ureteral obstruction
Stage D is metastatic disease.
D0: clinically localized disease (prostate only) but persistently elevated enzymatic serum acid phosphatase
D1: regional lymph nodes only
D2: distant lymph nodes, metastases to bone or visceral organs
D3: D2 prostate cancer patients who relapse after adequate endocrine therapy

Figure **1-30** Whitmore-Jewett stages.

**TNM STAGES:**

**Primary Tumor (T)**

TX: Primary tumor cannot be assessed

T0: No evidence of primary tumor

T1: Clinically inapparent tumor not palpable or visible by imaging

    T1a: Tumor incidental histologic finding in 5% or less of tissue resected

    T1b: Tumor incidental histologic finding in more than 5% of tissue resected

    T1c: Tumor identified by needle biopsy (e.g., because of elevated PSA)

T2: Tumor confined within the prostate

    T2a: Tumor involves half a lobe or less

    T2b: Tumor involves more than half of a lobe, but not both lobes

    T2c: Tumor involves both lobes; extends through the prostatic capsule

T3a: Unilateral extracapsular extension

T3b: Bilateral extracapsular extension

T3c: Tumor invades the seminal vesicle(s)

T4: Tumor is fixed or invades adjacent structures other than the seminal vesicle(s)

    T4a: Tumor invades any of bladder neck, external sphincter, or rectum

    T4b: Tumor invades levator muscles and/or is fixed to the pelvic wall

**Regional lymph nodes (N)**

NX: Regional lymph nodes cannot be assessed

N0: No regional lymph node metastasis

N1: Metastasis in a single lymph node, 2 cm or less in greatest dimension

N2: Metastasis in a single lymph node, more than 2 cm but not more than 5 cm in greatest dimension; or multiple lymph node metastases, none more than 5 cm in greatest dimension

N3: Metastasis in a single lymph node more than 5 cm in greatest dimension

**Distant metastases (M)**

MX: Presence of distant metastasis cannot be assessed

M0: No distant metastasis

M1: Distant metastasis

    M1a: Nonregional lymph node(s)

    M1b: Bone(s)

    M1c: Other site(s)

Figure **1-31** TNM stages.

# MALE GENITAL SYSTEM PATHOPHYSIOLOGY QUIZ

1. What is the condition in which testes do not descend?
   a. cryptorchidism
   b. Bowen's disease
   c. torsion
   d. hypospadias

2. Orchitis is most often caused by a:
   a. bacteria
   b. virus
   c. parasite
   d. fungus

3. A condition that can be either congenital or acquired through trauma and that involves twisting of testes is:
   a. hydrocele
   b. hypospadias
   c. cryptorchidism
   d. torsion

4. Cancer of the _____ is divided into two main groups of germ cell tumors and sex stromal cord tumors.
   a. testes
   b. penis
   c. scrotum
   d. prostate

5. This type of surgical technique involves excision of a lesion in layers until no further evidence of abnormality is seen:
   a. Bowen's
   b. Addison's
   c. Mohs
   d. laser

6. Epispadias is a disorder of urethra in which urethral meatus is located on the _____ side of penis:
   a. ventral
   b. dorsal
   c. lateral
   d. medial

7. Inflammation of glans is:
   a. phimosis
   b. paraphimosis
   c. urethritis
   d. balanitis

8. This disease is also known as bent nail syndrome:
   a. Bowen's
   b. Peyronie's
   c. Addison's
   d. Whitmore-Jewett

9. Condition in which multiple fibroadenomatous nodules form and lead to decreased urine flow. Condition is thought to be related to increased levels of estrogen/androgen.
   a. BPH
   b. DRE
   c. GCT
   d. TNM

10. Cancer of prostate is predominately this type of cancer:
   a. sex cord
   b. adenocarcinoma
   c. squamous cell
   d. seminoma

# ■ URINARY SYSTEM
## URINARY SYSTEM—ANATOMY AND TERMINOLOGY

Removes metabolic waste materials (nitrogenous waste: urea, creatinine, and uric acid)

Conserves nutrients and water

Balances: electrolytes (acids/bases balance)

Electrolytes are electrically charged molecules required for nerve and muscle function

Assists liver in detoxification

### Organs (Fig. 1–32)

Kidneys

Ureters

Urinary bladder

Urethra

### Kidneys (Fig. 1–33)
Electrolytes and fluid balance

Control pH balance (acid/base)

Figure **1-32** Urinary system.

Figure **1-33** Kidney.

Secrete berenin (which affects blood pressure) and erythropoietin (which stimulates red blood cell production in bone marrow)

Secrete active vitamin D required for calcium absorption from intestines

Two organs located behind peritoneum (retroperitoneal space)

### *Kidney Structure*

Cortex (outer layer)

Medulla (inner portion)

Hilum (depression on medial border through which blood vessels and nerves pass)

Pyramids (divisions of medulla)

Papilla (inner part of pyramids)

Pelvis (receptacle for urine within kidney)

Calyces surround top of renal pelvis

Nephrons (3 types) are operational units of kidney

## Ureters
Narrow tubes transporting urine from kidneys to bladder

## Urinary Bladder
Reservoir for urine

Shaped like an upside down pear with three surfaces

- Posterior (base)

- Anterior (neck)

- Superior (peritoneum)

Trigone

- Smooth triangular area inside bladder—size never changes

- Formed by openings of ureters and urethra

**Urethra**

Canal from bladder to exterior of body

Urinary meatus, outside opening of urethra

## COMBINING FORMS

|     |           |                              |
|-----|-----------|------------------------------|
| 1.  | albumin/o | albumin                      |
| 2.  | azot/o    | urea                         |
| 3.  | bacteri/o | bacteria                     |
| 4.  | cali/o    | calyx                        |
| 5.  | cyst/o    | urinary                      |
| 6.  | dips/o    | thirst                       |
| 7.  | glomerul/o| glomerulus                   |
| 8.  | glyc/o    | sugar                        |
| 9.  | glycos/o  | sugar                        |
| 10. | hydr/o    | water                        |
| 11. | ket/o     | ketone bodies/ketoacidosis   |
| 12. | lith/o    | stone                        |
| 13. | meat/o    | meatus                       |
| 14. | nephr/o   | kidney                       |
| 15. | noct/i    | night                        |
| 16. | olig/o    | scant, few                   |
| 17. | pyel/o    | renal pelvis                 |
| 18. | ren/o     | kidney                       |
| 19. | son/o     | sound                        |
| 20. | tripsy    | to crush                     |
| 21. | tryg/o    | trigone region/kidney        |
| 22. | ur/o      | urine                        |
| 23. | ureter/o  | ureter                       |
| 24. | urethr/o  | urethra                      |
| 25. | uria      | urination/urinary condition  |
| 26. | urin/o    | urine                        |
| 27. | vesic/o   | bladder                      |

## PREFIXES

| | | |
|---|---|---|
| 1. | dys- | painful |
| 2. | peri- | surrounding |
| 3. | poly- | many |
| 4. | retro- | behind |

## SUFFIXES

| | | |
|---|---|---|
| 1. | -eal | pertaining to |
| 2. | -lithiasis | condition of stones |
| 3. | -lysis | separation |
| 4. | -plasty | repair |
| 5. | -rrhaphy | suture |
| 6. | -tripsy | crush |

## MEDICAL ABBREVIATIONS

| | | |
|---|---|---|
| 1. | ARF | acute renal failure |
| 2. | BUN | blood urea nitrogen |
| 3. | ESRD | end-stage renal disease |
| 4. | HD | hemodialysis |
| 5. | IVP | intravenous pyelogram |
| 6. | KUB | kidney, ureter, bladder |
| 7. | pH | symbol for acid/base level |
| 8. | PKU | phenylketonuria |
| 9. | sp gr | specific gravity |
| 10. | UA | urinalysis |
| 11. | UPJ | ureteropelvic junction |
| 12. | UTI | urinary tract infection |

## MEDICAL TERMS

| | |
|---|---|
| Bulbocavernosus | Muscle that constricts vagina in a female and urethra in a male |
| Bulbourethral | Gland with duct leading to urethra |
| Calculus | Concretion of mineral salts, also called a stone |
| Calycoplasty | Surgical reconstruction of recess of renal pelvis |
| Calyx | Recess of renal pelvis |
| Cystolithectomy | Removal of a calculus (stone) from urinary bladder |
| Cystometrogram | CMG, measurement of pressures and capacity of urinary bladder |
| Cystoplasty | Surgical reconstruction of bladder |
| Cystorrhaphy | Suture of bladder |

| | |
|---|---|
| Cystoscopy | Use of a scope to view bladder |
| Cystostomy | Surgical creation of an opening into bladder |
| Cystotomy | Incision into bladder |
| Cystourethroplasty | Surgical reconstruction of bladder and urethra |
| Cystourethroscopy | Use of a scope to view bladder and urethra |
| Dilation | Stretching or expansion |
| Dysuria | Painful urination |
| Endopyelotomy | Procedure involving bladder and ureters, including insertion of a stent into renal pelvis |
| Extracorporeal | Occurring outside of body |
| Fundoplasty | Repair of the bottom of bladder |
| Hydrocele | Sac of fluid |
| Kock pouch | Surgical creation of a urinary bladder from a segment of the ileum |
| Nephrocutaneous fistula | An abnormal channel from kidney to skin |
| Nephrolithotomy | Removal of a kidney stone through an incision made into the kidney |
| Nephrorrhaphy | Suturing of kidney |
| Nephrostomy | Creation of a channel into renal pelvis of kidney |
| Transureteroureterostomy | Surgical connection of one ureter to other ureter |
| Transvesical ureterolithotomy | Removal of a ureter stone (calculus) through bladder |
| Ureterectomy | Surgical removal of a ureter, either totally or partially |
| Ureterocutaneous fistula | Channel from ureter to exterior skin |
| Ureteroenterostomy | Creation of a connection between intestine and ureter |
| Ureterolithotomy | Removal of a stone from ureter |
| Ureterolysis | Freeing of adhesions of ureter |
| Ureteroneocystostomy | Surgical connection of ureter to a new site on bladder |
| Ureteropyelography | Ureter and renal pelvis radiography |
| Ureterotomy | Incision into ureter |
| Urethrocystography | Radiography of bladder and urethra |
| Urethromeatoplasty | Surgical repair of urethra and meatus |
| Urethropexy | Fixation of urethra by means of surgery |
| Urethroplasty | Surgical repair of urethra |
| Urethrorrhaphy | Suturing of urethra |
| Urethroscopy | Use of a scope to view urethra |
| Vesicostomy | Surgical creation of a connection of viscera of bladder to skin |

# URINARY SYSTEM ANATOMY AND TERMINOLOGY QUIZ

1. The outer covering of kidney:
   a. medulla
   b. pyramids
   c. cortex
   d. papilla

2. Which is not a division of kidneys?
   a. pelvis
   b. pyramids
   c. cortex
   d. trigone

3. The inner portion of kidneys:
   a. medulla
   b. pyramids
   c. cortex
   d. papilla

4. The smooth area inside bladder:
   a. pyramids
   b. calyces
   c. trigone
   d. cystocele

5. The narrow tube connecting kidney and bladder:
   a. urethra
   b. ureter
   c. meatus
   d. trigone

6. Which of the following is NOT a surface of urinary bladder?
   a. posterior
   b. anterior
   c. superior
   d. inferior

7. Combining form that means "stone":
   a. azot/o
   b. cyst/o
   c. lith/o
   d. olig/o

8. Term meaning "painful urination":
   a. pyuria
   b. dysuria
   c. diuresis
   d. hyperemia

9. Combining form meaning "scant":
   a. glyc/o
   b. hydr/o
   c. meat/o
   d. olig/o

10. Term that describes renal failure that is acute:
    a. ARF
    b. ESRD
    c. HD
    d. BPH

# URINARY SYSTEM—PATHOPHYSIOLOGY

## Renal Failure

### Acute Renal Failure
Sudden onset of renal failure

**Cause**
Extreme hypotension

Trauma

Infection

Inflammation

Toxicity

Obstructed vascular supply

**Symptoms**
Uremia

Oliguria (decreased output) or anuria (no output)

Hyperkalemia (high potassium in blood)

Pulmonary edema

**Types**
Prerenal

- Associated with poor systemic perfusion
- Decreased renal blood flow
  - Such as with congestive heart failure

Intrarenal

- Associated with renal parenchyma disease (functional tissue of kidney)
  - Such as acute interstitial nephritis, glomerulopathies, and malignant hypertension

Postrenal

- Resulting from urine flow obstruction outside kidney (ureters or bladder neck)

**Treatment**
Underlying condition

Dialysis

Monitoring of fluid and electrolyte balance

### Chronic Renal Failure
Gradual loss of function

- Progressively more severe renal insufficiency until end stage of
  - Renal disease
  - Irreversible kidney failure

**Stages—based on level of creatinine clearance**
Stage I: Blood flow through kidney increases, kidney enlarges

Stage II (mild): Small amounts of blood protein (albumin) leak into urine (microalbuminuria)

Stage III (moderate): Albumin and other protein losses increase; patient may develop high blood pressure and kidney loses ability to filter waste

Stage IV (severe): Large amounts of urine pass through kidney; blood pressure increases

Stage V: End-stage renal failure. Ability to filter waste nearly stops; dialysis or transplant only option

### Cause
Long-term exposure to nephrotoxins

Diabetes

Hypertension

### Symptoms
No symptoms until well advanced

Polyuria

Nausea or anorexia

Dehydration

Neurologic manifestations

### Stages of nephron loss
Decreased reserve

- 60% loss

Renal insufficiency

- 75% loss

End-stage renal failure

- 90% loss

### Treatment
No cure

Dialysis

Kidney transplant

## Urinary Tract Infections (UTI)

### Cystitis—Bacterial
### Cause
Bacteria, usually *E. coli*

### Symptoms
Lower abdominal pain

Dysuria

Lower back pain

Urinary frequency and urgency

Cloudy, foul-smelling urine

### Systemic signs
Fever

Malaise

Nausea

**Treatment**

Antibiotics

Increased fluid intake

## Cystitis—Nonbacterial

**Cause**

Unknown

May later produce bacterial infection

**Symptoms**

Urinary frequency and urgency

Dysuria

Negative urine culture

**Treatment**

No known treatment

## Acute Pyelonephritis (Fig. 1–34)

Bacterial infection with multiple abcesses of renal pelvis and medullary tissue

• May involve one or both kidneys

Figure **1-34** Acute pyelonephritis. Cortical surface exhibits grayish white areas of inflammation and abscess formation. (From Kumar V, Abbas AK, Fausto N: *Robbins and Cotran Pathologic Basis of Disease*, ed 7, Philadelphia, 2005, Saunders.)

**Cause**
*E. coli*

*Proteus*

*Pseudomonas*

Obstruction and reflux of urine from bladder

**Symptoms**
Fever

Chills

Groin or flank pain

Dysuria

Pyuria

Nocturia

**Treatment**
Antibiotics

Surgical correction of obstruction

## Chronic Pyelonephritis
Recurrent infection that causes scarring of kidney

Cause is difficult to determine

- Repeated infections
- Obstructive conditions

**Symptoms**
Hypertension

Dysuria

Flank pain

Increased frequency of urination

**Treatment**
Antibiotics for extended periods when reoccurring

Surgical reduction of obstruction

# Glomerular Disorders

May be acute or chronic

Function of glomerulus is blood filtration

## Glomerulonephritis
Inflammation of glomerulus

**Cause**
Drugs or toxins

Systemic disorder affecting many organs or idiopathic

May follow acute infections—most commonly streptococcal infections

Vascular pathology

Immune disorders

### Treatment
Follows cause

## Nephrotic Syndrome (Nephrosis)
Disease of kidneys that includes damage to membrane of the glomerulus causing excessive protein loss to urine

Accompanied by

- Hypoalbuminemia
- Hypercholesterolemia
- Hypercoagulability (excessive clotting)
- Prone to infections
- Edema
- Protein loss of >3.5 g

Damage to glomerulus results from

- Infection
- Immune response
    - Most predominant cause of dysfunction is exposure to toxins

May be a manifestation of an underlying condition, such as diabetes

### Symptoms
Edema

Weight gain

Pallor

Proteinuria

Lipiduria

### Treatment
Glucocorticoids, such as prednisone

- Reduces inflammation

Sodium- and fat-reduced diet

Protein supplements

Careful monitoring for continued inflammation

## Acute Poststreptococcal Glomerulonephritis (APSGN)
### Cause
*Streptococcus* infection

- With certain types of group A beta-hemolytic *Streptococcus*

Creates an antigen-antibody complex

- Infiltrates glomerular capillaries
- Results in inflammation in kidneys
- Inflammation interferes with normal kidney function
- Fluid and waste build-up
- Can lead to acute renal failure and scarring

Usually occurs in children 3 to 7 years of age

- Most often in boys

**Symptoms**

Back and flank pain

Cloudy, dark urine

Oliguria (decreased output)

Edema

Elevated blood pressure

Fatigue

Malaise

Headache

Nausea

**Treatment**

Sodium reduction

Antibiotics

Careful monitoring for continued inflammation

## Urinary Tract Obstructions

Interference with urine flow

Causes urine backup behind obstruction of urinary system

Damage occurs to structures behind blockages

Increased urinary tract infection

Obstruction can be

- Functional

- Anatomic

  • Also known as obstructive uropathy

## Kidney Stones (nephrolithiasis—renal calculi)

Formed of mineral salts (uric and calcuim)

Develop anywhere in urinary tract

Tend to form in presence of excess salt and decreased fluid intake

- Most stones are formed of calcium salts

- Staghorn calculus forms in renal pelvis

**Symptoms**

Asymptomatic until obstruction occurs

Obstruction results in renal colic

  • Extremely intense pain in flank

  • Nausea

  • Vomiting

  • Cold, clammy skin

  • Increased pulse rate

### Treatment

Stone usually passes spontaneously

May use extracorporeal ultrasound or laser lithotripsy to break up stone (also known as extracorporeal shock wave lithotripsy, or ESWL)

Drugs may be used to dissolve stone

Preventative treatment to adjust pH level

- Increased fluid intake

## Bladder Carcinoma

### Malignant tumor

Most common site of malignancy in urinary system

Tumors originate in transitional epithelial lining

Tends to recur

Often metastatic to liver and bone

### Tumor staging for renal cancer

Stage I—Tumor of kidney capsule only

Stage II—Tumor invading renal capsule/vein but within fascia

Stage III—Tumor extending to regional lymph nodes/vena cava

Stage IV—Other organ metastasis

### Symptoms

Often asymptomatic in early stage

Hematuria

Dysuria

Frequent urination

Infections common

## Increased Risks

Cigarette smoking

Males age 50+

Working with industrial chemicals

Analgesics used in large amounts

Recurrent bladder infections

### Treatment

Immunotherapy (bacillus Calmette-Guérin [BCG] vaccine)

Excision

Chemotherapy

Radiation therapy

## Hydronephrosis

Distention of kidney with urine

- Due to an obstruction

- Usually as a result of a kidney stone

- May also be due to scarring, tumor, edema from infection, or other obstruction

### Symptoms

Usually asymptomatic

Mild flank pain

Infection may develop

May lead to chronic renal failure

### Treatment

Treat underlying condition, such as removal of stone or antibiotics for infection

Dilation of stricture

## Vascular Disorders

### Nephrosclerosis

Excessive hardening and thickening of vascular structure of kidney

- Reduces blood supply
  - Increases blood pressure
  - Results in atrophy and ischemia of structures
  - May lead to chronic renal failure

### Symptoms

Asymptomatic in early stages

### Treatment

Diuretics

ACE (angiotensin-converting enzyme) inhibitors

Beta blockers that block release of resin

Antihypertensive drugs

Sodium intake reduction

## Congenital Disorders

### Polycystic Kidney (PKD)

Numerous kidney cysts

Genetic disease

### Symptoms

Asymptomatic until 40s

Cysts progressive in development (both kidneys)

Nephromegaly, hematuria, URT, hypertension, uremia

Develops chronic renal failure

Cysts may spread to other organs, such as liver

### Treatment

As for chronic renal failure

## Wilms' Tumor—Nephroblastoma

Usually unilateral kidney tumors

Most common tumor in children

Usually advanced at time of diagnosis

- Metastasis to lungs at time of diagnosis is common

### Symptoms

Asymptomatic until abdominal mass becomes apparent at age 1 to 5

### Treatment

Excision

Radiation therapy

Chemotherapy

Usually a combination of above

# URINARY SYSTEM PATHOPHYSIOLOGY QUIZ

1. Which of the following is NOT a type of acute renal failure?
   a. prerenal
   b. intrarenal
   c. interrenal
   d. postrenal

2. The loss of nephron function in end-stage renal disease is:
   a. 60%
   b. 70%
   c. 80%
   d. 90%

3. The cause of bacterial cystitis is usually:
   a. *Proteus*
   b. *Pseudomonas*
   c. Staphylococcus
   d. *E. coli*

4. The primary treatment for acute pyelonephritis would be:
   a. prednisone
   b. sodium reduction
   c. antibiotics
   d. BCG

5. APSGN stands for:
   a. advanced poststaphylococcal glomerulonephritis
   b. acute poststreptococcal glomerulonephritis
   c. acute poststaphylococcal glomerulonephritis
   d. advanced poststreptococcal glomerulonephritis

6. Obstructive uropathy is also known as:
   a. pyelonephritis
   b. renal failure
   c. urinary tract obstruction
   d. nephrotic syndrome

7. A treatment for kidney stone may be:
   a. ESWL
   b. prednisone
   c. open surgical procedure
   d. diuretics

8. The treatment for hydronephrosis involves:
   a. an open surgical procedure
   b. use of diuretics
   c. treatment of the underlying condition
   d. BCG

9. This is a congential condition in which numerous cysts form in the kidney:
   a. Wilms' tumor
   b. polycystic kidney
   c. nephrosclerosis
   d. nephrotic syndrome

10. The treatment of Wilms' tumor would NOT include which of the following?
    a. excision
    b. chemotherapy
    c. diuretic
    d. radiation therapy

# ■ DIGESTIVE SYSTEM

## DIGESTIVE SYSTEM—ANATOMY AND TERMINOLOGY

**Function:** digestion, absorption, and elimination

Includes gastrointestinal tract (alimentary canal) and accessory organs

### Mouth (Fig. 1–35)

**Roof:** hard palate, soft palate, uvula (projection at back of mouth)

**Floor:** contains tongue (Fig. 1–36), muscles, taste buds, and lingual frenulum, which anchors tongue to floor of mouth

### Teeth

Thirty-two teeth (permanent)

Names of teeth: incisor, cuspid, bicuspid, and tricuspid

Tooth has crown (outer portion), neck (narrow part below gum line), root (end section), and pulp cavity (core)

### Salivary Glands (Fig. 1–37)

Surround mouth and produce saliva—1.5 liters daily

Parotid

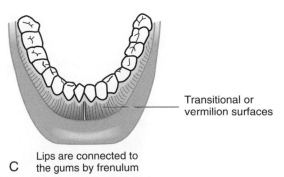

Figure **1-35** Anatomic structures of the mouth.

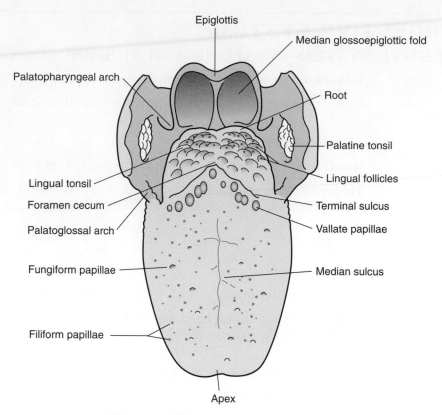

Figure **1-36** Dorsum of the tongue.

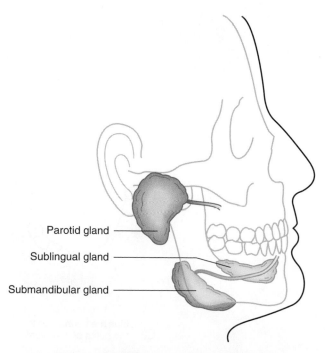

Figure **1-37** Major salivary glands.

Submandibular

Sublingual

## Pharynx or Throat (Fig. 1–38)

Muscular tube (5 inches long) lined with mucous membrane through which air and food/water travel

Epiglottis covers larynx/esophagus when swallowing

## Esophagus

Muscular tube (9-10 inches long) that carries food from pharynx to stomach by means of peristalsis (rhythmic contractions)

## Stomach

Sphincter (ring of muscles) at entry into stomach (gastroesophageal or cardiac)

Three parts of stomach:

   Fundus (upper part)

   Body (middle part)

   Antrum/pylorus (lower part)

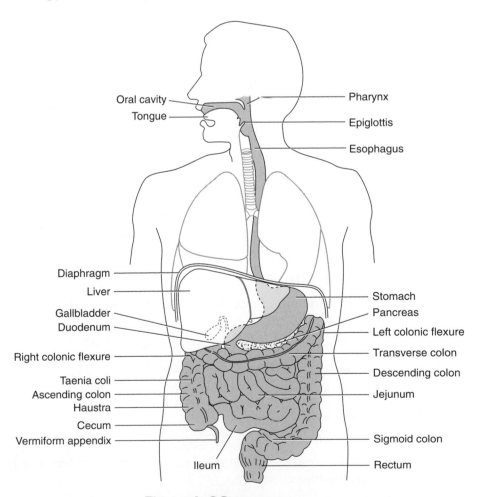

Figure **1-38** Digestive system.

Lined with rugae (folds of mucosal membrane)

Pyloric sphincter opens to allow chyme (thick liquid) to leave stomach and enter small intestine

## Small Intestine

Duodenum (2 inches long): first portion beyond stomach—bile and pancreatic juice delivered here

Jejunum (96 inches long): connects duodenum to ileum

Ileum (132 inches long): attaches to large intestine

## Large Intestine

Extends from ileum to anus

Cecum, from which appendix extends, connects ileum and colon

Colon (60 inches long), divided into:

Ascending

Transverse

Descending

Sigmoid

Sigmoid colon connected to rectum, which terminates at anus

## Accessory Organs

Liver produces bile, sent to gallbladder via hepatic duct and cystic duct

Gallbladder stores bile, sent to duodenum from cystic duct into common bile duct

Bile emulsifies fat (breaks up large globules)

Pancreas produces enzymes sent through pancreatic duct to hepatopancreatic ampulla (ampulla of Vater) then to duodenum

Pancreatic cells—islets of Langerhans produce insulin and glucagon

## Peritoneum

Serous membrane lines abdominal cavity and maintains organs in correct anatomic position

Food passes through digestive tract via:

Mouth—including salivary glands

Pharynx

Esophagus

Stomach

Duodenum—pancreatic enzymes and bile produced in liver and stored in gallbladder enter

Jejunum

Ileum

Cecum

Ascending colon

Transverse colon

Descending colon

Sigmoid colon

Rectum

Anus

## COMBINING FORMS

1. abdomin/o      abdomen
2. an/o      anus
3. appendic/o      appendix
4. bil/i      bile
5. bilirubin/o      bile pigment
6. bucc/o      cheek
7. cec/o      cecum
8. celi/o      abdomen
9. cheil/o      lip
10. chol/e      gall/bile
11. cholangio/o      bile duct
12. cholecyst/o      gallbladder
13. choledoch/o      common bile duct
14. col/o      colon
15. dent/i      tooth
16. diverticul/o      diverticulum
17. duoden/o      duodenum
18. enter/o      small intestine
19. esophag/o      esophagus
20. faci/o      face
21. gastr/o      stomach
22. gingiv/o      gum
23. gloss/o      tongue
24. hepat/o      liver
25. herni/o      hernia
26. ile/o      ileum
27. jejun/o      jejunum

| 28. labi/o | lip |
| 29. lapar/o | abdomen |
| 30. lingu/o | tongue |
| 31. lip/o | fat |
| 32. lith/o | stone |
| 33. or/o | mouth |
| 34. ordont/o | tooth |
| 35. palat/o | palate |
| 36. pancreat/o | pancreas |
| 37. peritone/o | peritoneum |
| 38. pharng/o | throat |
| 39. polyp/o | polyp |
| 40. proct/o | rectum |
| 41. pylor/o | pylorus |
| 42. rect/o | rectum |
| 43. sial/o | saliva |
| 44. sialaden/o | salivary gland |
| 45. sigmoid/o | sigmoid colon |
| 46. steat/o | fat |
| 47. stomat/o | mouth |
| 48. uvul/o | uvula |

## SUFFIXES

| 1. -ase | enzyme |
| 2. -cele | hernia |
| 3. -chezia | defecation |
| 4. -iasis | abnormal condition |
| 5. -phagia | eating |
| 6. -prandial | meal |

## MEDICAL ABBREVIATIONS

| 1. EGD | esophagogastroduodenoscopy |
| 2. EGJ | esophagogastric junction |
| 3. ERCP | endoscopic retrograde cholangiopancreatography |
| 4. GERD | gastroesophageal reflux disease |
| 5. GI | gastrointestinal |
| 6. HJR | hepatojugular reflux |

| | | |
|---|---|---|
| 7. | LLQ | left lower quadrant |
| 8. | LUQ | left upper quadrant |
| 9. | PEG | percutaneous endoscopic gastrostomy |
| 10. | RLQ | right lower quadrant |
| 11. | RUQ | right upper quadrant |

## MEDICAL TERMS

| | |
|---|---|
| Anastomosis | Surgical connection of two tubular structures, such as two pieces of intestine |
| Biliary | Refers to gallbladder, bile, or bile duct |
| Cholangiography | Radiographic recording of bile ducts |
| Cholecystectomy | Surgical removal of gallbladder |
| Cholecystoenterostomy | Creation of a connection between gallbladder and intestine |
| Colonoscopy | Fiberscopic examination of entire colon that may include part of terminal ileum |
| Colostomy | Artificial opening between colon and abdominal wall |
| Diverticulum | Protrusion in wall of an organ |
| Dysphagia | Difficulty swallowing |
| Enterolysis | Releasing of adhesions of intestine |
| Eventration | Protrusion of bowel through an opening in abdomen |
| Evisceration | Pulling viscera outside of the body through an incision |
| Exstrophy | Condition in which an organ is turned inside out |
| Fulguration | Use of electric current to destroy tissue |
| Gastrointestinal | Pertaining to stomach and intestine |
| Gastroplasty | Operation on stomach for repair or reconfiguration |
| Gastrostomy | Artificial opening between stomach and abdominal wall |
| Hernia | Organ or tissue protruding through wall or cavity that usually contains it |
| Ileostomy | Artificial opening between ileum and abdominal wall |
| Imbrication | Overlapping |
| Incarcerated | Regarding hernias, a constricted, irreducible hernia that may cause obstruction of an intestine |
| Intussusception | Slipping of one part of intestine into another part |
| Jejunostomy | Artificial opening between jejunum and abdominal wall |
| Laparoscopy | Exploration of the abdomen and pelvic cavities using a scope placed through a small incision in abdominal wall |
| Lithotomy | Incision into an organ or a duct for the purpose of removing a stone |
| Lithotripsy | Crushing of a stone by sound wave or force |

| | |
|---|---|
| Paraesophageal or hiatal hernia | Protrusion of any structure through esophageal hiatus of diaphragm |
| Proctosigmoidoscopy | Fiberscopic examination of sigmoid colon and rectum |
| Sialolithotomy | Surgical removal of a stone of salivary gland or duct |
| Varices | Varicose veins |
| Volvulus | Twisted section of intestine |

# DIGESTIVE SYSTEM ANATOMY AND TERMINOLOGY QUIZ

1. This is NOT a part of the small intestine:
   a. ileum
   b. cecum
   c. duodenum
   d. jejunum

2. Term meaning "ring of muscles":
   a. pyloric
   b. parotid
   c. epiglottis
   d. sphincter

3. The throat is also known as the:
   a. larynx
   b. epiglottis
   c. esophagus
   d. pharynx

4. The three parts of the stomach:
   a. pyloric, rugae, fundus
   b. fundus, body, antrum
   c. antrum, pyloric, rugae
   d. ilium, fundus, pyloric

5. The projection at the back of the mouth:
   a. palate
   b. sublingual
   c. uvula
   d. parotid

6. Mucosal membrane that lines the stomach:
   a. cecum
   b. rugae
   c. frenulum
   d. fundus

7. The parts of the colon are:
   a. ascending, transverse, descending, sigmoid
   b. ascending, descending, sigmoid
   c. transverse, descending, sigmoid
   d. descending, sigmoid

8. Combining form meaning "abdomen":
   a. an/o
   b. cec/o
   c. celi/o
   d. col/o

9. Term that means connecting two ends of a tube:
   a. anastomosis
   b. amylase
   c. aphthous stomatitis
   d. atresia

10. Abbreviation that means a scope placed through the esophagus, into the stomach, and to the duodenum:
    a. ERCP
    b. EGD
    c. GERD
    d. PEG

# DIGESTIVE SYSTEM—PATHOPHYSIOLOGY

## Disorders of Oral Cavity

### Cleft Lip and Cleft Palate (Orofacial Cleft) (Fig. 1–39)

Congenital defect

Cleft lip and palate

   Lip and palate do not properly join together

Causes feeding problems

- Infants cannot create sufficient suction for feeding

- Danger of aspirating food

- Results in speech defects

**Treatment**

   Surgical repair of defects

### Ulceration

Canker sore—caused by herpes simplex virus

- Ulceration of oral mucosa

Also known as

- Aphthous ulcer (aphtha: small ulcer)

- Aphthous stomatitis

Heals spontaneously

### Infections

**Candidiasis**

*Candida albicans* is naturally found in mouth

Thrush (oral candidiasis) is overarching infection

Figure **1-39** Cleft palate.

*Causes*

Antibiotic regimen

Chemotherapy

Glucocorticoids

Common in diabetics and AIDS patients

*Treatment*

Nystatin (topical fungal agent)

**Herpes simplex type 1**

Herpetic stomatitis

- Viral cold sores and blisters

- Associated with herpes simplex virus type 1 (HSV-1)

*Treatment*

No cure

May be alleviated somewhat by antiviral medications

### Cancer of Oral Cavity

Most common type is squamous cell carcinoma

- Kaposi's sarcoma is type seen in AIDS patients

Increased in smokers

    Lip cancer also increased in smokers, particularly pipe

Poor prognosis

Usually asymptomatic until later stages

Metastasis through lymph nodes

## Esophageal Disorders

### Scleroderma

Also known as progressive systemic sclerosis

Atrophy of smooth muscles of lower esophagus

Lower esophageal sphincter (LES) does not close properly

- Leads to esophageal reflux

- Strictures form

**Symptom**

Predominantly dysphagia

### Esophagitis

Inflammation of esophagus

**Types**

*Acute*

Most common type is that caused by hiatal hernia

Infectious esophagitis is common in patients with AIDS

Ingestion of strong alkaline or acid substances

• Such as those in household cleaners

Inflammation leads to scarring

### Chronic
Most common type is that caused by LES reflux

## Cancer of Esophagus
Most common type is squamous cell or secondary adenocarcinoma

Usually caused by continued irritation

• Smoking

• Alcohol

• Hiatal hernia

• Chronic esophagitis/GERD

Poor prognosis

## Hiatal Hernia (Diaphragmatic hernia)
Diaphragm goes over stomach

• Esophagus passes through diaphragm at natural opening (hiatus)

• Part of the stomach protrudes (herniates) through opening in diaphragm into thorax

### Types (Fig. 1–40)
Sliding

• Stomach and gastroesophageal junction protrude through the hiatus

Paraesophageal/rolling hiatal

• Part of fundus protrudes

### Symptoms
Heartburn

Reflux

Belching

Lying down causes discomfort

Figure **1-40** Sliding and paraesophageal hernias (hiatal hernias).

Dysphagia

Substernal pain after eating

## Gastroesophageal Reflux Disease (GERD)
Associated with hiatal hernias

- Reflux of gastric contents

Lower esophageal sphincter does not constrict properly

### Treatment
Reduce irritants, such as

- Smoking
- Spicy foods
- Alcohol

Antacids

Elevate head of bed

Avoid tight clothing

## Stomach and Duodenum Disorders

### Gastritis
Inflammation of stomach mucosa

### Acute superficial gastritis
Mild, transient irritation

### Causes
Excessive alcohol

Infection

Food allergies

Spicy foods

Aspirin

*H. pylori (Helicobacter pylori)*

### Symptoms
Nausea

Vomiting

Anorexia

Bleeding in more severe cases

Epigastric pain

### Treatment
Usually spontaneous remission in 2 to 3 days

Removal of underlying irritation

Antibiotics for infection

### Chronic atrophic gastritis
Progressive atrophy of epithelium

*Types*

**Type A,** atrophic or fundal

- Involves fundus of stomach
- Autoimmune disease
  - Decreases acid secretion
  - Results in high gastrin levels

**Type B,** antral

- Involves antrum region of stomach
- Often associated with elderly
  - May be associated with pernicious anemia
- Low gastrin levels
- Usually caused by infection
- Irritated by alcohol, drugs, and tobacco

Symptom abatement

- Bland diet
- Alcohol avoidance
- ASA avoidance
- Antibiotics for *H. pylori*

## Peptic Ulcers

Erosive area on mucosa

- Extends below epithelium
- Chronic ulcers have scar tissue at base of erosive area

Ulcers can occur anywhere on gastrointestinal tract but typically are found on the

- Lower esophagus
- Stomach
- Proximal duodenum

**Some causes**

Alcohol

Smoking

Aspirin

Severe stress

Bacterial infection caused by *Helicobacter pylori (H. pylori)*, 90% of the time

Genetic factor

Constant use of anti-inflammatory drugs

**Symptoms**

Epigastric pain when stomach is empty

- Relieved by food or antacid

Burning

May include

- Vomiting blood
- Nausea
- Weight loss
- Anorexia

Severe cases may include

- Obstruction
- Hemorrhage
- Perforation

**Treatment**

Surgical intervention

Antacids

Dietary restrictions

Rest

Antibiotics

## Gastric Cancer (malignant tumor of stomach)

Most often occurs in men over 40

Cause is unknown, but often associated with *Helicobacter pylori* (bacterial infection)

### Predisposing Factors

Atrophic gastritis

Pernicious anemia

History of nonhealing gastric ulcer

Blood type A

Geographic factors

Environmental factors

Carcinogenic foods

- Smoked meats
- Nitrates
- Pickled foods

**Symptoms**

Usually asymptomatic in early stages

**Treatment**

Excision

Chemotherapy

Radiation (poor response)

Prognosis is poor

## Pyloric Stenosis

Narrowing of the pyloric sphincter

Signs appear soon after birth

- Failure to thrive
- Projectile vomiting

**Treatment**
Surgery to relieve stenosis (pyloromyotomy)

## Intestinal Disorders

### ■ Small Intestine

### Malabsorption Conditions

**Celiac disease**
Most important malabsorption condition

Villi atrophy in response to food containing gluten and lose ability to absorb

- Gluten is a protein found in wheat, rye, oats, and barley

*Symptoms*
Malnutrition

Muscle wasting

Distended abdomen

Diarrhea

Fatigue

Weakness

Steatorrhea (excess fat in feces)

*Treatment*
Gluten-free diet

Steroids when necessary

**Lactase deflciency**
Enzyme deficiency

- Secondary to gastrointestinal damage, such as
  - Regional enteritis
  - Infection
- Common in African Americans, occurring in adulthood

*Symptoms*
Intolerance to milk

Intestinal cramping

Diarrhea

Flatulence

*Treatment*
Elimination of milk products

**Crohn's disease (regional enteritis)**
Inflammatory bowel disease (IBD)—affects terminal ileum and colon

*Cause*
Unknown

*Symptoms*
- Vary greatly
- Inflammation of GI tract

Diarrhea

Gas

Fever

Abdominal pain

Malaise

Anorexia

Weight loss

*Treatment*

No specific treatment

Palliative medications to control symptoms

Resection of affected section of intestine with anastomosis

Diet modifications

## Duodenal Ulcers

Most common ulcer

Develop in younger population

Common in type O blood types

## Appendicitis

Inflammation of vermiform appendix that projects from cecum

Obstruction of lumen leads to infection

- Appendix becomes hypoxic (decreased oxygen levels)
- May cause gangrene
- May rupture, causing peritonitis

*Symptoms*

Periumbilical (around umbilicus) pain, initially

Right lower quadrant (RLQ) pain as inflammation progresses

Nausea

Vomiting

Possible diarrhea

*Treatment*

Appendectomy

Management of any perforation or abscess

## Meckel's Diverticulum—an appendage of ileum near cecum derived from an unobliterated yolk stalk in fetal development. Symptoms can mimic appendicitis.

## Peritonitis

Inflammation of peritoneum (membrane that lines abdominal cavity)

Usually a result of

- Spread of infection from abdominal organ
- Puncture wound to abdomen
- Rupture of gastrointestinal tract—appendicitis or Meckel's diverticulum

Abscesses form, resulting in adhesions

- May result in obstruction

*Types*

Acute

Chronic

**Symptoms**
Abdominal pain

Vomiting

Rigid abdomen

Fever

Leukocytosis (increased white cells in blood)

**Treatment**
Antibiotics

Suction of stomach and intestines

If possible, surgical removal of origin of infection, such as appendix

Fluid replacement

Bed rest

## Obstruction
Any interference with passage of intestinal contents

May be

- Acute
- Chronic
- Partial
- Total

**Types**
Nonmechanical

- Paralytic ileus
- Result of trauma or toxin

Mechanical

- Result of tumors, adhesions, hernias
- Simple mechanical obstruction
  - One point of obstruction
- Closed-loop obstruction
  - At least two points of obstruction

Diverticulosis

Twisted bowel (volvulus)

Telescoping bowel (intussception)

**Symptoms**
Abdominal distention

Pain

Vomiting

Total constipation

**Treatment**
Surgical intervention

Symptomatic treatment

## ■ Large Intestine

### Diverticulosis

Herniation of intestinal mucosa

- Forms sacs in lining, called diverticula

### Diverticulitis

Sacs fill and become inflamed

- Common in aged

#### Symptoms

Diarrhea or constipation

Gas

Abdominal discomfort

#### Complications

Perforation

Bleeding

Peritonitis

Abscess

Obstruction

#### Treatment

Antimicrobials as necessary

High-fiber diet (greater than 20 g daily)

Stool softeners

Dietary restrictions of solid foods

Surgical intervention if necessary

### Ulcerative Colitis (Fig. 1-41)

Inflammation of rectum that progresses to sigmoid colon

Intermittent exacerbations and remissions

May develop into toxic megacolon

- Leads to obstruction and dilation of colon

Increased risk for colorectal cancer

Figure **1-41** Ulcerative colitis. (From Damjanov I: *Pathology for the Health Professions,* ed 3, St. Louis, 2006, Saunders.)

**Symptoms**

Diarrhea

- Blood and mucus may be present

Cramping

Fever

Weight loss

**Treatment**

Remove physical or emotional stressors

Anti-inflammatory medications

Antimotility agents

Nutritional supplementation

Surgical intervention, if necessary

## Colorectal Cancer

Usually develop from polyp

- In those 55 and older

**Increased risks**

Genetic factors

40 years of age and older

Diets high in

- Fat
- Sugar
- Red meat

Low-fiber diets

**Symptoms**

Asymptomatic until advanced

Some may experience

- Cramping
- Ribbon stools
- Feeling of incomplete evacuation
- Fatigue
- Weight loss
- Change in bowel habits
- Blood in stool

**Treatment**

Surgical excision

Radiation

Chemotherapy

Combination of above

## Disorders of Liver, Gallbladder, and Pancreas

### ■ Disorders of Liver

### Jaundice (Hyperbilirubinemia)
A symptom of biliary disease, not a disease itself

- Results in yellow eyes (sclera) and skin

**Types**
Prehepatic

- Excess destruction of red blood cells
- Result of hemolytic anemia or reaction to transfusion

Intrahepatic

- Impaired uptake of bilirubin and decreased blending of bilirubin by hepatic cells
- Result of liver disease, such as cirrhosis or hepatitis

Posthepatic

- Excess bile flows into blood
- Result of obstruction
    - Due to conditions such as inflammation of liver, tumors, cholelithiasis

**Treatment**
Removal of cause

### Cancer of Liver
Most commonly a metastasis; primary CA rare

Risk for primary liver CA

- Hepatitis B, C, and D
- Cirrhosis
- Myotoxins
- Heavy smoking/alcohol use

**Treatment**
Surgical resection if localized

Survival typically 3 or 4 months

### Viral Hepatitis
Liver cells are damaged

Results in inflammation and necrosis

Damage can be mild or severe

Scar tissue forms in liver

- Leads to ischemia

**Hepatitis A (HAV)**
Infectious hepatitis—caused by hepatitis A virus

Transmission

- Most commonly fecal-oral route—contaminated food or water

Does not have a chronic state

Slow onset—complete recovery characteristic

Vaccine available for those who are traveling

Gamma globulin may be administered to those just exposed

**Hepatitis B (HBV)**
Serum hepatitis

Carrier state is common

Caused by hepatitis B virus

• Asymptomatic but contagious

Long incubation period

Transmission

• Intravenous drug users

• Transfusion

• Exposure to blood and bodily fluids

• Sexual transmission

• Mother-to-fetus transmission

• Immune globulin is temporary prophylactic

• Vaccine is now routine for children and is given to those at risk

Severe forms cause liver cell destruction, cirrhosis, death

**Hepatitis C (HCV)**
Transmission of virus

• Most commonly by transfusion

• IV drug users

Half of cases develop into chronic hepatitis

Increases risk of hepatocellular cancer

Carrier state may develop

**Hepatitis D (HDV)**
Transmission of hepatitis D virus

• Blood

• Intravenous drug users

Hepatitis B is present for this type to develop

**Hepatitis E (HEV)**
Transmission of hepatitis E virus

• Fecal-oral route

Does not develop into chronic or carrier

**Hepatitis G**
Transmission of hepatitis G virus

• IV drug use

• Sexual transmission

**Symptoms of hepatitis**

*Stages*

Preicteric

- Anorexia

- Nausea and vomiting

Liver enzymes may be elevated—indication of liver cell damage

- Fatigue

- Malaise

- Generalized pain with low grade fever

- Cough

Icteric

- Jaundice

- Hepatomegaly (enlarged liver)

- Biliary obstruction

- Light-colored stools and dark urine

- Pruritus

- Abdominal pain

Posticteric (recovery)

- Reduction of symptoms

**Treatment**

None

In early stages gamma globulins may be used

Interferon may be used for cases of chronic hepatitis B and C

**Nonviral hepatitis**

Hepatitis that results from hepatotoxins

Symptoms

- Similar to viral hepatitis

Treatment

- Removal of hepatotoxin

## Cirrhosis

Profuse liver damage

- Extensive fibrosis

  - Results in inflammation

Progressive disorder

Leads to liver failure

**Types**

Alcoholic liver

- Known as Laënnec's cirrhosis or portal cirrhosis

- Largest group

Biliary

- Associated with immune disorders

- Obstructions (intrahepatic or extrahepatic blood vessels) occur and disrupt normal function

Postnecrotic

- Associated with chronic hepatitis (A or C) and exposure to toxins

**Symptoms**
Asymptomatic in early stages

Nausea

Vomiting

Fatigue

Weight loss

Pruritus

Jaundice

Edema

**Treatment**
Symptomatic

Dietary restrictions

- Reduced protein and sodium

- Increased vitamins and carbohydrates

Diuretics

Antibiotics

Liver transplant

## ■ Disorders of Gallbladder

### Cholecystitis
Inflammation of gallbladder and cystic duct

### Cholangitis
Inflammation of bile duct

### Cholelithiasis
Formation of gallstones (Fig. 1–42)

- Consists of cholesterol or bilirubin

Figure **1-42** Resected gallbladder containing mixed gallstones. (From Kissane JM, editor: *Anderson's Pathology,* ed 9, St Louis, 1990, Mosby.)

- Occurs most often in those with high levels of cholesterol, calcium, or bile salts

Stones cause irritation and inflammation

- May lead to infection
- Obstruction
  - May result in pancreatitis
  - Rupture is possible

**Symptoms**

Often asymptomatic

Dietary intolerance particularly to fat

Right upper quadrant (RUQ) pain

Pain in back and/or shoulder

Epigastric discomfort

Bloating heartburn, flatulence

**Treatment**

Surgical intervention (laparoscopic cholecystectomy)

Lithotripsy

Medical management by use of drugs that break down stone

## ■ Disorders of Pancreas

### Pancreatitis

Inflammation of pancreas resulting from digestive enzyme attack to pancreas

Acute and chronic forms

Commonly associated with alcoholism, biliary tract obstruction, drug toxicity, gallstone obstruction of common bile duct, and viral infections

**Symptoms**

Severe pain

Fever

Acute form is a medical emergency

Neurogenic shock

Septicemia

General sepsis

**Complications**

Adult respiratory distress syndrome (ARDS)

Renal failure

**Treatment**

No oral intake

- IV fluids given and carefully monitored

Analgesics

Stop process of autodigestion

Prevent systemic shutdown

## Pancreatic Cancer

**Increased risk**

Cigarette smoking

Diet high in fat and protein

**Symptoms**

Weight loss

Jaundice

Anorexia

Most types of pancreatic cancer are asymptomatic until well advanced

**Treatment**

Palliative

Pain management

# DIGESTIVE SYSTEM PATHOPHYSIOLOGY QUIZ

1. This type of hyperbilirubinemia is hallmarked by excess bile flow into the blood:
   a. intrahepatic
   b. prehepatic
   c. posthepatic
   d. jaundice

2. This type of hepatitis is transmitted by the fecal-oral route:
   a. A
   b. B
   c. C
   d. D

3. Which of the following is the recovery stage of hepatitis?
   a. prehepatic
   b. posthepatic
   c. preicteric
   d. posticteric

4. This type of cirrhosis is also known as portal cirrhosis:
   a. biliary
   b. alcoholic liver
   c. postnecrotic
   d. traumatic

5. This condition is the inflammation of the bile ducts:
   a. cholangitis
   b. cholecystitis
   c. cholelithiasis
   d. cholangioma

6. Formation of gallstones most often occurs with high levels of the following:
   a. bile salts and toxins
   b. cholesterol and toxins
   c. cholesterol and bile salts
   d. toxins

7. The primary factor that increases the risk of pancreatic cancer is:
   a. smoking
   b. alcohol
   c. intravenous drug use
   d. hepatitis

8. A potential complication of this condition is ARDS:
   a. hyperbilirubinemia
   b. hepatitis
   c. pancreatitis
   d. pancreatic cancer

9. The primary treatment for jaundice is:
   a. removal of cause
   b. antibiotics
   c. dialysis
   d. vaccine

10. This condition has as the largest group of those who abuse alcohol:
    a. cirrhosis
    b. hepatitis
    c. pancreatitis
    d. pancreatic cancer

# ■ MEDIASTINUM AND DIAPHRAGM

## MEDIASTINUM AND DIAPHRAGM—ANATOMY AND TERMINOLOGY

Not an organ system

### Mediastinum

That area between lungs that a median (partition) divides (Fig. 1–43) into

- Superior
- Anterior
- Posterior
- Middle

Space that houses heart, thymus gland, trachea, esophagus, nerves, lymph and blood vessels and major blood vessels

- Aorta
- Inferior vena cava

### Diaphragm

A dome-shaped muscular partition that separates abdominal cavity from thoracic cavity

- Assists in breathing
  - Expands to assist lungs in exhalation/relaxation of diaphragm
  - Flattens out during inspiration/contraction of diaphragm
- Diaphragmatic hernia: esophageal hernia

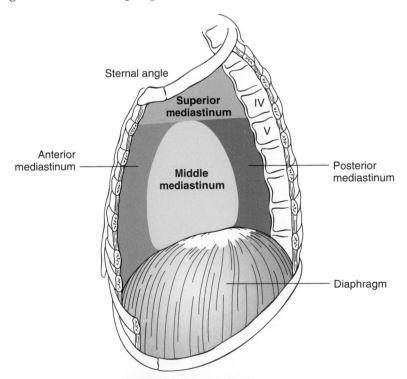

Figure **1-43** Mediastinum and diaphragm.

# MEDIASTINUM AND DIAPHRAGM ANATOMY AND TERMINOLOGY QUIZ

1. The mediastinum is NOT an organ system.
   a. true
   b. false

2. The mediastinum is divided into:
   a. superior, anterior, posterior
   b. superior, anterior, posterior, middle
   c. anterior, posterior, middle
   d. middle, anterior, superior

3. During inspiration, the diaphragm:
   a. expands
   b. moves upward
   c. collapses
   d. flattens out

4. Term meaning "partition":
   a. middle
   b. aspect
   c. median
   d. diaphragm

5. The diaphragm is said to be this shape:
   a. square
   b. flat
   c. dome
   d. round

6. This separates the abdominal cavity from the thoracic cavity:
   a. mediastinum
   b. diaphragm
   c. superior
   d. inferior

7. This is the area between the lungs:
   a. mediastinum
   b. diaphragm
   c. superior
   d. inferior

8. This is an esophageal hernia:
   a. mediastinal
   b. diaphragmatic
   c. paraesophageal
   d. hiatal

9. A diaphragmatic hernia is also known as:
   a. esophageal
   b. epiglottis
   c. partitional
   d. medial

10. The diaphragm assists in:
    a. percussion
    b. auscultation
    c. contraction
    d. breathing

# ■ HEMIC AND LYMPHATIC SYSTEM
## HEMIC AND LYMPHATIC SYSTEM—ANATOMY AND TERMINOLOGY

Hemic refers to blood

Lymphatic system removes excess tissue fluid

- Lymph tissue is scattered throughout body

- Composed of lymph nodes, vessels, and organs

### Lymph

Colorless fluid containing lymphocytes and monocytes

Originates from blood and after filtering, returns to blood

Transports interstitial fluids and proteins that have leaked from blood system into venous system

Absorbs and transports fats from villi of small intestine to venous system

Assists in immune function

### Lymph Vessels

Similar to veins

Organized circulatory system throughout body

### Lymph Organs

Lymph nodes, spleen, bone marrow, thymus, tonsils, and Peyer's patches (lymphoid tissue on mucosa of small intestine)

Lymph nodes, areas of concentrated tissue (Fig. 1–44)

Spleen, located in left upper quadrant (LUQ) of abdomen

- Composed of lymph tissue

  - Function is to filter blood; activates lymphocytes and B cells to filter antigens

  - Stores blood

Thymus secretes thymosin, causing T cells to mature

- Larger in infants and shrinks with age

Tonsils

- Palatine tonsils

- Pharyngeal tonsils/adenoids

### Hematopoietic Organ

Bone marrow, contains tissue that produces RBCs, WBCs, and platelets

- Produces stem cells

## COMBINING FORMS

1. aden/o            gland
2. adenoid/o         adenoids

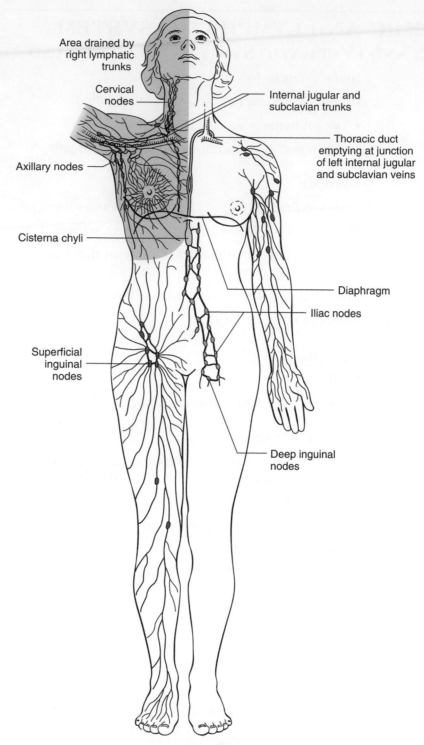

Area drained by right lymphatic trunks

Cervical nodes

Internal jugular and subclavian trunks

Thoracic duct emptying at junction of left internal jugular and subclavian veins

Axillary nodes

Cisterna chyli

Diaphragm

Iliac nodes

Superficial inguinal nodes

Deep inguinal nodes

Figure **1-44** Lymphatic system.

3. axill/o          armpit

4. cervic/o         neck/cervix

5. immun/o          immune

6. inguin/o         groin

7. lymph/o          lymph

8. lymphaden/o      lymph gland

9. splen/o          spleen

10. thym/o          thymus gland

11. tonsill/o       tonsil

12. tox/o           poison

## PREFIXES

1. hyper-           excess

2. inter-           between

3. retro-           behind

## SUFFIXES

1. -ectomy          removal

2. -edema           swelling

3. -itis            inflammation

4. -megaly          enlargement

5. -oid             resembling

6. -oma             tumor

7. -penia           deficient

8. -pexy            fixation

9. -phylaxis        protection

10. -poiesis        production

## MEDICAL TERMS

Axillary nodes        Lymph nodes located in armpit

Cloquet's node        Also called a gland; it is highest of deep groin lymph nodes

Inguinofemoral        Referring to groin and thigh

Jugular nodes         Lymph nodes located next to large vein in neck

Lymph node            Station along lymphatic system

Lymphadenectomy       Excision of a lymph node or nodes

Lymphadenitis         Inflammation of a lymph node

Lymphangiography      Radiographic recording of lymphatic vessels and nodes

| | |
|---|---|
| Lymphangiotomy | Incision into a lymphatic vessel |
| Lymphangitis | Inflammation of lymphatic vessel or vessels |
| Parathyroid | Produces a hormone to mobilize calcium from bones to blood |
| Splenectomy | Excision of spleen |
| Splenography | Radiographic recording of spleen |
| Splenoportography | Radiographic procedure to allow visualization of splenic and portal veins of spleen |
| Stem cell | Immature blood cell |
| Thoracic duct | Largest lymph vessel; it collects lymph from portions of body below diaphragm and from left side of body above diaphragm |
| Transplantation | Grafting of tissue from one source to another |

# HEMIC AND LYMPHATIC SYSTEM ANATOMY AND TERMINOLOGY QUIZ

1. The spleen is located in this quadrant of the abdomen:
   a. RUQ
   b. LUQ
   c. LLQ
   d. LRQ

2. Produces RBCs and platelets:
   a. thymus
   b. tonsils
   c. lymph node
   d. bone marrow

3. Which of the following is NOT a lymph organ?
   a. adrenal
   b. spleen
   c. thymus
   d. tonsil

4. Lymph transports fluids and _____ that have leaked from the blood system back to veins.
   a. stem cells
   b. lymphocytes
   c. B cells
   d. proteins

5. This is largest in infants and shrinks with age:
   a. tonsils
   b. spleen
   c. thymus
   d. bone marrow

6. Combining form meaning "gland":
   a. axill/o
   b. thym/o
   c. aden/o
   d. tox/o

7. Prefix meaning "excess":
   a. hyper-
   b. hypo-
   c. inter-
   d. retro-

8. Suffix meaning "enlargement":
   a. -edema
   b. -poiesis
   c. -penia
   d. -megaly

9. Lymph node located on neck:
   a. thoracic
   b. jugular
   c. Cloquet's
   d. axillary

10. These cells originate in the bone marrow:
   a. B cells
   b. antigens
   c. erythrocytes
   d. stem cells

# HEMIC AND LYMPHATIC SYSTEM—PATHOPHYSIOLOGY

## Anemia

Reduction in number of erythrocytes or decrease in quality of hemoglobin

- Less oxygen is transported in the blood

## Aplastic Anemia

Diverse group of anemias

Characterized by bone marrow failure with reduced numbers of red and white blood cells and platelets

### Causes

Genetic or acquired (primary or secondary)

Toxins/chemical agents

    Benzene and antibiotics such as chloramphenicol

Irradiation

Immunologic

Idiopathic (unknown)

### Treatment

Blood transfusion

Bone marrow transplant

## Iron Deficiency Anemia

Characterized by small erythrocytes and a reduced amount of hemoglobin

Caused by low or absent iron stores or serum iron concentrations

- Blood loss
- Decreased intake of iron
- Malabsorption of iron

### Symptoms

Pallor

Headache

Stomatitis

Oral lesions

Gastrointestinal complaints

Retinal hemorrhages

Thinning, brittle nails and hair

### Treatment

Iron supplement

## Pernicious Anemia

Megaloblastic anemia (large stem cells)

Inability to absorb vitamin $B_{12}$ due to a lack of intrinsic factor (found in gastric juices)

Usually in older adults

Caused by impaired intestinal absorption of vitamin $B_{12}$

**Symptoms**
Pallor

Weakness

Neurologic manifestations

Gastric discomfort

**Treatment**
Injections of vitamin $B_{12}$

Transfusions

## Hemolytic Anemia
May be acute or chronic

Shortened survival of mature erythrocytes—excessive destruction of RBC

- Inability of bone marrow to compensate for decreased survival of erythrocytes

**Treatment**
Treat cause

## Sickle Cell Anemia
Occurs primarily in those of West African descent

Abnormal sickle-shaped erythrocytes (sickle cell) caused by an abnormal type of hemoglobin (hemoglobin S)

**Symptoms**
Abdominal pain

Arthralgia

Ulceration of lower extremities

Fatigue

Dyspnea

Increased heart rate

**Treatment**
Symptomatic

## Granulocytosis

Increase in granulocytes

- Neutrophils
- Eosinophils
- Basophils

## Eosinophilia

Increase in number of eosinophilic granulocytes

**Cause**

Allergic disorders

Dermatologic disorders

Parasitic invasion

Drugs

Malignancies

## Basophilia

Increase in basophilic granulocytes seen in leukemia

## Monocytosis

Increased number of monocytes

**Cause**

Infection

Hematologic factors

## Leukocytosis

Increased number of leukocytes

**Cause**

Acute viral infections, such as hepatitis

Chronic infections, such as syphilis

## Leukocytopenia

Decreased number of leukocytes

**Cause**

Neoplasias

Immune deficiencies

Drugs

Virus

Radiation

## Infectious Mononucleosis

### Acute Infection of B Cells

Epstein-Barr virus most common cause

**Symptoms**

Fatigue

Fever

Weakness (asthenia)

Pharyngitis

Atypical lymphocytes in blood

Lymph node enlargement

Splenomegaly

Hepatomegaly

## Transmission
Saliva

- Known as kissing disease

### Treatment
Rest

Treatment of symptoms

## Leukemia

Malignant disorder of blood and blood-forming organs

Leads to dysfunction of cells

- Primarily leads to proliferation of abnormal leukocytes—filling bone marrow and bloodstream

### Acute Myelogenous Leukemia (AML)
Rapid onset

Short survival time

#### Symptoms
Abrupt onset

Fatigue

Lymphadenopathy

Bone pain and tenderness

Anemia

Bleeding

Fever

Infection

Anorexia

Splenomegaly

Hepatomegaly

Headache, vomiting, paralysis

#### Treatment
Chemotherapy

Bone marrow transplant following high-dose chemotherapy eradicating leukemic cells

### Acute Lymphocytic Leukemia (ALL)
Immature lymphocytes (lymphoblasts)

Most cases occur in children and adolescents

Sudden onset

**Treatment**
> Chemotherapy with drugs that suppress cell division and destroy rapidly dividing cells

> Remission

> Relapse—leukemia cells in bone marrow and blood requiring treatment

## Chronic Myelogenous Leukemia (CML)

Mature and immature granulocytes in bone marrow and blood

Slow progressive disease (those over 55 years live many years without life threat)

Cells are more differentiated

Gradual onset with milder symptoms

- Majority of cases are in adults

**Symptoms**

Extreme fatigue

Weight loss

Splenomegaly

Night sweats

Fever

Infections

**Treatment**
> Chemotherapy—target abnormal proteins

> Bone marrow transplant—following high-dose chemotherapy

## Chronic Lymphocytic Leukemia (CLL)

Increased numbers of mature lymphocytes in marrow, lymph nodes, spleen

Most common form seen in elderly

Slowly progressive

**Treatment**
> Chemotherapy

## Lymph

### Lymphadenopathy

Any abnormality of lymph node

Enlargement of lymph node

### Lymphangitis

Inflammation of lymphatic vessel

### Lymphadenitis

Inflammation of lymph node

Localized inflammation associated with inflamed lesion

Generalized inflammation associated with disease

Inflammation can occur as result of

- Trauma
- Infection
- Drug reaction
- Autoimmune disease
- Immunologic disease

## Malignant Lymphoma

### Hodgkin Disease

Initial sign is a painless mass commonly located on neck

Giant Reed-Sternberg cells are present in lymphatic tissue

**Presentation**

Enlarged spleen (splenomegaly)

Abdominal mass

Mediastinal mass

Localized node involvement

- Orderly spreading of node involvement
- Cervical, axillary, inguinal, and retroperitoneal lymph node involvement

**Symptoms**

Night sweats

Fever

Weight loss

Itching (pruritus)

Anorexia

Weakness

**Treatment**

If localized: radiation therapy and chemotherapy

If systemic: chemotherapy alone

High probability of cure with new treatments

### Non-Hodgkin Lymphoma

No giant Reed-Sternberg cells present

Involves multiple nodes scattered throughout body (follicular lymphoma)

Large cell lymphoma (large lymphocytes in diffuse nodes and lymph tissue)

- Noncontiguous spread of node involvement
- Not localized

Usually begins as a painless enlargement of node

**Symptoms**
Presents similar to Hodgkin disease

**Treatment**
Chemotherapy cures or stops disease progression

## Burkitt's Lymphoma
Type of non-Hodgkin lymphoma

Usually found in Africa and New Guinea

Characterized by lesions in jaw and face

Epstein-Barr (herpes virus) has been found in Burkitt's lymphoma

**Treatment**
Radiation and chemotherapy for African type

# Myeloma

## Multiple Myeloma
B-cell cancer—lymphocytes that produce antibodies destroying bone tissue

• Also known as plasma cell myeloma

Increased plasma cells replace bone marrow

Overproduction of immunoglobulins—Bence Jones protein (found in urine)

Multiple tumor sites cause bone destruction

Results in weakened bone

Hypercalcemia

Anemia

Renal damage

Increased susceptibility to infections

**Cause**
Unknown

**Treatment**
Chemotherapy

Radiotherapy

Autologous bone marrow transplant (ABMT) prolongs remission—may be a cure

Palliative treatments

# HEMIC AND LYMPHATIC SYSTEM PATHOPHYSIOLOGY QUIZ

1. This condition involves a reduced number of erythrocytes and decreased quality of hemoglobin:
   a. monocytosis
   b. eosinophilia
   c. anemia
   d. leukocytosis

2. This condition is hallmarked by a shortened survival of mature erythrocytes and inability of bone marrow to compensate for decreased survival:
   a. hemolytic anemia
   b. granulocytosis
   c. eosinophilia
   d. monocytosis

3. The most common cause of this disease is Epstein-Barr virus:
   a. leukocytopenia
   b. infectious mononucleosis
   c. leukocytosis
   d. hemolytic anemia

4. Inflammation of the lymphatic vessels is:
   a. lymphadenitis
   b. lymphoma
   c. lymphadenopathy
   d. lymphangitis

5. What giant cell is present in Hodgkin disease?
   a. B cell
   b. Reed-Sternberg
   c. T cell
   d. C cell

6. This condition increases plasma cells, which replace bone marrow:
   a. Burkitt's lymphoma
   b. Multiple myeloma
   c. Hodgkin disease
   d. leukemia

7. Injection of vitamin B may be prescribed for this type of anemia:
   a. pernicious
   b. aplastic
   c. sideroblastic
   d. sickle cell

8. These are large stem cells:
   a. megaloblasts
   b. leukocytes
   c. erythrocytes
   d. granulocytes

9. This is known as the kissing disease:
   a. monocytosis
   b. leukocytopenia
   c. infectious mononucleosis
   d. granulocytosis

10. This lymphoma is usually found in Africa:
    a. multiple
    b. Burkitt's
    c. B-cell
    d. T-cell

# ■ ENDOCRINE SYSTEM
## ENDOCRINE SYSTEM—ANATOMY AND TERMINOLOGY

Regulates body through hormones (chemical messengers)

Ductless endocrine glands secrete hormones directly to bloodstream

Affects growth, development, and metabolism

### Endocrine Glands (Fig. 1–45)

### Pituitary (Hypophysis): Master Gland
Located at base of brain in a depression in skull (sella turcica)

Anterior pituitary (adenohypophysis)

- Adrenocorticotropic hormone (ACTH)—stimulates adrenal cortex and increases production of cortisol

- Follicle-stimulating hormone (FSH)—males, stimulates sperm and testosterone production; females, with luteinizing hormone (LH) stimulates secretion of estrogen and follicle development and ovulation

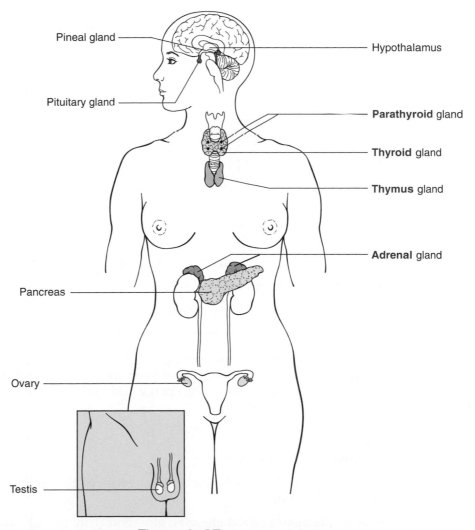

Figure **1-45** Endocrine system.

- Growth hormone (GH or somatotropin STH)—stimulates protein processing resulting in growth of bones, muscle, and fat metabolism, and maintains blood glucose levels

- Luteinizing hormone (LH)—males, stimulates testosterone production; females, stimulates secretion of progesterone and estrogen

- Melanocyte-stimulating hormone (MSH)—increases skin pigmentation

- Prolactin (PRL)—secreted by anterior pituitary, stimulates milk production and breast development

- Thyroid-stimulating hormone (TSH or thyrotropin)—stimulates thyroid gland

Posterior pituitary (neurohypophysis)—stores and releases hormones

- Antidiuretic hormone (ADH) or vasopressin—stimulates reabsorption of water by kidney tubules and increases blood pressure by constricting arterioles

- Oxytocin (OT)—stimulates contractions during childbirth, production and release of milk

## Thyroid
Two lobes overlying trachea

Secretes two hormones that increase cell metabolism—thyroxine ($T_4$) and triiodothyronine ($T_3$)—synthesized from iodine

Secretes one hormone that decreases blood calcium—thyrocalcitonin (nasal spray used to treat osteoporosis)

## Parathyroid Glands (4)
Located on posterior side of thyroid

Secretes PTH (parathyroid hormone) or parathoromone

Promotes calcium homeostasis in bloodstream

## Adrenal Gland (Pair)
Located on top of each kidney

Adrenal cortex—outer region that secretes corticosteroids

- Cortisol—increases blood glucose

- Aldosterone—increases reabsorption of sodium (salt)

- Androgen, estrogen, progestin—sexual characteristics

Adrenal medulla—inner region that secretes catecholamines (epinephrine to dilate blood vessels to lower blood pressure, increase heart rate, dilate bronchial tubes, and release glycogen for energy and norepinephrine to constrict blood vessels to raise blood pressure)

## Pancreas
Located behind stomach

Contains specialized cells (islets of Langerhans) that produce insulin and glycogen hormones

Insulin (decreases blood glucose), glucagon (converts glycogen to glucose, raising blood sugar), and somatostatin (regulates other cells of pancreas)

### Thymus
Located behind sternum

Atrophies during adolescence

Produces thymosin—stimulates T-lymphocytes, effecting a positive immune response

### Hypothalamus (Part of Brain)
Located below thalamus and above pituitary gland

Stimulates anterior pituitary to release hormones and posterior hypothalamus to store and release horomones

### Pineal
Located between two cerebral hemispheres and above third ventricle

Secretes melatonin—more so at night, which affects sleep cycle

Also responsible for delaying sexual maturation in children

Also has neurotransmitters such as somatostatin, norepinephrine, seratonin, and histamine

### Ovaries (Pair, Females)
Estrogen production stimulates ova production and secondary female sex characteristics

Progesterone—prepares the uterus for and maintains pregnancy

### Placenta
Produces HCG (human chorionic gonadotropin) to sustain a pregnancy

### Testes (Pair, Males)
Testosterone—male sex characteristics

## COMBINING FORMS

| | | |
|---|---|---|
| 1. | aden/o | in relationship to a gland |
| 2. | adren/o | adrenal gland |
| 3. | adrenal/o | adrenal gland |
| 4. | andr/o | male |
| 5. | calc/o, calc/i | calcium |
| 6. | cortic/o | cortex |
| 7. | crin/o | secrete |
| 8. | dips/o | thirst |
| 9. | estr/o | female |
| 10. | gluc/o | sugar |
| 11. | glyc/o | sugar |
| 12. | gonad/o | ovaries and testes |
| 13. | home/o | same |
| 14. | hormon/o | hormone |

| 15. kal/i | potassium |
|-----------|-----------|
| 16. lact/o | milk |
| 17. myx/o | mucus |
| 18. natr/o | sodium |
| 19. pancreat/o | pancreas |
| 20. parathyroid/o | parathyroid gland |
| 21. phys/o | growing |
| 22. pituitar/o | pituitary gland |
| 23. somat/o | body |
| 24. ster/o, stere/o | solid, having three dimensions |
| 25. thry/o | thyroid gland |
| 26. thyroid/o | thyroid gland |
| 27. toc/o | child birth |
| 28. toxic/o | poison |
| 29. ur/o | urine |

## PREFIXES

| 1. eu- | good/normal |
|--------|-------------|
| 2. oxy- | sharp, oxygen |
| 3. pan- | all |
| 4. tetra- | four |
| 5. tri- | three |
| 6. tropin- | act upon |

## SUFFIXES

| 1. -agon | assemble |
|----------|----------|
| 2. -drome | run, relationship to conducting, to speed |
| 3. -emia | blood condition |
| 4. -in | a substance |
| 5. -ine | a substance |
| 6. -tropin | act upon |
| 7. -uria | urine |

## MEDICAL TERMS

| Adrenals | Glands, located at top of kidneys, that produce steroid hormones (cortex) and catecholamines (medulla) |
|----------|--------|
| Contralateral | Opposite side |
| Hormone | Chemical substance produced by body's endocrine glands |

214

| | |
|---|---|
| Isthmus | Connection of two regions or structures |
| Isthmus, thyroid | Tissue connection between right and left thyroid lobes |
| Isthmusectomy | Surgical removal of isthmus |
| Lobectomy | Removal of a lobe |
| Thymectomy | Surgical removal of thymus |
| Thymus | Gland that produces hormones important to immune response |
| Thyroglossal duct | A duct in embryo between thyroid and posterior tongue which occasionally persists into adult life and causes cysts, fistulas, or sinuses |
| Thyroid | Part of endocrine system that produces hormones that regulate metabolism |
| Thyroidectomy | Surgical removal of thyroid |

## ENDOCRINE SYSTEM ANATOMY AND TERMINOLOGY QUIZ

1. Which of the following is NOT affected by the endocrine system?
   a. digestion
   b. development
   c. progesterone
   d. metabolism

2. Gland that overlies the trachea:
   a. parathyroid
   b. adrenal
   c. pancreas
   d. thyroid

3. Gland that is located on the top of each kidney:
   a. parathyroid
   b. adrenal
   c. pancreas
   d. thyroid

4. The outer region of the adrenal gland that secretes corticosteroids:
   a. cortex
   b. medulla
   c. sternum
   d. medullary

5. Located on the thyroid:
   a. hypophysis
   b. thymus
   c. pineal
   d. parathyroid

6. Located at the base of the brain in a depression in the skull:
   a. pituitary
   b. thymus
   c. adrenal
   d. pineal

7. Stimulates contractions during childbirth:
   a. cortisol
   b. PTH
   c. ADH
   d. oxytocin

8. Produced only during pregnancy by the placenta:
   a. estrogen and progesterone
   b. melatonin
   c. thymosin
   d. adrenocorticotropic hormone

9. Combining form meaning "secrete":
   a. dips/o
   b. crin/o
   c. gluc/o
   d. kal/i

10. Prefix meaning "good":
   a. tri-
   b. tropin-
   c. pan-
   d. eu-

# ENDOCRINE SYSTEM—PATHOPHYSIOLOGY

## Diabetes Mellitus

Caused by a deficiency in insulin production or poor use of insulin by body cells

Islets of Langerhans (pancreatic cells) secrete glucagon and insulin to regulate fat, carbohydrate, and protein metabolism

### Types of Diabetes Mellitus

**Type 1, IDDM (insulin-dependent diabetes mellitus), immune mediated**
Onset before age 30—peak onset age 12

Includes beta islet cell destruction, insulin deficiency

Acute onset

Positive family history

Requires insulin

Ketoacidosis (fats improperly burned leads to ketones and acids circulating)

**Type 2, NIDDM (non–insulin-dependent diabetes mellitus)**
Adult onset, after age 30, but it is now occurring earlier

Insidious onset/asymptomatic

Positive in immediate family

Dietary management and/or oral hypoglycemics and/or insulin

Most common type—85% are obese at onset

Insulin is present

Ketoacidosis does not occur

**Symptoms**
Polyuria

Polydipsia

Glycosuria

Hyperglycemia

Polyphagia

Unexplained weight loss

**Acute complications**
Hypoglycemia

Diabetic ketoacidosis

**Chronic complications**
Diabetic neuropathy (Fig. 1–46)

Retinopathy

Coronary artery disease (atherosclerosis)

Stroke

Peripheral vascular disease

Infection

Figure **1-46** Patient with diabetes mellitus and neuropathy had severe claw toes, and shear forces across plantar surface of first metatarsal head caused recurrent ulceration. (From Canale ST, Beaty JH, *Campbell's Operative Orthopaedics,* ed 11, Philadelphia, 2008, Mosby.)

**Gestational diabetes mellitus—predisposition to diabetes**
Most often recognized in third trimester

Glucose intolerance may be temporary, occurring only during pregnancy

Majority will develop diabetes mellitus within 15 years

## Pituitary Disorders

Tumors

Most common cause of pituitary disorders

May secrete hormone

Such as prolactin and ACTH

### Anterior Pituitary
**Dwarfism (hypopituitarism)**
Can be caused by deficiency of somatotrophin (growth hormone)

**Gigantism (Fig. 1–47) (hyperpituitarism)**
Can be caused by excess of somatotrophin (growth hormone) in childhood

**Treatment**
Resection of tumor or irradiation of pituitary

**Acromegaly (hyperpituitarism)**
Increased GH in adulthood

Enlargement of facial bones, feet, and hands

**Treatment**
Pituitary adenoma is irradiated or removed

Figure **1-47** Gigantism. A pituitary giant and dwarf contrasted with normal-size men. (From Thibodeau GA, Patton KT: *Anatomy & Physiology,* ed 5, St Louis, 2003, Mosby.)

## Posterior Pituitary

### Diabetes insipidus
Insufficient antidiuretic hormone—kidney tubules fail to retain needed water and salts

Causes polyuria, polydipsia, and dehydration

ADH or SIADH—syndrome of inadequate antidiuretic hormone

Excessive secretion of antidiuretic hormone

Causes excessive water retention

### Treatment
Some types have no treatment

Others can be controlled with vasopressin (drugs)

## Thyroid Disorders

### Goiter (Fig. 1–48)
Enlargement of thyroid gland in the neck

### Cause
Hypothyroid disorders

Hyperthyroid disorders

## Hyperthyroidism—Thyrotoxicosis
Excessive thyroid hormone production

Most common form: Graves' disease (familial)—results of autoimmune process

Figure **1-48** Goiter is an enlargement of thyroid gland.

**Characterized by**
Goiter

Tachycardia

Atrial fibrillation

Dyspnea

Palpitations

Fatigue

Tremor

Nervousness

Weight loss

Exophthalmos (protruding eyes)

• Decreased blinking

**Treatment**
Medication (antithyroid drugs)

Radioactive iodine

Surgical excision

Thyrotoxicosis storm/crisis

Thyroid storm/crisis is an acute, life-threatening hypermetabolic state induced by excessive release of thyroid horomones

Most extreme state of thyrotoxicosis

## Hypothyroidism
Primary: inadequate thyroid hormone production

Resulting in increasing levels of thyroid-stimulating hormone (TSH) production

Secondary: inadequate amounts of thyroid-stimulating hormone synthesized

**Types**
Cretinism

- Congenital
- Occurs in children
- If not treated, it will cause a severe delay in physical/mental development

**Treatment**
Thyroid hormone

Myxedema

- Severe form
- Occurs in adults
  - Atherosclerosis
- Symptoms
  - Cold intolerance
  - Weight gain
  - Mental sluggishness
  - Fatigue

**Treatment**
Thyroid hormone

Hashimoto's thyroiditis

- Autoimmune disorder

**Treatment**
Medication (levothyroxine synthetic hormone replacement)

## Parathyroid Disorders

### Hyperparathyroidism—Excessive Parathyroid Hormone (PTH)
Leads to hypercalcemia

- Affects heart and bones and damages kidneys

**Symptoms**
Brittle bones

Kidney stones

Cardiac disturbances

**Treatment**
Surgical excision

### Hypoparathyroidism—Abnormally Low PTH
Leads to hypocalcemia

**Symptoms**
Nerve irritability—twitching or spasms

Muscle cramps

Tingling and burning (parathesias) of fingertips, toes, and lips

Anxiety, nervousness

Tetany (constant muscle contraction)

**Treatment**
Calcium and vitamin D

## Adrenal Gland Disorders

### Cushing Syndrome—Hypercortisolism
Excess levels of adrenocorticotropic hormone (ACTH)

**Cause**
Hyperfunction of adrenal cortex

Long-term use of steroid medications

**Symptoms**
Weight gain

• Fat deposits on face (moonface) and trunk (buffalo hump)

Glucose intolerance

Hypernaturemia

Hypokalemia

Virilization

Hypertension

• Diabetes may develop (20%)

Muscle wasting

Osteoporosis

Change in mental status

Delayed healing

**Treatment**
Medication

Radiation therapy

Surgical intervention

### Addison's Disease—Primary Adrenal Insufficiency
Deficiency of adrenocortical hormones resulting from destruction of adrenal glands
• Glucocorticoids

• Mineralocorticoids

**Cause**
Tumors

Autoimmune disorders

Viral

Tuberculosis

Infection

**Symptoms**
Decreased blood glucose levels

Elevated serum ACTH

Fatigue

Lack of ability to handle stress

Weight loss

Infections

Hypotension

Decreased body hair

Hyperpigmentation

**Treatment**
Hormone (glucocorticoid) replacement

## Hyperaldosteronism
Excess aldosterone secreted by adrenal cortex

**Types**
Primary hyperaldosteronism (Conn's syndrome)

- Caused by an abnormality of adrenal cortex
  - Usually an adrenal adenoma

Secondary hyperaldosteronism

- Caused by other than adrenal stimuli

**Symptoms**
Hypertension

Hypokalemia

Neuromuscular disorders

**Treatment**
Treat the underlying condition that caused hyperaldosteronism

- Such as adrenal adenoma

## Adrenal Medulla
Hypersecretion

Pheochromocytoma—benign tumor of medulla

Excessive production of epinephrine and norepinephrine

**Symptoms**
Severe headaches

Sweating

Flushing

Hypertension

Muscle spasms

**Treatment**
Antihypertensive drugs

Remove tumor

### Androgen and Estrogen Hypersecretion

Androgen, male characteristic hormone

- Virilization, development of male characteristics

Feminization, hypersecretion of estrogen, female characteristic hormone

**Cause**

Underlying condition

- Adrenal tumor

- Cushing syndrome

- Adenomas or carcinomas

- Defects in steroid metabolism

**Treatment**

Surgical intervention for tumor

Underlying condition

# ENDOCRINE SYSTEM PATHOPHYSIOLOGY QUIZ

1. This type of diabetes typically occurs before age 30:
   a. type 1
   b. type 2

2. The acronym that indicates that insulin is not required is:
   a. IDDM
   b. NIDDM
   c. PIDDM
   d. NDDMI

3. The most common cause of pituitary disorders is:
   a. hypersecretion
   b. hyposecretion
   c. tumor
   d. infection

4. In excess, this hormone can cause gigantism:
   a. somatotrophin
   b. thyroid
   c. mineralocorticoids
   d. adrenocortical

5. Goiter can be caused by which of the following:
   a. hypothyroidism
   b. parathyroidism
   c. hyperthyroidism
   d. both a and c

6. This type of hypothyroidism is an autoimmune disorder:
   a. myxedema
   b. Hashimoto's
   c. cretinism
   d. hypokalemia

7. Tetany can be caused by:
   a. hypoparathyroidism
   b. hyperthyroidism
   c. hyperparathyroidism
   d. hyperaldosteronism

8. Conn's syndrome is also known as:
   a. primary hypoparathyroidism
   b. primary hyperthyroidism
   c. primary hyperparathyroidism
   d. primary hyperaldosteronism

9. Development of male characteristics is known as:
   a. virilization
   b. feminization
   c. hypertrophy
   d. hyperaldosteronism

10. The treatment for Addison's disease is often:
    a. chemotherapy
    b. radiation
    c. hormone replacement
    d. all of the above

# ■ NERVOUS SYSTEM
## NERVOUS SYSTEM—ANATOMY AND TERMINOLOGY

Controlling, regulating, and communicating system

Organization

- Central nervous system (CNS), brain and spinal cord
- Peripheral nervous system (PNS), cranial and spinal nerves
  - Autonomic nervous system—motor and sensory nerves of viscera (involuntary)
  - Somatic nervous system—motor and sensory nerves of skeletal muscles

### Cells of the Nervous System (Fig. 1–49)

### Neurons—Primary Cells of Nervous System
Classified according to function (afferent [sensory], efferent [motor], interneurons [associational])

- Dendrites (receive signals)
- Cell body (nucleus, within cell body)
- Axon (carries signals from cell body)
- Myelin sheath (insulation around axon)

### Glia
Astrocytes

Star shaped—transport water and salts between capillaries and neurons

Microglia

Multiple branching processes—protect neurons from inflammation

Figure **1-49** Myelinated axon.

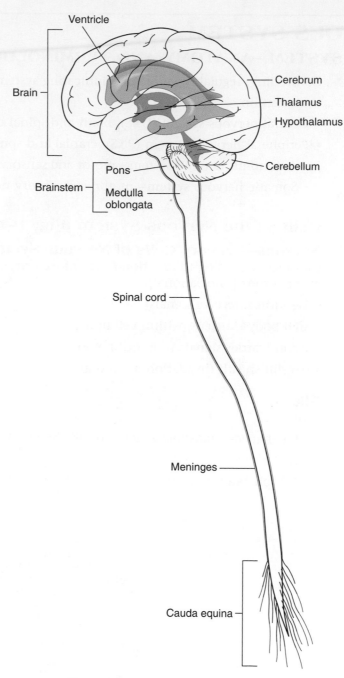

Figure **1-50** Brain and spinal cord.

Oligodendrocytes

　Form myelin sheath

Ependymal

　Lining membrane of brain and spinal cord where central spinal fluid circulates

## Divisions of Central Nervous System (CNS) (Fig. 1–50)

### Brain—Housed in Cranium (Box Comprised of 8 Bones)—Functioning to Enclose and Protect

Listing from inferior to superior

**Brainstem**

Medulla oblongata—crossover area left to right and center of respiratory and cardiovascular systems

Pons—connection of nerves (face and eyes)

Midbrain

**Diencephalon**

Hypothalamus controls autonomic nervous system, body temperature, sleep, appetite, and control of pituitary

Thalamus relays impulses to cerebral cortex for sensory system (pain)

**Cerebellum**

Controls voluntary movement and balance

**Cerebrum**

Largest part of brain

**Functions**

Mental processes, personality, sensory interpretation, movements, and memory

**Two hemispheres**

Right controls left side of body

Left controls right side of body

**Divided into five lobes**

- Frontal

- Parietal

- Temporal

- Occipital

- Insula

## Vertebral Column—33 Vertebrae

7 cervical

12 thoracic

5 lumbar

5 sacrum (fused)

4 coccygeal (fused)—tailbone

## Spinal Cord—housed within vertebrae from medulla oblongata to second lumbar

Spinal and brain meninges (coverings—dura mater [external], archnoid, pia mater [internal])

Spine and brain spaces bathed by cerebrospinal fluid (CSF) (subarachnoid space)

Cavities within brain contain cerebrospinal fluid (ventricles)

## Peripheral Nervous System (PNS)

Cranial nerves, 12 pair

Spinal nerves, 31 pair

## Autonomic Nervous System (ANS)—Housed within Both PNS and CNS

Two divisions

- Sympathetic system—functions in fight and flight (stress)
- Parasympathetic system—functions to restore and conserve energy

## COMBINING FORMS

| | | |
|---|---|---|
| 1. | cephal/o | head |
| 2. | cerebell/o | cerebellum |
| 3. | cerebr/o | cerebrum |
| 4. | crani/o | cranium |
| 5. | dur/o | dura mater |
| 6. | encephal/o | brain |
| 7. | gangli/o | ganglion |
| 8. | ganglion/o | ganglion |
| 9. | gli/o | glial cells |
| 10. | lept/o | slender |
| 11. | mening/o | meninges |
| 12. | meningi/o | meninges |
| 13. | ment/o | mind |
| 14. | mon/o | one |
| 15. | myel/o | bone marrow, spinal cord |
| 16. | neur/o | nerve |
| 17. | phas/o | speech |
| 18. | phren/o | mind |
| 19. | poli/o | gray matter |
| 20. | pont/o | pons |
| 21. | psych/o | mind |
| 22. | quadr/i | four |
| 23. | radic/o | nerve root |
| 24. | radicul/o | nerve root |
| 25. | rhiz/o | nerve root |
| 26. | vag/o | vagus nerve |

## PREFIXES

| | | |
|---|---|---|
| 1. | hemi- | half |
| 2. | per- | through |

3. quadri-        four

4. tetra-         four

## SUFFIXES

1. -algesia        pain sensation
2. -algia         pain
3. -cele          hernia
4. -esthesia     feeling
5. -iatry         medical treatment
6. -ictal          pertaining to
7. -kines/o      movement
8. -paresis      incomplete paralysis
9. -plegia       paralysis

## MEDICAL ABBREVIATIONS

1. ANS       autonomic nervous system
2. CNS       central nervous system
3. CSF        cerebrospinal fluid
4. CVA       stroke/cerebrovascular accident
5. EEG       electroencephalogram
6. LP         lumbar puncture
7. PNS       peripheral nervous system
8. TENS     transcutaneous electrical nerve stimulation
9. TIA        transient ischemic attack

## MEDICAL TERMS

| | |
|---|---|
| Burr | Drill used to create an entry into the cranium |
| Central nervous system | Brain and spinal cord |
| Craniectomy | Permanent, partial removal of skull |
| Craniotomy | Opening of the skull |
| Cranium | That part of the skeleton that encloses the brain |
| Discectomy | Removal of a vertebral disc |
| Electroencephalography | Recording of the electric currents of the brain by means of electrodes attached to the scalp |
| Laminectomy | Surgical excision of posterior arch of vertebra—includes spinal process |
| Peripheral nerves | 12 pairs of cranial nerves, 31 pairs of spinal nerves, and autonomic nervous system; connects peripheral receptors to the brain and spinal cord |

| | |
|---|---|
| Shunt | An artificial passage |
| Skull | Entire skeletal framework of the head |
| Somatic nerve | Sensory or motor nerve |
| Stereotaxis | Method of identifying a specific area or point in the brain |
| Sympathetic nerve | Part of the peripheral nervous system that controls automatic body function and sympathetic nerves activated under stress |
| Trephination | Surgical removal of a disk of bone |
| Vertebrectomy | Removal of vertebra |

# NERVOUS SYSTEM ANATOMY AND TERMINOLOGY QUIZ

1. Portion of nervous system that contains cranial and spinal nerves:
   a. central
   b. peripheral
   c. autonomic
   d. parasympathetic

2. Part of neuron that receives signals:
   a. dendrites
   b. cell body
   c. axon
   d. myelin sheath

3. NOT associated with glia:
   a. monocytes
   b. astrocytes
   c. microglia
   d. oligodendrocytes

4. Largest part of brain:
   a. cerebellum
   b. cerebrum
   c. cortex
   d. pons

5. Divided into two hemispheres:
   a. cerebellum
   b. cerebrum
   c. cortex
   d. pons

6. Number of pairs of cranial nerves:
   a. 10
   b. 11
   c. 12
   d. 13

7. Controls right side of body:
   a. left cerebrum
   b. right cerebrum
   c. right cortex
   d. left cortex

8. Combining form that means "brain":
   a. mening/o
   b. mon/o
   c. esthesi/o
   d. encephal/o

9. Prefix that means "four":
   a. per-
   b. tetra-
   c. para-
   d. bi-

10. Combining form that means "speech":
    a. phas/o
    b. rhiz/o
    c. poli/o
    d. myel/o

# NERVOUS SYSTEM—PATHOPHYSIOLOGY

## Dementias—Classified by Causative Factor

Cognitive deficiencies

### Causes

Alzheimer's disease

Vascular disease

Head trauma

Tumors

Infection

Toxins

Substance abuse

AIDS

## Alzheimer's Disease

Most common type of dementia

Progressive intellectual impairment

- Results in damage to neurons (neurofibrillary tangles)

- Fatal within 3 to 20 years

### Causes

Mostly unknown

Perhaps genetic defect, autoimmune reaction, or virus

### Symptoms

Behavior change

Memory loss

Confusion

Disorientation

Restlessness

Speech disturbances

Personality change—anxiety, depression

Irritability

Inability to complete activities of daily living

### Treatment

- No cure

- Aricept (drug has modest effect in early stages)

- Symptomatic treatment

- Support for family

## Vascular Dementia

Result of brain infarctions (vascular occlusion resulting in loss of brain function)

## Nutritional Degenerative Disease
Deficiency

- B vitamins

- Niacin

- Pantothenic acid

Associated with alcoholism

## Amyotrophic Lateral Sclerosis (ALS)
Motor neuron disease (MND)

Also known as Lou Gehrig's disease

- Baseball player who died of ALS

Deterioration of neurons of spinal cord and brain

Results in atrophy of muscles and loss of fine motor skills

Difficulty walking, talking, and breathing

Mental functioning remains normal

Survival is 2 to 5 years after diagnosis

Genetic cause/familial chromosome 21 aberration

- Death usually results from respiratory failure

**Treatment**
Symptomatic only

Emotional support

No cure

## Huntington's Disease—Chorea
Inherited progressive atrophy of cerebrum

**Symptoms**
Restlessness

Rapid, jerky movements in arms and face (uncontrollable jerking and facial grimacing)

Rigidity

Intellectual impairment/bradyphrenia/apathy

**Treatment**
Genetic defect of chromosome 4

No cure

Symptomatic

## Parkinson's Disease (Parkinsonism)
Decreased secretion of dopamine

Typically occurs after age 40

Cause unknown

**Symptoms**
Muscle rigidity and weakness

Bradykinesia—slow voluntary movements

Postural instability, stooped

Shuffling gait

Tremors at rest

Masklike facial appearance

Depression

**Treatment**
Medications to reduce symptoms

Dopamine replacement

## Multiple Sclerosis (MS)
Common neurologic condition

- Demyelination of central nervous system—replaced by sclerotic tissue

Affects young adults 20–40 years old

Results in myelin destruction and gliosis of white matter of central nervous system

Speculation that it is an autoimmune condition or result of a virus

Exacerbations and remission patterns

**Symptoms**
Precipitated by "an event," e.g., infection, pregnancy, stress

Loss of feeling (paresthesias)

Vision problems

Bladder disorder

Mood disorders

Weakness of limbs—unsteady gait and paralysis

**Treatment**
Symptomatic

Management of relapses

Reducing relapses and disease progression—disease-modifying drugs (DMDs)

## Myasthenia Gravis (MG)
Means grave muscle weakness

Autoimmune neuromuscular condition—antibodies block neurotransmission to muscle cells

Most have pathologic changes of thymus

**Symptoms**
Insidious

Muscle weakness and fatigability

May be localized or generalized

Often affects

- Swallowing

- Breathing

- Compromised swallowing and breathing may lead to crisis

**Treatment**
Anticholinesterase drugs

- Restores normal muscle strength and recoverability after fatigue

Corticosteroids (prednisone) and immunosuppressive drugs

Thymectomy

## Tourette syndrome

**Symptoms**

Spasmodic, twitching movements, uncontrollable vocal sounds, inappropriate words

Begins with twitching eyelids and facial muscles (tics)

Verbal outbursts

**Cause**

Unknown

Excess dopamine or hypersensitivity to dopamine

**Treatment**

Antipsychotic drugs

Antidepressant drugs

Mood-elevating drugs

## Poliomyelitis
Contagious viral disease

Affects motor neurons

Causes paralysis and respiratory failure

Prevent with vaccination

## Postpolio Syndrome (PPS)
Also known as postpoliomyelitis neuromuscular atrophy

Progressive muscle weakness

- Past history of paralytic polio

**Symptoms**
Muscle weakness and fatigability

- May include atrophy and muscle twitching

**Treatment**
Symptomatic

Maintenance of respiratory function

### Guillain-Barré Syndrome

Also known as

- Idiopathic polyneuritis
- Acute inflammatory polyneuropathy
- Landry's ascending paralysis

Demyelination of peripheral nerves—acquired disease

**Symptoms**

Primary ascending motor paralysis

Variable sensory disturbances

**Treatment**

Supportive

## Congenital Neurologic Disorders

### Hydrocephalus

Excessive amounts circulating of cerebrospinal fluid in ventricles of brain

Circulation is impaired in brain or spinal cord

Compresses brain

**Treatment**

Surgical placement of a shunt

### Spina Bifida (Fig. 1–51)

Developmental birth defect that causes incomplete development of spinal cord and its coverings

Vertebrae overlying open portions of spinal cord do not fully form and remain unfused and open

- Spina bifida occulta—may not be noticed, no protrusion through defect
- Spina bifida manifesta, which includes:
  - Myelomeningocele (spina bifida cystica)
    - Meninges and spinal cord protrude through defect
  - Meningocele
    - Meninges herniated through defect

Results in neurologic deficiencies

**Treatment**

Surgical repair

## Mental, Behavioral and Neurodevelopmental Disorders

### Schizophrenia

Variety of syndromes

Results in changes in brain

Hereditary factors are considered a cause

- Also, fetal brain damage caused by viral infections, complications of pregnancy, nutritional deficiences

Stress usually precipitates onset

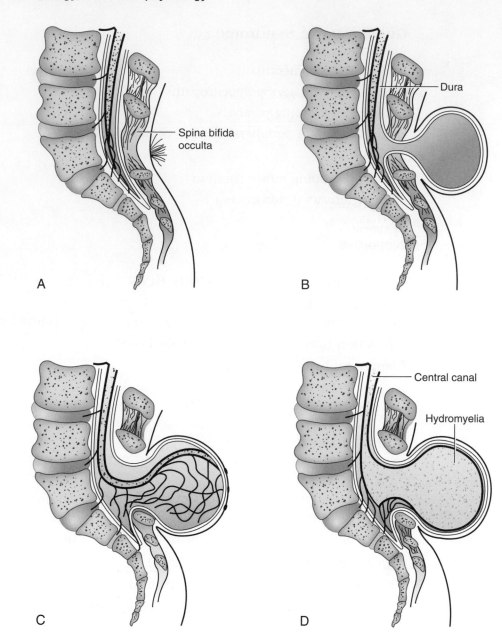

Figure **1-51** **A,** Spina bifida occulta. **B,** Meningocele. **C,** Myelomeningocele. **D,** Myelocystocele or hydromyelia.

**Symptoms**

Delusions of persecution and/or grandeur

Disorganized thought

Repetitive behaviors

Behavior issues

Decreased speech

Decreased ability to solve problems

Loss of emotions/flat affect

Hallucinations

Types are based on characteristics

**Treatment**
Antipsychotic drugs

Drugs have very unpleasant side effects such as tardive dyskinesia, with symptoms as follows:

- Excessive movement
- Grimacing
- Jerking
- Tremors
- Shuffling gait
- Dry mouth
- Blurred vision

## Depression
Mood (sustained emotional state) disorder

Exact cause is unknown

**Symptoms**
Sadness

Hopelessness

Lethargy

Insomnia

Anorexia

## Treatment
Antidepressant drugs

Electroconvulsive therapy

## Central Nervous System (CNS) Disorders
### ■ Vascular Disorder
### Transient Ischemic Attack (TIA)
Temporary reduction of blood flow to brain that produces strokelike symptoms but no lasting damage

Often a warning sign of cerebrovascular accident

**Symptoms**
Depend on location of ischemia

- Usual recovery within 24 hours

No loss of consciousness

Slurred, indiscernible speech

May display muscle weakness in legs/arms

Paresthesia (numbness) of face

Mental confusion may be present

Repeated attacks common in the presence of atherosclerotic disease

## Cerebrovascular Accident (CVA) or Stroke
Infarction of brain due to lack of blood/oxygen flow

Necrosis of tissue with total occlusion of vessel

### Causes
Atherosclerotic disease—thrombus formation

Embolus

Hemorrhage—arterial aneurysm

### Symptoms
Depend on location of obstruction

- Thrombus
  - Gradual onset
  - Often occurs at rest
  - Intracranial pressure (ICP) minimal
  - Localized damage
- Embolus
  - Sudden onset
  - Occurs anytime
  - ICP minimal
  - Localized damage unless multiple emboli
- Hemorrhage
  - Sudden onset
  - Occurs most often with activity
  - ICP high
  - Widespread damage
  - May be fatal

### Treatment
Anticoagulant drugs (clot dissolving) if caused by thrombus or embolus—tissue plasminogen activator (tPA)

Carotid endarterectomy (removes artherosclerotic plaque)

Oxygen treatment

Underlying condition treated, such as

- Hypertension
- Atherosclerosis
- Thrombus

## Aneurysm—Cerebral
Dilation of artery

- May be localized or multiple

Rupture possible, often on exertion

- Fatal if rupture is massive

**Symptoms**

May display visual effects, such as

- Loss of visual fields

- Photophobia

- Diplopia

Headache

Confusion

Slurred speech

Weakness

Stiff neck (nuchal rigidity)

**Treatment**

Dependent on diagnosis prior to rupture

Surgical intervention

## Encephalitis

Infection of parenchymal tissue of brain or spinal cord

- Often viral

Accompanying inflammation

Usually results in some permanent damage

**Symptoms**

Stiff neck

Headaches

Vomiting

Fever

May have seizure

Lethargy

**Some types of encephalitis**

Herpes simplex

Lyme disease

West Nile fever

Western equine

**Treatment**

Symptomatic

Supportive

## Reye's Syndrome

Associated with viral infection

- Especially when aspirin has been administered

Changes occur in brain and liver

- Leads to increased intracranial pressure

**Symptoms**

Headaches

Vomiting

Lethargy

Seizures

**Treatment**

Symptomatic treatment

## Brain Abscess

Localized infection

Necrosis of tissue

Usually spread from infection elsewhere, such as ears or sinus

**Symptoms**

Neurologic deficiencies

Increased intracranial pressure

**Treatment**

Antibiotics for bacterial infections

Surgical drainage

## ■ Epilepsies

Chronic seizure disorder

## Types

**Partial seizures (focal)**

State of altered focus but conscious—simple

Impaired consciousness—complex

Specialized epileptic seizures

Aura

- Auditory or visual sign that precedes a seizure

**Generalized seizures**

Absence seizures—petit mal

- Brief loss of awareness
- Most common in children (febrile causation)

Tonic-clonic—grand mal or ictal event

- Loss of consciousness
- Alternate contraction and relaxation
- Incontinence
- No memory of seizure

**Causes**

Tumor

Hemorrhage

Trauma

Edema

Infection

Excessive cerebrospinal fluid

High fever

**Treatment**

Correct cause

Anticonvulsant drugs

Neurosurgery

Postictal event—after seizure—neurologic symptoms (weakness, etc.)

## ■ Trauma

### Head Injury—Traumatic Brain Injury (TBI)
**Concussion**
Mild blow to head

Temporary axonal disturbances

Grade 1: temporary confusion and amnesia (brief)

Grade 2: memory loss for very recent events and confusion

Grade 3: amnesia for recent events and disorientation (longer duration)

Results in reversible interference with brain function

• Recovery within 24 hours with no residual damage

**Contusion**
Bruising of brain

Force of blow determines outcome

**Hematomas—blood accumulation (clot)**
Compresses surrounding structures

Classified based on location

• Epidural
  • Develops between dura and skull
• Subdural
  • Develops between dura and arachnoid
    · Development within 24 hours is acute
    · Development within a week is subacute
  • ICP increases with enlargement of hematoma
• Subarachnoid
  • Develops between pia and arachnoid
  • Blood mixes with cerebrospinal fluid
    · No localized hematoma forms

- Intracerebral
  - As a result of a contusion

*Symptoms*

Increased ICP

Others dependent on location and severity of injury

*Treatment*

Identification of the location of hematoma

Medications to decrease edema

Antibiotics

Surgical intervention—burr hole if necessary to decrease the ICP

## Spinal Cord Injury

Result of trauma to vertebra, cord, ligaments, intervertebral disc

**Vertebral injuries classified as**

- Simple—affects spinous or transverse process
- Compression—anterior fracture of vertebrae
- Comminuted—vertebral body is shattered
- Dislocation—vertebrae are out of alignment
- Flexion injury in which hyperflexion compresses vertebra

Dislocation

Rotation

**Symptoms**

Depend on vertebral level and severity

Paralysis

Loss of sensation

Drop in blood pressure

Loss of bladder and rectal control

Decreased venous circulation

**Treatment**

Identification of area of injury

Immobilization

Corticosteroids to decrease edema

Bladder and bowel management

Rehabilitation

# ■ Tumors of Brain and Spinal Cord

Increases ICP

Life threatening

Rarely metastasize outside of central nervous system

Secondary brain tumors are common

Metastasis from lung or breast

## Gliomas Common Type

Primary malignant tumor—encapsulated and invasive

Types based on cell from which tumor arises and location of tumor

### Glioblastoma
Located in cerebral hemispheres (deep in white matter)

Highly aggressive

### Oligodendrocytoma
Usually located in frontal lobes

Oligodendroblastoma, more aggressive form

### Ependymoma
Located in ventricles

Most often occurs in children

Ependymoblastoma, more aggressive form

### Astrocytoma
Located anywhere in brain and spinal cord

Invasive but slow growing

## Pineal Region
### Germ cell tumors
Usually in adolescents

Rare

Variable growth rate

### Several other pineal tumors
Pineocytoma

Teratoma

Germinoma

## Blood Vessel
### Angioma
Usually located in posterior cerebral hemispheres

Slow growing

### Hemangioblastoma
Located in cerebellum

Slow growing

### Medulloblastoma
Aggressive tumor

Located in posterior cerebellar vermis (fourth ventricle roof)

### Meningioma
Originates in arachnoid

Slow growing

### Pituitary Tumor
Related to aging

Slow growing

- Such as macroadenomas

### Cranial Nerve Tumors
Neurilemmomas most common location: cranial nerve VIII

Slow growing

Metastatic

### Spinal Cord Tumors

Symptoms are based on location of spinal compression

Intramedullary

- Originates in neural tissue

Extramedullary

- Originates outside the spinal cord

Metastatic tumors of spinal cord are more common

- Myeloma—marrow

- Lymphoma—lymph

- Carcinomas—lung, breast, prostate

Most common type of primary extramedullary tumor

- Meningiomas—anyplace in spine

- Neurofibromas—common in thoracic and lumbar regions

# NERVOUS SYSTEM PATHOPHYSIOLOGY QUIZ

1. Most common dementia is:
   a. Alzheimer's disease
   b. secondary
   c. nutritional degenerative disease
   d. Lou Gehrig's disease

2. MND stands for:
   a. maximal neuron disorder
   b. migrating niacin disorder
   c. motor neuron disease
   d. motor neuropathic disorder

3. Dopamine replacement is useful in treating:
   a. multiple sclerosis
   b. Parkinson's disease
   c. Huntington's disease
   d. CVA

4. Condition in which primary symptoms are muscle weakness and fatigability:
   a. amyotrophic lateral sclerosis
   b. multiple sclerosis
   c. dyskinesis
   d. myasthenia gravis

5. Another name for idiopathic polyneuritis is:
   a. Guillain-Barré syndrome
   b. multiple sclerosis
   c. amyotrophic lateral sclerosis
   d. postpolio syndrome

6. This condition is thought to be caused by genetic factors and possibly fetal brain damage:
   a. Parkinson's
   b. schizophrenia
   c. spina bifida
   d. Guillain-Barré syndrome

7. This condition is associated with viral infection, especially when aspirin has been administered:
   a. Reye's syndrome
   b. Guillain-Barré syndrome
   c. Lou Gehrig's disease
   d. Conn's syndrome

8. Concussion is a mild blow to the head in which recovery is expected within
   _____.
   a. 12 hours
   b. 24 hours
   c. 48 hours
   d. 1 week

9. ICP means:
   a. intercranial pressure
   b. intracranial pressure
   c. interior cranial pressure
   d. intensive cranial pressure

10. In this type of hematoma, blood mixes with cerebrospinal fluid:
   a. epidural
   b. subdural
   c. subarachnoid
   d. intracerebral

# ■ SENSES

## SENSES—ANATOMY AND TERMINOLOGY

| | |
|---|---|
| Sight | Eyes |
| Hearing | Ears |
| Smell | Nose |
| Taste | Tongue |
| Touch | Skin |

### Sight: Three Layers of Eye (Fig. 1–52)

### Cornea (Outer Layer)
Fibrous, transparent layer that extends over dome of eye

Refracts (bends) light to focus on receptor cells (posterior eye)

Avascular (nourished by sclera)

### Sclera (Extension of Outer Layer)
White of eye

Extends from cornea (anterior or surface) to optic nerve (posterior surface)

- Lies over iris

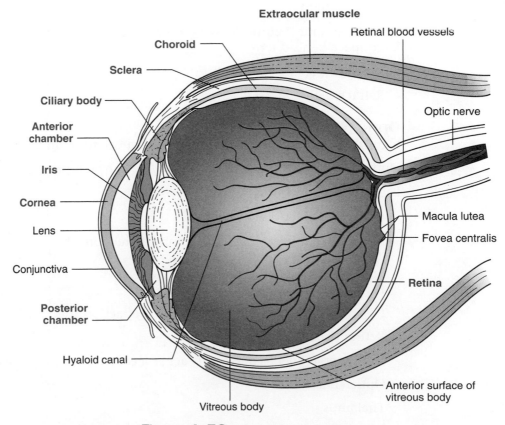

Figure **1-52** Eye and ocular adnexa.

### Choroid (Middle Layer)
Pigment layer

Ciliary muscle and iris on front portion of layer

• Contracts

### Retina (Inner Layer)
Contains rods and cones

• Rods provide night and peripheral vision

• Cones provide day and color vision and are stimulated by primary colors of red, green, and blue

### Conjunctiva
Covers front of sclera and lines eyelid (contiguous layer)

### Lens
Behind pupil

Lens is connected by zonules to ciliary body

Ciliary body muscles cause lens to change shape to refract light rays (accommodation)

### Fluids
Aqueous humor (front of lens)—watery substance secreted by ciliary body

    Maintains shape of front portion of eye

    Refracts light

Vitreous humor (behind lens)—gel-like substance (not readily re-formed) filling large space behind lens

    Maintains shape of eyeball

    Refracts light

### Optic Nerve
Light rays from rods and cones travel from eye to brain via optic nerve

Optic nerve meets retina in optic disc (no light receptors)—blind spot

Pathway of light ray

    Cornea—refraction site

    Anterior chamber (aqueous humor)—refraction site

    Pupil

    Lens—refraction site

    Posterior chamber (vitreous humor)—refraction site

    Retina (rods and cones)

    Optic nerve fibers—nerve cells act as a cable connecting the eye with the brain

    Optic chiasm

    Thalamus

    Cerebral cortex (occipital lobe)—light is interpreted

## Hearing, Three Divisions of Ear

### External Ear

Auricle (pinna)—sound waves enter ear

External auditory canal—tunnel from auricle to middle ear

### Middle Ear

Begins with tympanic membrane (eardrum)

Ossicles—small bones conducting sound waves from middle to inner ear

- Malleus

- Incus

- Stapes

Eustachian tube—leads to pharynx

### Inner Ear (Labyrinth)

Vestibule

Semicircular canals/vestibular apparatus

Cochlea contains perilymph and endolymph (liquids through which sound waves are conducted)

Organ of Corti—auditory receptor area

Auditory nerve—electrical impulse is conducted to cerebral cortex for interpretation (hearing)

Pathway of sound vibration (exterior to brain)

Pinna

External auditory canal

Tympanic membrane

Malleus

Incus

Stapes

Oval window

Cochlea

Auditory fluid/receptors in organ of Corti

Auditory nerve

Cerebral cortex

## Smell

### Olfactory Sense Receptors

Located in nasal cavity

Closely related to sense of taste

Cranial nerve I

## Taste

Gustatory sense—sweet, salty, and sour differentiated

Taste buds located on anterior portion of tongue

Cranial nerves VII and IX

## Touch

### Mechanoreceptors
Widely distributed throughout body

Reacts to touch and pressure

- Meissner corpuscles (touch)

- Pacinian corpuscles (pressure)

### Proprioceptors
Position and orientation

Dysfunctions

- Vestibular nystagmus—involuntary movement of eyes

- Vertigo—sense of spinning/dizziness

### Thermoreceptors
Under skin

Sense temperature changes

### Nociceptors
Pain sensors

In skin and internal organs

## COMBINING FORMS

| | | |
|---|---|---|
| 1. | ambly/o | dim, dullness |
| 2. | aque/o | water |
| 3. | audi/o | hearing |
| 4. | blephar/o | eyelid |
| 5. | conjunctiv/o | conjunctiva |
| 6. | cor/o, core/o | pupil |
| 7. | corne/o | cornea |
| 8. | cycl/o | ciliary body |
| 9. | dacry/o | tear |
| 10. | essi/o, esthesi/o | sensation |
| 11. | glauc/o | gray |
| 12. | ir/o | iris |
| 13. | irid/o | iris |

14. kerat/o          cornea
15. lacrim/o         tear
16. mi/o             smaller
17. myring/o         eardrum
18. ocul/o           eye
19. ophthalm/o       eye
20. opt/o            eye, vision
21. optic/o          eye
22. ot/o             ear
23. palpebr/o        eyelid
24. papill/o         optic nerve
25. phac/o           eye lens
26. phak/o           eye lens
27. phot/o           light
28. presby/o         old age
29. pupill/o         pupil
30. retin/o          retina
31. scler/o          sclera
32. scot/o           darkness
33. staped/o         stapes
34. tympan/o         eardrum
35. uve/o            uvea
36. vitre/o          glassy
37. xer/o            dry

## PREFIXES

1. audi-             hearing
2. eso-              inward
3. exo-              outward

## SUFFIXES

1. -opia             vision
2. -omia             smell
3. -tropia           to turn

## MEDICAL ABBREVIATIONS

1. AD                right ear
2. AS                left ear
3. AU                both ears

| | | |
|---|---|---|
| 4. | H or E | hemorrhage or exudate |
| 5. | IO | intraocular |
| 6. | IOL | intraocular lens |
| 7. | OD | right eye |
| 8. | OS | left eye |
| 9. | OU | each eye |
| 10. | PERL | pupils equal and reactive to light |
| 11. | PERRL | pupils equal, round, and reactive to light |
| 12. | PERRLA | pupils equal, round, and reactive to light and accommodation |
| 13. | REM | rapid eye movement |
| 14. | TM | tympanic membrane |

## MEDICAL TERMS

| | |
|---|---|
| Anterior segment | Those parts of eye in the front of and including lens, orbit, extraocular muscles, and eyelid |
| Apicectomy | Excision of a portion of temporal bone |
| Astigmatism | Condition in which refractive surfaces of eye are unequal |
| Aural atresia | Congenital absence of external auditory canal |
| Blepharitis | Inflammation of eyelid |
| Cataract | Opaque covering on or in lens |
| Chalazion | Granuloma around sebaceous gland |
| Cholesteatoma | Tumor that forms in middle ear |
| Conjunctiva | The lining of eyelids and covering of sclera |
| Dacryocystitis | Blocked, inflamed infection of nasolacrimal duct |
| Dacryostenosis | Narrowing of lacrimal duct |
| Ectropion | Eversion (outward sagging) of eyelid |
| Entropion | Inversion of eyelid (lashes rubbing cornea) |
| Enucleation | Removal of an organ or organs from a body cavity |
| Episclera | Connective covering of sclera |
| Exenteration | Removal of an organ all in one piece, commonly used to describe radical excision |
| Exophthalmos | Protrusion of eyeball |
| Exostosis | Bony growth |
| Fenestration | Creation of a new opening in inner wall of middle ear |
| Glaucoma | Eye diseases that are characterized by an increase of intraocular pressure |
| Hordeolum | Stye—infection of sebaceous gland (nodule on lid margin) |
| Hyperopia | Farsightedness, eyeball is too short from front to back |
| Keratomalacia | Softening of cornea associated with a deficiency of vitamin A |

| | |
|---|---|
| Keratoplasty | Surgical repair of the cornea |
| Labyrinth | Inner connecting cavities, such as internal ear |
| Labyrinthitis | Inner ear inflammation |
| Lacrimal | Related to tears |
| Mastoidectomy | Removal of mastoid bone |
| Ménière's disease | Condition that causes dizziness, ringing in ears, and deafness |
| Myopia | Nearsightedness, eyeball too long from front to back |
| Myringotomy | Incision into tympanic membrane |
| Ocular adnexa | Orbit, extraocular muscles, and eyelid |
| Ophthalmoscopy | Examination of the interior of eye by means of a scope, also known as funduscopy |
| Otitis media | Noninfectious inflammation of middle ear; serous otitis media produces liquid drainage (not purulent), and suppurative otitis media produces purulent (pus) matter |
| Otoscope | Instrument used to examine ear |
| Papilledema | Swelling of optic disc (papilla) |
| Posterior segment | Those parts of eye behind lens |
| Ptosis | Drooping of upper eyelid |
| Sclera | Outer covering of eye |
| Strabismus | Extraocular muscle deviation resulting in unequal visual axes |
| Tarsorrhaphy | Suturing together of eyelids |
| Tinnitus | Ringing in the ears |
| Transmastoid | Creates an opening in mastoid for drainage antrostomy |
| Tympanolysis | Freeing of adhesions of the tympanic membrane |
| Tympanometry | Test of the inner ear using air pressure |
| Tympanostomy | Insertion of ventilation tube into tympanum |
| Uveal | Vascular tissue of the choroid, ciliary body, and iris |
| Vertigo | Dizziness |
| Xanthelasma | Yellow plaque on eyelid (lipid disorder) |

# SENSES ANATOMY AND TERMINOLOGY QUIZ

1. The middle layer of the eye:
   a. sclera
   b. retina
   c. episclera
   d. choroid

2. The covering of the front of sclera and lining of eyelid:
   a. aqueous humor
   b. ossicles
   c. vitreous
   d. conjunctiva

3. Which of the following is NOT a bone of the middle ear?
   a. cochlea
   b. stapes
   c. malleus
   d. incus

4. This cranial nerve controls the sense of smell:
   a. I
   b. II
   c. III
   d. IV

5. Which of the following is NOT part of the inner ear?
   a. pinna
   b. vestibule
   c. semicircular canals
   d. cochlea

6. These receptors react to touch:
   a. nociceptors
   b. mechanoreceptors
   c. proprioceptors
   d. thermoreceptors

7. These receptors react to position and orientation:
   a. nociceptors
   b. mechanoreceptors
   c. proprioceptors
   d. thermoreceptors

8. Combining form meaning "eyelid":
   a. aque/o
   b. blephar/o
   c. optic/o
   d. uve/o

9. Combining form meaning "eye lens":
   a. cor/o
   b. irid/o
   c. ocul/o
   d. phak/o

10. Abbreviation meaning the pupils are equal, round, and reactive to light and accommodation:
    a. PERRLA
    b. PERRL
    c. PERL
    d. PURL

# SENSES—PATHOPHYSIOLOGY

## Eye

### Visual Disturbances

#### Astigmatism
Irregular curvature of refractive surfaces (cornea or lens) of eye

Can be congenital or acquired (as a result of disease or trauma)

Image is distorted

#### Treatment
Corrected with cylindrical lens

#### Diplopia
Double vision

#### Amblyopia
Dimness of vision—impairment of vision without detectable organic lesion of eye

#### Hyperopia
Farsightedness

Shortened eyeball

- Can see objects in distance, not close up

#### Treatment
Corrected with convex lens

#### Presbyopia
Age-related farsightedness

#### Treatment
Magnification (reading glasses or bifocals)

#### Myopia
Nearsightedness

Elongated eyeball

- Can see objects up close, not in distance

#### Treatment
Corrected with concave lens thicker at periphery

#### Nystagmus—unilateral or bilateral
Rapid, involuntary eye movements

Movements can be

- Vertical
- Horizontal
- Rotational
- Combination of above

**Cause**
Brain tumor or inner ear disease

Normal in newborns

Due to underlying condition or adverse effect of drug

Various types, such as

- Vestibular nystagmus
- Rhythmic eye movements

**Strabismus**
Cross-eyed

Due to muscle weakness or neurologic defect

Forms of strabismus

- Hypotropia (downward deviation of one eye)
- Hypertropia (upward deviation of one eye)
- Estropia (one eye turns inward)
- Exotropia (one eye turns outward)

**Treatment**
- Eye exercises/patching of normal eye
- Surgery to establish muscle balance

## Infections
**Conjunctivitis (pink eye)**
Inflammation of conjunctival lining of eyelid or covering of sclera

Due to

- Infection
- Allergy
- Irritation

**Treatment**
- Varies with cause
- Antibiotic eye drops

**Hordeolum (stye)**
Bacterial infection of eyelid hair follicle

- Usually *Staphylococcus*

Results in mass on eyelid

**Treatment**
- Antibiotics
- Incision and drainage may be necessary

**Keratitis**
Corneal inflammation

Caused by herpes simplex virus

Causes tearing and photophobia

## Macular Degeneration

Destruction of fovea centralis

- Fovea centralis is small pit in center of retina (fovea centralis retinae)

Usually age related—leading cause of blindness in elderly

Results from exposure to ultraviolet rays or drugs

- Also may have a genetic component

Central vision is lost

Two types of macular degeneration

- Wet—development of new vascularization and leaking blood vessels near macula

- Dry (85% of cases)—atrophy and degeneration of retinal cells and deposits of drusen (clumps of extracellular waste)

### Treatment

None for "dry" macular degeneration

Surgical intervention with laser for "net" macular degeneration to coagulate leaking vessels; success is limited

Medications

## Detached Retina

Retinal tear—two layers of retina separate from each other

- Vitreous humor then leaks behind retina

- Retina then pulls away from choroid

Results in increasing blind spot in visual field

Condition is painless

Pressure continues to build if left unattended

Final result is blindness

### Treatment

Surgical intervention with laser to repair tear (emergency/urgency)—photocoagulation for small tears

Scleral buckle for large retinal detachments

Pneumatic retinopexy for medium to large retinal detachment. Gas bubble is injected into vitreous cavity; pressure to tear resulting in retinal reattachment.

## Cataracts

Lens becomes opaque with protein aggregates

### Classified by morphology

Size

Shape

Location

Also may be classified by etiology (cause) or time cataract occurs

**Examples of classification**
Congenital cataract

- Bilateral opacity present at birth

- Also known as developmental cataract

Heat cataract

- Also known as glassblowers' cataract

- Caused by exposure to radiation

Traumatic cataract (Fig. 1–53)

- Result of injury to eye

Senile cataract

- Age related

- Usually forms on corneal area of lens

**Symptoms**
Blurring of vision

Halos around lights

**Treatment**
Removal of cataract with intraocular lens implantation

If no intraocular lens implant, then glasses or contact lenses for refraction

## Glaucoma
Excess accumulation of intraocular aqueous humor

- Results in decreased blood flow and edema

- Damages retinal cells and optic nerve

**Narrow-angle glaucoma**
Acute type of glaucoma

**Chronic glaucoma**
Also known as

- Wide-angle glaucoma

- Open-angle glaucoma

Figure **1-53** A concussion injury that resulted in a traumatic cataract. (From Yanoff M, Duker J: *Ophthalmology,* ed 2, St Louis, 2004, Mosby.)

Asymptomatic

Diagnosed in eye examination using tonometry to test anterior chamber pressure

**Treatment**

Medications that decrease output of aqueous humor and decrease intraocular pressure (IOP)

Laser treatment to provide drainage

# Ear

## ■ Infections

### Otitis Media

Infection or inflammation of middle ear cavity

Chronic infection produces adhesions

Results in loss of hearing

Often occurs in children in combination with URI (upper respiratory infection)

Causes severe ear pain (otalgia)

**Treatment**

Antibiotics

Surgical intervention with placement of tubes to allow for drainage

- Useful in patients with recurrent infection

### Otitis Externa

Also known as swimmer's ear

Infection of external auditory canal and pinna (exterior ear)

Caused by bacteria or fungus

Results in pain and discharge

**Treatment**

Antibiotic

Encouraged to keep ear dry

## ■ Hearing Loss

### Conductive Hearing Loss

Due to a defect of sound-conducting apparatus

- Accumulation of wax
- Scar tissue on tympanic membrane

Also known as:

- Transmission hearing loss
- Conduction deafness

**Treatment**
- Hearing aids

### Sensorineural

Due to a lesion of cochlea or central neural pathways

Also known as

• Perceptive deafness

May be divided into

• Cochlear hearing loss
  • Due to a defect in receptor or transducing mechanisms of cochlea
• Retrocochlear hearing loss
  • Due to defect located proximal to cochlea (vestibulocochlear nerve or auditory area of brain)

Presbycusis is age-related sensorineural hearing loss

**Treatment**
• Unknown

### Ototoxic Hearing Loss

Caused by ingestion of toxic substance

Also known as toxic deafness

### Ménière's Disease

Inner ear disturbance

  Also known as idiopathic endolymphatic hydrops

Cause unknown

Most common cause of vertigo (dizziness)

Other symptoms include hearing loss and tinnitus

## SENSES PATHOPHYSIOLOGY QUIZ

1. This condition can be acquired or congenital and results in an irregular curvature of the refractive surfaces of the eye:
   a. diplopia
   b. hyperopia
   c. nystagmus
   d. astigmatism

2. In this condition the eyeball is shorter than normal and results in being able to see objects in the distance but not close up:
   a. diplopia
   b. hyperopia
   c. nystagmus
   d. astigmatism

3. Rapid, involuntary eye movement is the predominant symptom of this condition:
   a. diplopia
   b. hyperopia
   c. nystagmus
   d. astigmatism

4. Age-related farsightedness is:
   a. presbyopia
   b. hyperopia
   c. diplopia
   d. myopia

5. Another name for a stye is:
   a. keratitis
   b. hordeolum
   c. hyperopia
   d. strabismus

6. An inflammation of the cornea that is caused by herpes simplex virus is:
   a. keratitis
   b. hordeolum
   c. hyperopia
   d. strabismus

7. In this condition there is destruction of the fovea centralis:
   a. macular degeneration
   b. detached retina
   c. glaucoma
   d. cataract

8. This is an infection that occurs in the middle ear cavity:
   a. otitis media
   b. otitis externa
   c. ototoxic hearing loss
   d. retrocochlear disease

9. The hearing loss that can be due to a lesion on the cochlea is:
   a. conductive
   b. sensorineural
   c. ototoxic
   d. transmission

10. This condition is also known as perceptive deafness:
    a. conductive
    b. sensorineural
    c. otitis media
    d. transmission

# UNIT I QUIZ ANSWERS

## Integumentary System

### Anatomy and Terminology Quiz

| | |
|---|---|
| 1. c | 6. c |
| 2. d | 7. d |
| 3. a | 8. b |
| 4. b | 9. c |
| 5. d | 10. c |

### Pathophysiology Quiz

| | |
|---|---|
| 1. c | 6. c |
| 2. c | 7. d |
| 3. a | 8. b |
| 4. d | 9. d |
| 5. b | 10. a |

## Musculoskeletal System

### Anatomy and Terminology Quiz

| | |
|---|---|
| 1. b | 6. d |
| 2. c | 7. b |
| 3. a | 8. d |
| 4. c | 9. a |
| 5. a | 10. c |

### Pathophysiology Quiz

| | |
|---|---|
| 1. d | 6. d |
| 2. c | 7. a |
| 3. b | 8. c |
| 4. a | 9. b |
| 5. d | 10. d |

### Respiratory System

#### Anatomy and Terminology Quiz

| | |
|---|---|
| 1. b | 6. c |
| 2. d | 7. c |
| 3. c | 8. b |
| 4. a | 9. d |
| 5. a | 10. d |

#### Pathophysiology Quiz

| | |
|---|---|
| 1. b | 6. a |
| 2. a | 7. c |
| 3. d | 8. b |
| 4. d | 9. a |
| 5. d | 10. c |

### Cardiovascular System

#### Anatomy and Terminology Quiz

| | |
|---|---|
| 1. d | 6. b |
| 2. a | 7. d |
| 3. c | 8. a |
| 4. a | 9. d |
| 5. d | 10. d |

#### Pathophysiology Quiz

| | |
|---|---|
| 1. b | 6. a |
| 2. c | 7. c |
| 3. c | 8. c |
| 4. c | 9. a |
| 5. d | 10. d |

## Female Genital System and Pregnancy

### Anatomy and Terminology Quiz

| | |
|---|---|
| 1. d | 6. a |
| 2. a | 7. b |
| 3. a | 8. b |
| 4. b | 9. c |
| 5. c | 10. d |

### Pathophysiology Quiz

| | |
|---|---|
| 1. b | 6. a |
| 2. d | 7. a |
| 3. a | 8. c |
| 4. c | 9. b |
| 5. b | 10. c |

## Male Genital System

### Anatomy and Terminology Quiz

| | |
|---|---|
| 1. c | 6. a |
| 2. a | 7. a |
| 3. d | 8. d |
| 4. b | 9. d |
| 5. a | 10. b |

### Pathophysiology Quiz

| | |
|---|---|
| 1. a | 6. b |
| 2. b | 7. d |
| 3. d | 8. b |
| 4. a | 9. a |
| 5. c | 10. b |

## Urinary System

### Anatomy and Terminology Quiz

| | |
|---|---|
| 1. c | 6. d |
| 2. d | 7. c |
| 3. a | 8. b |
| 4. c | 9. d |
| 5. b | 10. a |

### Pathophysiology Quiz

| | |
|---|---|
| 1. c | 6. c |
| 2. d | 7. a or c |
| 3. d | 8. c |
| 4. c | 9. b |
| 5. b | 10. c |

## Digestive System

### Anatomy and Terminology Quiz

| | |
|---|---|
| 1. b | 6. b |
| 2. d | 7. a |
| 3. d | 8. c |
| 4. b | 9. a |
| 5. c | 10. b |

### Pathophysiology Quiz

| | |
|---|---|
| 1. c | 6. c |
| 2. a | 7. a |
| 3. d | 8. c |
| 4. b | 9. a |
| 5. a | 10. a |

## Mediastinum and Diaphragm

### Anatomy and Terminology Quiz

| | |
|---|---|
| 1. a | 6. b |
| 2. b | 7. a |
| 3. d | 8. b |
| 4. c | 9. a |
| 5. c | 10. d |

## Hemic and Lymphatic System

### Anatomy and Terminology Quiz

| | |
|---|---|
| 1. b | 6. c |
| 2. d | 7. a |
| 3. a | 8. d |
| 4. d | 9. b |
| 5. c | 10. d |

### Pathophysiology Quiz

| | |
|---|---|
| 1. c | 6. b |
| 2. a | 7. a |
| 3. b | 8. a |
| 4. d | 9. c |
| 5. b | 10. b |

## Endocrine System

### Anatomy and Terminology Quiz

| | |
|---|---|
| 1. c | 6. a |
| 2. d | 7. d |
| 3. b | 8. a |
| 4. a | 9. b |
| 5. d | 10. d |

### Pathophysiology Quiz

| | |
|---|---|
| 1. a | 6. b |
| 2. b | 7. a |
| 3. c | 8. d |
| 4. a | 9. a |
| 5. d | 10. c |

### Nervous System

#### Anatomy and Terminology Quiz

| | |
|---|---|
| 1. b | 6. c |
| 2. a | 7. a |
| 3. a | 8. d |
| 4. b | 9. b |
| 5. b | 10. a |

#### Pathophysiology Quiz

| | |
|---|---|
| 1. a | 6. b |
| 2. c | 7. a |
| 3. b | 8. b |
| 4. d | 9. b |
| 5. a | 10. c |

## Senses

#### Anatomy and Terminology Quiz

| | |
|---|---|
| 1. d | 6. b |
| 2. d | 7. c |
| 3. a | 8. b |
| 4. a | 9. d |
| 5. a | 10. a |

#### Pathophysiology Quiz

| | |
|---|---|
| 1. d | 6. a |
| 2. b | 7. a |
| 3. c | 8. a |
| 4. a | 9. b |
| 5. b | 10. b |

# Reimbursement Issues

Make sure to check
**⊖volve**
learning system
**for the latest
content updates**

## REIMBURSEMENT ISSUES

### Your Responsibility

Ensure accurate coding based upon services provided and documented

Obtain correct reimbursement for services rendered

Recognize upcoding (maximizing) or downcoding is never appropriate

Stay abreast of current and changing

- Reimbursement policies
- Coding guidelines

**H**ealth **I**nsurance **P**ortability and **A**ccountability **A**ct of 1996 (HIPAA)

- HIPAA changes are based on various resources such as
  - Centers for Medicare and Medicaid Policy Manuals
  - National Correct Coding Guidelines

### Population Changing = Reimbursement Change

In 2010, the Administration on Aging (AOA) of Department of Health and Human Services published a population survey

- In 1900 persons 65 and older were only 4.1% of population in United States
- In 2010 that same group had grown to 13%
- By 2050, elderly will be over 20% of the population

Medicare primarily for elderly

### Medicare

### Getting Bigger All the Time!

- In 2010, 21 percent of federal spending went to Medicare and Medicaid; by 2020 it's expected to reach 31 percent
- By 2018, national health spending expected to reach $4.4 trillion

Health care will continue to expand to meet enormous future demands

- Job security for coders!

### Those Covered

Originally established for those 65 and older, and implemented in 1966

Later disabled and permanent renal disease (end-stage renal disease or transplant) added in 1972

Persons covered are called "beneficiaries"

### Basic Structure

Medicare program established in 1965

**Part A:** Hospital and Institutional Care Coverage

- This is the part that most inpatient coders will work with

**Part B:** Supplemental—nonhospital

   *Example:* Physician services and medical equipment

- This is the part that most outpatient coders will work with

**Part C:** Medicare Advantage Organizations (MAO) plans—combines part A and B (added later)

Plans include

    Medicare Health Maintenance Organization (HMOs)

    Medicare Preferred Provider Organizations (PPO)

    Medicare Private Fee-for-Service (PPFS) plans

    Medicare Special Needs plans

    Medicare Medical Savings Accounts (MSAs) plans

**Part D:** Prescription Drug Plan (PDP) (added January 1, 2006)

Plans include

- Medicare Advantage Plans (MA-PD)
- Private prescription drug plans (PDPs)
- Premium paid by beneficiary

## Officiating Office

Department of Health and Human Services (DHHS) (http://www.dhhs.gov)

Delegated to Centers for Medicare and Medicaid Services (CMS) (formerly HCFA)

- CMS runs Medicare and Medicaid
- CMS delegates daily operation to Medicare Administrative Contractors (MACs)
- MACs are usually insurance companies
- The Medicare Prescription Drug Improvement and Modernization Act of 2003 allowed CMS to reduce the current 48 Fiscal Intermediaries to 19 Medicare Administrative Contractors (MACs); 15 Part A and B, and 4 DME
    - The final 19 MACs were replaced with 10 MACs in 2011

## Funding for Medicare

Social security taxes

Equal match from government

CMS sends money to MACs

MACs handle paperwork and pay claims

## Medicare Covers

**Medical necessity and frequency limitations**

Defined in

- LCDs (Local Coverage Determinations)
- NCDs (National Coverage Determinations)

**Beneficiary pays**

20% of Medicare-approved amount after deductible is met

Part A and B annual deductible

**Medicare pays**

Part A all covered costs except deductible

Part B 80% of Medicare-allowed amount of covered services after deductible is met

## Participating Providers

Signed Quality Improvement Organization (QIO) agreement with MACs to accept assignment on Medicare claims

Provider agrees to accept the Medicare Fee Schedule amount as payment in full

- Accepting assignment

Block 27 on CMS-1500 (Figure 2-1)

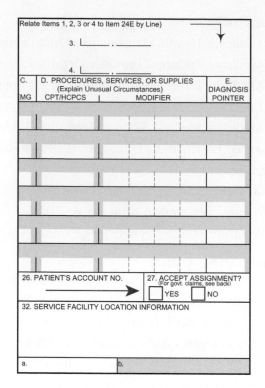

Figure **2-1** Block 27, Accept Assignment on the CMS-1500 (08-05) Health Insurance Claim Form. (Courtesy U.S. Department of Health and Human Services, Centers for Medicare and Medicaid Services.)

### National Provider Identification (NPI)
10-digit number assigned to all covered healthcare providers
- Designed to provide one unique identifier for all providers as part of HIPAA
- Eliminates the need for additional numbers by other carriers
- Block 17b on CMS-1500

### Good reasons to participate
- Significant decrease in reimbursement amount for nonparticipating providers

Participating providers receive approximately 5% more from Medicare than non-PAR providers

Check sent directly from MACs to QIO providers

Faster claims processing

Provider names listed in QIO directory
- Sent to all beneficiaries

## Part A, Hospital Inpatient
Hospitals submit charges electronically or, if an exempt facility, on UB-04 form

MS-DRG basis for payment for Medicare patients
- Using principal diagnosis or principal procedure

### Covered in-hospital expenses
Semiprivate room

Meals and special diets in hospital

All medically necessary services

**Noncovered in-hospital expenses**
Personal convenience items

> ***Example:*** Slippers, TV

Any service or procedure determined to be "not medically necessary"

**Types of covered expenses**
Rehabilitation

Skilled nursing

Some personal convenience items for long-term illness or disabilities

Home health visits

Hospice care

- Not automatically covered

- Must meet certain criteria

### Part B, Supplemental
Part B pays services and supplies not covered under Part A

Not automatic

Beneficiaries purchase

- Pay monthly premiums

**Types of items covered in part B**
Physician services

Outpatient hospital services

Ambulatory surgical services

Home health care

Medically necessary supplies and equipment

**Coding for Medicare Part B services**
Three coding systems used to report Part B

- CPT (procedures and service)

- HCPCS (drugs, supplies, equipment, and special services)

- ICD-9-CM (diagnosis codes)

## NATIONAL CORRECT CODING INITIATIVE (NCCI)

Developed by the Centers for Medicare and Medicaid Services to

- Promote national correct coding methods

- Control improper coding that result in inappropriate payment of Part B claims (physician) and hospital outpatient claims

- Complete list may be found at http://www.cms.gov/NationalCorrectCodInitEd/

### Unbundling

CMS defines unbundling as

- Billing multiple procedure codes for a group of procedures that are covered by a single comprehensive code

    ***Example:*** Dividing one service into parts and coding for each part separately, such as:

    - Reporting bilateral procedures unilaterally

        Reporting 31231, bilateral or unilateral diagnostic nasal endoscopy, with Modifier -50 (bilateral procedure), rather than correctly as 31231

    - Downcoding to use an additional code

        Reporting one of two lacerations of the same complexity and site with a lesser code to enable reporting two separate repairs

    - Separating the surgical approach from the major surgical service

        Coding separately for a thoracic approach during an anterior spine procedure

## *FEDERAL REGISTER*

Government publishes updates, revisions (changes), deletions in laws (Figure 2-2) (http://www.gpo.gov/fdsys/)

November and December issues contain outpatient facility updates

## QUALITY IMPROVEMENT ORGANIZATIONS (QIO)

Social Security Act (SSA) was amended to establish QIO

Purpose:

- To ensure quality of patient care
- Protect beneficiaries by addressing complaints
- Ensure Medicare pays only for reasonable and necessary services

### QIO Reviews (Formerly Referred to as the Medicare Utilization and Quality Control Peer Review Organization)

Admission

Discharge

Quality of care

MS-DRG (Medicare Severity Diagnosis-Related Groups) validation

Coverage

Procedure

### The Review

Begins with nurse who screens records based on QIO guidelines

Out-of-compliance cases forwarded to physician reviewer

Violations can result in severe sanctions

1. Issuing Office →
2. Subject →
3. Agency →
4. Action →
5. Summary →
6. Dates →
7. Further Information →
8. Supplementary Information →

**1366**   Federal Register / Vol. 76, No. 6 / Monday, January 10, 2011 / Rules and Regulations

**DEPARTMENT OF HEALTH AND HUMAN SERVICES**

**Centers for Medicare & Medicaid Services**

**42 CFR Part 410**

**[CMS–1503–F2]**

**RIN 0938–AP79**

**Medicare Program; Amendment to Payment Policies Under the Physician Fee Schedule and Other Revisions to Part B for CY 2011**

**AGENCY:** Centers for Medicare & Medicaid Services (CMS), HHS.

**ACTION:** Final rule.

**SUMMARY:** This amendment rescinds the addition and definition of voluntary advance care planning as a specified element of the annual wellness visit that was finalized in the "Medicare Program; Payment Policies Under the Physician Fee Schedule and Other Revisions to Part B for CY 2011" that appeared in the November 29, 2010 **Federal Register**.

**DATES:** *Effective Date:* This amendment is effective on January 10, 2011.

**FOR FURTHER INFORMATION CONTACT:** Dennis Wagoner, (410) 786–6841.

**SUPPLEMENTARY INFORMATION:**

**I. Background**

The final rule with comment period entitled "Medicare Program; Payment Policies Under the Physician Fee Schedule and Other Revisions to Part B for CY 2011" appeared in the November 29, 2010 **Federal Register** (75 FR 73170). The November 29, 2010 final rule with comment period included the agency's responses to comments made by the public in response to its Notice of Proposed Rulemaking (NPRM) published on July 13, 2010. In that NPRM, CMS sought to define the new annual wellness visit providing personalized prevention plan services as provided by the Patient Protection and Affordable Care Act (the Affordable Care Act or the Act). CMS proposed that the specified elements of the "first annual wellness visit" and the "subsequent annual wellness visit" be only those identified in the Act. In response, a number of commenters urged CMS to include voluntary advance care planning as an additional specified element of the annual wellness visit in the final rule. As described more fully below, we are rescinding this part of the final rule.

**II. Provisions of the Amendment**

In the July 13, 2010 **Federal Register** (75 FR 40039), we published the

proposed rule entitled "Medicare Program; Payment Policies Under the Physician Fee Schedule and Other Revisions to Part B for CY 2011." In response to this publication, we received comments from health care providers, and others urging us to add voluntary advance care planning as a specified element of the definitions of both the "first annual wellness visit" and the "subsequent annual wellness visit." The commenters stated that their recommendations were based upon a number of recent research studies, and the inclusion by the Medicare initial preventive physical examination (IPPE) provisions of a similar element in the existing IPPE benefit.

CMS agreed with the commenters that voluntary advance care planning should be added as a specified element in the definitions of both the "first annual wellness visit" and the "subsequent annual wellness visit" based on the evidence provided and the inclusion of a similar element in the IPPE benefit (also referred to as the Welcome to Medicare exam) since January 1, 2009, and incorporated it into the final rule.

It has since become apparent that we did not have an opportunity to consider prior to the issuance of the final rule the wide range of views on this subject held by a broad range of stakeholders (including members of Congress and those who were involved with this provision during the debate on the Affordable Care Act). Therefore, we are rescinding the provision of the final rule that includes voluntary advance care planning as a specified element of the annual wellness visits providing personalized prevention plan services, and returning to the policy that was proposed, which was limited to the elements specified in the Act. We are revising our regulation at § 410.15(a) to remove voluntary advance care planning as a specified element from the definitions of "first annual wellness visit providing personalized prevention plan services" and "subsequent annual wellness visit providing personalized prevention plan services" and to remove the definition of "voluntary advance care planning."

**III. Waiver of Proposed Rulemaking and Delay in Effective Date**

We ordinarily publish a notice of proposed rulemaking in the **Federal Register** and invite public comment on the proposed rule before the provisions of the rule take effect in accordance with section 553(b) of the Administrative Procedure Act (5 U.S.C. 553(b)). The Physician Fee Schedule notice of proposed rulemaking includes a reference to the legal authority under

which the rule is proposed, and the terms and substance of the proposed rule or a description of the subjects and issues involved. This notice and comment procedure can be waived, however, if an agency finds good cause that the procedure is impracticable, unnecessary, or contrary to the public interest, and incorporates a statement of the finding and its reasons for it in the rule. Section 553(d) of the APA ordinarily requires a 30-day delay in the effective date of final rules after the date of their publication. This 30-day delay in effective date can be waived, however, if an agency finds for good cause that the delay is impracticable, unnecessary, or contrary to the public interest, and the agency incorporates a statement of the findings and its reasons in the rule issued.

As noted earlier, a number of commenters suggested in response to the NPRM that we should include voluntary advance care planning as an additional specified element of the new annual wellness visit. While we believe that we acted within our authority in including voluntary advance care planning as an additional specified element of the new annual wellness visit in the final rule, it has become apparent that we did not have an opportunity to consider prior to the issuance of the final rule the wide range of views on this subject held by a broad range of stakeholders (including members of Congress and those who were involved with this provision during the debate on the Affordable Care Act). Because we believe it is in the public interest to specify contemporaneous with the January 1, 2011 effective date the scope of the new "annual wellness visit for personalized prevention plan services" benefit, we believe it would be contrary to the public interest to provide for a 30-day delay in effective date. Therefore, we find good cause, based on the public interest, both to waive the notice of proposed rulemaking and the 30-day delay in effective date, and to issue this amendment effective January 1, 2011.

**IV. Collection of Information Requirements**

This document does not impose information collection and recordkeeping requirements. Consequently, it need not be reviewed by the Office of Management and Budget under the authority of the Paperwork Reduction Act of 1995.

**V. Regulatory Impact Statement**

We have examined the impact of this amendment as required by Executive Order 12866 on Regulatory Planning

Figure **2-2** Example of page from the *Federal Register*. (From *Federal Register*, January 10, 2011, Vol. 76, No. 6, Rules and Regulations.)

# RESOURCE-BASED RELATIVE VALUE SCALE (RBRVS)

Physician payment reform implemented in 1992

Prior to reform, physicians were paid lowest of

- Physician's charge for service
- Physician's customary charge
- Prevailing charge in locality

## National Fee Schedule (NFS)

RBRVS payment method

Termed Medicare Fee Schedule (MFS)

Payment 80% of MFS, after patient deductible

Used for physicians and suppliers

## Relative Value Units (RVUs)

Assigns national unit values to each CPT code

Local adjustments made

- Work and skill required
- Overhead costs
- Malpractice costs

Often referred to as fee schedule

Annually, CMS updates RVU based on national and local factors

# MEDICARE FRAUD AND ABUSE

Program established by Medicare

- To decrease and eliminate fraud and abuse

Beneficiary signatures on file

- Service, charges submitted without need for patient signature

Presents opportunity for fraud

## Fraud

Intentional deception to benefit

   ***Example:*** Submitting for services not provided

Anyone who submits for Medicare services can be violator

- Physicians
- Hospitals
- Laboratories
- Billing services
- YOU

### Fraud Can Be

Billing for services not provided

Misrepresenting diagnosis or CPT/HCPCS codes

Kickbacks

Unbundling services

Falsifying medical necessity

Systematic waiver of copayment or deductible

## Office of the Inspector General (OIG)

Develops and publishes Work Plan annually

Outlines Medicare monitoring program

MACs monitor those areas identified in plan

## Complaints of Fraud or Abuse

Submitted orally or in writing to MACs or QIG

Allegations made by anyone against anyone

Allegations followed up by MACs or QIG
(www.oig.hhs.gov/reports-and-publications/workplan/index.asp)

## Abuse

Generally involves

- Impropriety
- Lack of medical necessity for services reported

Review takes place after claim submitted

- MACs do historical review of claims

## Kickbacks

Bribe or rebate for referring patient for any service covered by Medicare

Any personal-gain kickback

A felony

- $25,000 fine or
- 5 years in jail or
- Both

## Protect Yourself

Use your common sense

Submit only truthful and accurate claims

- Stay current with all coding changes

If you are unsure about charges, services, or procedures

- Check with physician or supervisor

## MANAGED HEALTH CARE

Network health care providers that offer health care services under one organization

Group hospitals, physicians, or other providers

Majority of people with health care coverage are covered by a Managed Health Care Organization (e.g., HMO, PPO, POS)

### Managed Care Organizations

Responsible for health care services to an enrolled group or person

Coordinate various health care services

Negotiate with providers and groups

### Preferred Provider Organization (PPO)

Providers form network to offer health care services as group

Enrollees who seek health care outside PPO pay more

### Point of Service (POS)

In-network or out-of-network providers may be used

Benefits are paid at a higher rate to in-network providers

Subscribers are not limited to providers, but to amount covered by plan

### Health Maintenance Organization (HMO)

Total package health care

Out-of-pocket expenses minimal

Assigned physician that acts as gatekeeper to refer patient outside organization

## REIMBURSEMENT TERMINOLOGY

| | |
|---|---|
| Advance Beneficiary Notice | ABN, notification in advance of services that Medicare probably will not pay for and the estimated cost to patient (Figure 2-3) (formerly WOL, waiver of liability) |
| Ancillary Service | A service that is supportive of care of a patient, such as laboratory services |
| Assignment | A legal agreement that allows the provider to receive direct payment from a payer and the provider to accept payment as payment in full for covered services |
| Attending Physician | The physician legally responsible for oversight of an inpatient's care (in residency programs, the teaching physician that monitors the resident's work) |
| Beneficiary | The person who benefits from insurance coverage; also known as subscriber, dependent, enrollee, member, or participant |

*(A)* Notifier(s):

*(B)* Patient Name: _____     *(C)* Identification Number: _____

## ADVANCE BENEFICIARY NOTICE OF NONCOVERAGE (ABN)

*NOTE:* If Medicare doesn't pay for *(D)*_____ below, you may have to pay.

Medicare does not pay for everything, even some care that you or your health care provider have good reason to think you need. We expect Medicare may not pay for the *(D)*_____ below.

| *(D)*_____ | *(E)* Reason Medicare May Not Pay: | *(F)* Estimated Cost: |
|---|---|---|
| | | |

**WHAT YOU NEED TO DO NOW:**

- Read this notice, so you can make an informed decision about your care.
- Ask us any questions that you may have after you finish reading.
- Choose an option below about whether to receive the *(D)*_____ listed above.
  **Note:** If you choose Option 1 or 2, we may help you to use any other insurance that you might have, but Medicare cannot require us to do this.

| *(G)* OPTIONS:          Check only one box.  We cannot choose a box for you. |
|---|

❑ **OPTION 1.** I want the *(D)*_____ listed above.  You may ask to be paid now, but I also want Medicare billed for an official decision on payment, which is sent to me on a Medicare Summary Notice (MSN). I understand that if Medicare doesn't pay, I am responsible for payment, but **I can appeal to Medicare** by following the directions on the MSN. If Medicare does pay, you will refund any payments I made to you, less co-pays or deductibles.

❑ **OPTION 2.** I want the *(D)*_____ listed above, but do not bill Medicare.  You may ask to be paid now as I am responsible for payment. **I cannot appeal if Medicare is not billed**.

❑ **OPTION 3.** I don't want the *(D)*_____ listed above. I understand with this choice I am **not responsible for payment,** and **I cannot appeal to see if Medicare would pay.**

*(H)* Additional Information:

**This notice gives our opinion, not an official Medicare decision.** If you have other questions on this notice or Medicare billing, call **1-800-MEDICARE** (1-800-633-4227/**TTY**: 1-877-486-2048).

Signing below means that you have received and understand this notice. You also receive a copy.

| *(I)* Signature: | *(J)* Date: |
|---|---|
| | |

According to the Paperwork Reduction Act of 1995, no persons are required to respond to a collection of information unless it displays a valid OMB control number. The valid OMB control number for this information collection is 0938-0566. The time required to complete this information collection is estimated to average 7 minutes per response, including the time to review instructions, search existing data resources, gather the data needed, and complete and review the information collection. If you have comments concerning the accuracy of the time estimate or suggestions for improving this form, please write to: CMS, 7500 Security Boulevard, Attn: PRA Reports Clearance Officer, Baltimore, Maryland 21244-1850.

Form CMS-R-131 (03/08)                                      Form Approved OMB No. 0938-0566

Figure **2-3** Centers for Medicare and Medicaid Services Advance Beneficiary Notice of Noncoverage (ABN).

| | |
|---|---|
| Birthday Rule | When both parents have insurance coverage, the parent with the birthday earlier in the year carries the primary coverage for a dependent |
| Certified Registered Nurse Anesthetist | CRNA, an individual with specialized training and certification in nursing and anesthesia |
| "Clean Claim" | A properly completed CMS-1500 form submitted to a payer with all data boxes containing current and accurate information and submitted within the timely filing period required by the insurer |
| Coinsurance | Cost-sharing of covered services |

| | |
|---|---|
| Compliance Plan | Written strategy developed by medical facilities to ensure appropriate, consistent documentation within the medical record and ensure compliance with third-party payer guidelines and the Office of the Inspector General (OIG) Workplan guidelines |
| Concurrent Care | More than one physician providing care to a patient at the same time |
| Coordination of Benefits | COB, management of multiple third-party payments to ensure overpayment does not occur |
| Co-payment | Cost-sharing between beneficiary and payer |
| Deductible | That portion of covered services paid by the beneficiary before third-party payment begins |
| Denial | Statement from a payer that coverage is denied |
| Documentation | Detailed chronology of facts and observations, procedures, services, and diagnoses relative to the patient's health |
| Durable Medical Equipment | DME, medically related equipment that is not disposable, such as wheelchairs, crutches, and vaporizers |
| Electronic Data Interchange | EDI, computerized submission of health care insurance information exchange |
| Employer Identification Number | EIN, Internal Revenue Service (IRS)–issued identification number used on tax documents |
| Encounter Form Superbill | Medical document that contains information regarding a patient visit for health care services, can serve as a billing and/or coding document |
| Explanation of Benefits | EOB or EOMB, written, detailed listing of medical service payments by third-party payer to inform beneficiary and provider of payment |
| Fee Schedule | List of established payment for medical services arranged by CPT and HCPCS codes |
| Follow-up Days | FUD, established by third-party payers and listing the number of days after a procedure for which a provider must provide services to a patient for no fee. Also known as *global days*, *global package*, and *global period* |
| Group Provider Number | GPN, a numeric designation for a group of providers that is used instead of the individual provider number |
| HMO | Health Maintenance Organization |
| Invalid Claim | Claim that is missing necessary information and cannot be processed or paid |
| Medical Record | Documentation about the health care of a patient to include diagnoses, services, and procedures rendered |
| Noncovered Services | Any service not included by a third-party payer in the list of services for which payment is made |

| | |
|---|---|
| National Provider Identifier | NPI, 10-digit number assigned to provider by CMS and National Plan and Provider Enumeration System (NPPES) and used for identification purposes when submitting services to third-party payers |
| Point of Service | POS, a plan in which either an in-network or out-of-network provider may be used with a higher rate paid to in-network providers |
| Preferred Provider Organization | PPO, providers form a network to offer health care services to a group |
| Prior Authorization | Also known as preauthorization, which is a requirement by the payer to receive written permission prior to patient services in order to be considered for payment by the payer |
| Provider Identification Number | PIN, a number assigned by a third-party payer to providers to be used for identification purposes when submitting claims |
| Reimbursement | Payment from a third-party payer for services rendered to a patient covered by the payer's health care plan |
| Rejection/Denial | A claim that did not pass the edits and is returned to the provider as rejected |
| Resource-Based Relative Value Scale | RBRVS, a list of physician services with assigned units of monetary value |
| State License Number | Identification number issued by a state to a physician who has been granted the right to practice in that state |
| UPIN | Unique provider identification number was replaced by the NPI |
| Usual, Customary, and Reasonable | UCR, used by some third-party payers to establish a payment rate for a service in an area with the usual (standard fee in area), customary (standard fee by the physician), and reasonable (as determined by payer) fee amounts |

## REIMBURSEMENT QUIZ

1. Any person who is identified as receiving life or medical benefits:
   a. primary
   b. beneficiary
   c. participant
   d. recipient

2. According to the Birthday Rule, if both parents are covered by an employer-provided health policy, the insurance policy that would be primary for reporting their child's health services is:
   a. parent with the birthday earlier in the year
   b. parent with the birthday later in the year
   c. either parent
   d. parent whose birthday is closer to the child's

3. Abbreviation for reusable medical equipment is:
   a. DRG
   b. CRN
   c. DME
   d. DIM

4. Management of multiple third-party payments to ensure that overpayment does not occur:
   a. PRO
   b. COB
   c. DME
   d. FUD

5. CMS delegates the daily operation of the Medicare program to:
   a. DHHS
   b. QIO
   c. RVU
   d. MACs

6. A QIO provider is one who:
   a. signs an agreement with the MACs
   b. submits charges directly to CMS
   c. receives 5% less than some other physicians
   d. can bill the patient the total remaining balance after payment from Medicare

7. This part of Medicare covers the inpatient portion of covered costs after the deductible has been paid:
   a. Part A
   b. Part B
   c. Part C
   d. Part D

8. This issue of the *Federal Register* contains outpatient facility changes for CMS programs for the coming year:
   a. October/November
   b. November/December
   c. December/October
   d. November/August

9. This is the RBRVS payment method:
   a. RAI
   b. OPPS
   c. APC
   d. NFS

10. Entity responsible for development of the plan that outlines monitoring of the Medicare program:
    a. MACs
    b. OIG
    c. DHSS
    d. HEW

## REIMBURSEMENT QUIZ ANSWERS

| | |
|---|---|
| 1. b | 6. a |
| 2. a | 7. a |
| 3. c | 8. b |
| 4. b | 9. d |
| 5. d | 10. b |

# Overview of CPT, ICD-9-CM, and HCPCS Coding

Make sure to check Evolve learning system for the latest content updates

# ■ INTRODUCTION TO MEDICAL CODING

Translates services/procedures/supplies/drugs into CPT/HCPCS codes

Translates diagnosis(es) into ICD-9-CM codes

## Three Levels of Service Codes

1. Level I CPT

2. Level II HCPCS, National Codes

3. Level III Local Codes—phased out with implementation of HIPAA code sets

## Diagnosis Codes, ICD-9-CM

ICD-9-CM, Volumes 1 and 2, *International Classification of Diseases,* 9th ed., Clinical Modification

Volume 1, Tabular

Volume 2, Index

Volume 3, Index and Tabular of Procedures (hospital version)

- Classification system
- Translates diagnosis(es) (dx) into standardized codes that explain why service was provided
- Very specific in nature
- May be up to five numeric or alphanumeric places
- Example: Diabetes becomes 250.XX

# ■ CPT

Developed by the AMA in 1966

Five-digit codes to report services provided to patients

Updated each November for use January 1

Resequencing was a 2010 new initiative for CPT

- Historically in numerical order
- Not the case for 43 codes
- Pound symbol (#) appears before the resequenced codes

  ***Example:*** In the 51725-51798 range, code 51797 follows 51729 (in numeric order). Code 51797 also appears in correct numeric order in the CPT, but next to the code a note states "Code is out of numerical sequence. See 51725-51798."

See Appendix N of the CPT for a complete list of the resequenced codes.

## Types of CPT Codes

- Medical
- Surgical
- Diagnostic services
- Anesthesia
- Evaluation and Management

## CPT Codes

Allow communication that is both effective and efficient

Inform third-party payers of services/procedures provided

Used as a basis of payment

## Incorrect Coding
Results in providers being paid inappropriately (either overpayment or underpayment)

## Outpatient Physician (Non-Hospital) Services
Reported on standardized insurance form

CMS-1500 = Health Insurance Claim Form (Figure 3-1)

## CPT Format

**Symbols.** Used to convey information

- Bullet = New code symbol

▲ Triangle = Revised Code

►◄ Right and left triangles = Beginning and ending of text change

+ Plus = Add-on code

  • Full list in Appendix D of CPT

⊘ Circle with line = Modifier -51 exempt code

  • Modifier -51 cannot be used with these codes

  • Full list in Appendix E of CPT

⊙ Bullseye = Codes that include moderate (conscious) sedation

  • Such as 45391, flexible colonoscopy

  • Full list in Appendix G of CPT

⚡ Lightning bolt symbol = Codes for which the FDA status pending

  • Full list in Appendix K of CPT

# Number sign = Resequenced CPT codes

  • Such as 21552, excision of tumor, 3 cm or greater, resequenced code in 2010

  • Full text in Appendix N

## CPT Sections
1. Evaluation & Management (E/M)

2. Anesthesia

3. Surgery

4. Radiology

5. Pathology and Laboratory

6. Medicine

> **TIP:** During your examination, the front section of the CPT (Introduction and Illustrations) is an excellent resource on the format, definitions of terms, medical terms, and instructions in the CPT. Review these well before the examination to familiarize yourself with where to find the information that is contained in the front section.
>
> Also, flag the different sections of the CPT for easy access during the examination—for example, the list of illustrations section, E/M Guidelines, Appendices, and other major sections of the manual.

## Categorized by
Sections

Subsections

**1500**

**HEALTH INSURANCE CLAIM FORM**

APPROVED BY NATIONAL UNIFORM CLAIM COMMITTEE 08/05

PICA

| 1. MEDICARE | MEDICAID | TRICARE CHAMPUS | CHAMPVA | GROUP HEALTH PLAN | FECA BLK LUNG | OTHER | 1a. INSURED'S I.D. NUMBER (For Program in Item 1) |
| --- | --- | --- | --- | --- | --- | --- | --- |
| (Medicare #) | (Medicaid #) | (Sponsor's SSN) | (Member ID#) | (SSN or ID) | (SSN) | (ID) | |

2. PATIENT'S NAME (Last Name, First Name, Middle Initial)

3. PATIENT'S BIRTH DATE MM DD YY   SEX  M  F

4. INSURED'S NAME (Last Name, First Name, Middle Initial)

5. PATIENT'S ADDRESS (No., Street)

6. PATIENT RELATIONSHIP TO INSURED   Self  Spouse  Child  Other

7. INSURED'S ADDRESS (No., Street)

CITY   STATE

8. PATIENT STATUS   Single  Married  Other

CITY   STATE

ZIP CODE   TELEPHONE (Include Area Code) ( )

Employed   Full-Time Student   Part-Time Student

ZIP CODE   TELEPHONE (Include Area Code) ( )

9. OTHER INSURED'S NAME (Last Name, First Name, Middle Initial)

10. IS PATIENT'S CONDITION RELATED TO:

11. INSURED'S POLICY GROUP OR FECA NUMBER

a. OTHER INSURED'S POLICY OR GROUP NUMBER

a. EMPLOYMENT? (Current or Previous)  YES  NO

a. INSURED'S DATE OF BIRTH MM DD YY   SEX  M  F

b. OTHER INSURED'S DATE OF BIRTH MM DD YY   SEX  M  F

b. AUTO ACCIDENT?  YES  NO   PLACE (State)

b. EMPLOYER'S NAME OR SCHOOL NAME

c. EMPLOYER'S NAME OR SCHOOL NAME

c. OTHER ACCIDENT?  YES  NO

c. INSURANCE PLAN NAME OR PROGRAM NAME

d. INSURANCE PLAN NAME OR PROGRAM NAME

10d. RESERVED FOR LOCAL USE

d. IS THERE ANOTHER HEALTH BENEFIT PLAN?  YES  NO   If yes, return to and complete item 9 a-d.

**READ BACK OF FORM BEFORE COMPLETING & SIGNING THIS FORM.**

12. PATIENT'S OR AUTHORIZED PERSON'S SIGNATURE I authorize the release of any medical or other information necessary to process this claim. I also request payment of government benefits either to myself or to the party who accepts assignment below.

SIGNED _____   DATE _____

13. INSURED'S OR AUTHORIZED PERSON'S SIGNATURE I authorize payment of medical benefits to the undersigned physician or supplier for services described below.

SIGNED _____

14. DATE OF CURRENT: MM DD YY   ILLNESS (First symptom) OR INJURY (Accident) OR PREGNANCY(LMP)

15. IF PATIENT HAS HAD SAME OR SIMILAR ILLNESS. GIVE FIRST DATE MM DD YY

16. DATES PATIENT UNABLE TO WORK IN CURRENT OCCUPATION FROM MM DD YY TO MM DD YY

17. NAME OF REFERRING PROVIDER OR OTHER SOURCE

17a.
17b.

18. HOSPITALIZATION DATES RELATED TO CURRENT SERVICES FROM MM DD YY TO MM DD YY

19. RESERVED FOR LOCAL USE

20. OUTSIDE LAB?  YES  NO   $ CHARGES

21. DIAGNOSIS OR NATURE OF ILLNESS OR INJURY (Relate Items 1, 2, 3 or 4 to Item 24E by Line)

1. ____ . ____   3. ____ . ____
2. ____ . ____   4. ____ . ____

22. MEDICAID RESUBMISSION CODE   ORIGINAL REF. NO.

23. PRIOR AUTHORIZATION NUMBER

| 24. A. DATE(S) OF SERVICE From MM DD YY   To MM DD YY | B. PLACE OF SERVICE | C. EMG | D. PROCEDURES, SERVICES, OR SUPPLIES (Explain Unusual Circumstances) CPT/HCPCS   MODIFIER | E. DIAGNOSIS POINTER | F. $ CHARGES | G. DAYS OR UNITS | H. EPSDT Family Plan | I. ID. QUAL. | J. RENDERING PROVIDER ID. # |
| --- | --- | --- | --- | --- | --- | --- | --- | --- | --- |
| 1 | | | | | | | | | |
| 2 | | | | | | | | | |
| 3 | | | | | | | | | |
| 4 | | | | | | | | | |
| 5 | | | | | | | | | |
| 6 | | | | | | | | | |

25. FEDERAL TAX I.D. NUMBER   SSN  EIN

26. PATIENT'S ACCOUNT NO.

27. ACCEPT ASSIGNMENT? (For govt. claims, see back)  YES  NO

28. TOTAL CHARGE $

29. AMOUNT PAID $

30. BALANCE DUE $

31. SIGNATURE OF PHYSICIAN OR SUPPLIER INCLUDING DEGREES OR CREDENTIALS (I certify that the statements on the reverse apply to this bill and are made a part thereof.)

SIGNED _____   DATE _____

32. SERVICE FACILITY LOCATION INFORMATION

a.   b.

33. BILLING PROVIDER INFO & PH # ( )

a.   b.

NUCC Instruction Manual available at: www.nucc.org

**PLEASE PRINT OR TYPE**

APPROVED OMB-0938-0999 FORM CMS-1500 (08-05)

CARRIER

PATIENT AND INSURED INFORMATION

PHYSICIAN OR SUPPLIER INFORMATION

Figure **3-1** The CMS-1500 (08-05) Health Insurance Claim Form was revised from the CMS-1500 (12-90) form to accommodate reporting of the National Provider Identifier (NPI) number mandated for May 2007. The CMS-1500 (08-05) version was mandated for use on February 1, 2007. For more information: http://www.cms.gov/transmittals/downloads/R899CP.pdf. (Courtesy U.S. Department of Health and Human Services, Centers for Medicare and Medicaid Services.)

Subheadings

Categories

    Anatomy

        Knee or Shoulder

    Procedure

        Incision or Excision

    Condition

        Fracture or Dislocation

    Description

        Cast or Strap

    Surgical approach

        Anterior Cranial Fossa or Middle Cranial Fossa

## Guidelines

Section-specific information begins each section

Provides instruction pertinent to entire section

## Notes

Located throughout CPT

Provides instruction pertinent to specific subsection

## Two Types of Code Descriptions

**1. Stand-alone:** Full description

   *Example:* 10080 Incision and drainage of pilonidal cyst; simple

**2. Indented:** Dependent on preceding stand-alone for meaning

   *Example:* 10080 Incision and drainage of pilonidal cyst; simple

        10081     complicated

## Semicolon

- Description preceding semicolon is the common part of the description and applies to any indented codes under it

- You must return to stand-alone for full description

   *Example:* 10081 Incision and drainage of pilonidal cyst; complicated

## Modifiers Add Information

### CPT Modifier

Appended to the end of the CPT/HCPCS code

Some modifiers are informational; others affect reimbursement

   *Example:* 43820 gastrojejunostomy

- -62 two primary surgeons

- 43820-62 two surgeons performed a gastrojejunostomy

- Only used if both surgeons submit same CPT code and both surgeons dictate a separate operative report

### Level II HCPCS Modifiers

"-AS" physician's assistant

"-F1" Left hand, second digit

All modifiers used on CPT or HCPCS codes

All HCPCS modifiers begin with a letter

Modifiers are placed in 24D field on CMS-1500 (see Figure 3-1)

## Unlisted Services

Codes usually end in "99" = "no specific code" in Category I or Category III

Used when a more specific code cannot be assigned

Written report must accompany claim form indicating

- Nature
- Extent
- Need
- Time
- Effort
- Equipment used

## Category II Codes—Supplemental Tracking Codes

Used for performance measurements

- Optional unless practice participating in Physician Quality Reporting System (PQRS), formerly the PQRI (Physician Quality Improvement Reporting Initiative)

These codes collect data concerning the quality of care and test results

Alphanumeric and end in the letter "F" (0005F)

Located after the Medicine section in CPT

## Category III Codes—New Technology

Temporary codes—may be included in this section up to 3 years

Identify emerging technology, services, and procedures

Located after Category II codes

Alphanumeric and end in the letter "T" (0055T)

- May or may not receive future Category I code status
- Category I codes (00100-99607)
- Approved by AMA and the Food and Drug Administration (FDA)
- Proven clinical effectiveness (efficacy)
- Category III has not been approved and has no proven clinical effectiveness (efficacy)
- Use Category III code instead of unlisted code if no Category I code appropriate
- Use unlisted code if no Category III code exists

## The Index

Used to locate service/procedure terms and codes

Speeds up code location

Uses dictionary format

- First entries and last entries on top of page
- Code display in index
  - Single code: 38115
  - Multiple codes: 26645, 26650
  - Range of codes: 22305-22325

## Location Methods

**Service/procedure:** Repair, excision

**Anatomic site:** Meniscus, knee

**Condition or disease:** Cleft lip, clot

**Synonym:** Toe and interphalangeal joint

**Eponym:** Jones procedure, Heller operation

**Abbreviation:** ECG, PEEP (positive end-expiratory pressure)

**"See" in index**

**Cross-reference terms:** "Look here for code"

**Index:** Stem, Brain: *See* Brainstem

## Appendices of CPT

Appendix A: Modifiers

Appendix B: Summary of Additions, Deletions, and Revisions

Appendix C: Clinical Examples (E/M Codes)

Appendix D: Summary of CPT Add-on Codes

Appendix E: Summary of CPT Codes Exempt from Modifier 51

Appendix F: Summary of CPT Codes Exempt from Modifier 63

Appendix G: Summary of CPT Codes That Include Moderate (Conscious) Sedation

Appendix H: Alphabetical Clinical Topics Listing (AKA—Alphabetical Listing)—moved to AMA website

Appendix I: Genetic Testing Code Modifiers

Appendix J: Electrodiagnostic Medicine Listing of Sensory, Motor, and Mixed Nerves

Appendix K: Product Pending FDA Approval

Appendix L: Vascular Families

Appendix M: Summary of Crosswalked Deleted CPT Codes

Appendix N: Summary of Resequenced CPT Codes

Review information in the CPT appendices prior to examination

# ■ EVALUATION AND MANAGEMENT (E/M) SECTION (99201-99499)

> **Your job is to code only from what is documented in medical record**
> **Optimize—never maximize**
> **Accurately report documented services**
> **Coding for services not provided is a punishable CRIME**

Subsections by type of service

Types of service

- Consultation

- Office Services

- Hospital Services, etc.

## Integral Factors When Selecting E/M Codes

### 1. Place of Service

Explains setting of service

- Office

- Emergency Department

- Nursing Home

### 2. Type of Service

Physicians provide many types of service

- Consultations (not reported for Medicare)

- Admissions

- Office visits

### 3. Patient Status

The four status types are

1. New patient

2. Established patient

3. Outpatient

4. Inpatient

**New patient**

Has not received any professional service in last 3 years from the same physician or another physician of the same specialty and in the same group

New patients are more labor-intensive for physician, medical staff, and clerical staff

**Established patient**

Has received professional services in last 3 years from the same physician or another physician of the same specialty in the same group

Medical record available with current, relevant information

**Outpatient**
One who has not been formally admitted to a health care facility

> *Example:* Patient receives services at clinic or same-day surgery center

**Inpatient**
One who has been formally admitted to a health care facility

> *Example:* Patient admitted to a hospital or nursing home

Physician dictates:

- Admission orders

- H&P (history and physical)

- Requests for consultations

## Levels of E/M Service Based on

Skill required to provide service

Time spent

Level of knowledge necessary to treat the patient

Effort required

Responsibility required/assumed

## E/M Levels Divided Based on

### Key Components (KC)

- History (Hx)

- Physical examination (PE)

- Medical decision making (MDM)

### Contributory Factors (CF)

- Counseling

- Coordination of care

- Nature of presenting problem

### Every Encounter Contains Varying Amount of KC and CF

More extensive component/factor

- Higher level of service

  - Less extensive component/factor

- Lower level of service

## KEY COMPONENTS

### Four Elements of a History

1. Chief Complaint (CC)

2. History of Present Illness (HPI)

3. Review of Systems (ROS)

4. Past, Family, or Social History (PFSH)

### Chief Complaint (CC)—Subjective

Reason for encounter or presenting problem: Patient's current complaint in patient's own words

Documented in medical record for each encounter

### History of Present Illness (HPI)—Subjective

Description of development of current illness, e.g., date of onset

Patient describes HPI

Provider must personally document

## PHYSICIAN AND PATIENT DIALOGUE

Development of a CC of Abdominal Pain (HPI):

"Started Thursday night and was mild. During the night, it got worse. Friday morning I went to work but had to leave because the pain got so bad."

**Location.** Specific source of pain

"Pain was in lower left-hand side, a little toward back."

**Quality.** Is pain sharp, intermittent, burning?

"Pain is really sharp and constant."

**Severity.** Is pain intense, moderate, mild?

"Pain is terrible, worst pain I have ever had." (intensity of pain or on a scale of 1 to 10)

**\*Duration.** How long has pain been present?

"Pain has been going on now for 3 days."

**Timing.** Is pain constant or does it come and go?

"Pain just continues. It just doesn't go away."

**Context.** When does it hurt most?

"Pain is just there, it doesn't matter what I am doing."

**Modifying factors.** Does anything make it better or worse?

"Nothing I do makes it any better or any worse."

**Associated signs and symptoms.** Does anything else feel different when pain is present?

"Yes, I have nausea when pain is worst."

---

*Duration not in CPT as HPI element

## Review of Systems (ROS)—Subjective

Questions posed to the patient to identify signs and symptoms that have been or are being experienced relating to the HPI

**Organ systems (OS),** e.g., respiratory system, cardiovascular system

**Extent of ROS depends on CC and patient status (new, established, inpatient, outpatient)**

### ROS Elements

Constitutional—General, Fever, Weight loss or gain

Eyes—Organ System (OS)

Ears, Nose, Mouth, Throat (OS)

Cardiovascular (OS)

Respiratory (OS)

Gastrointestinal (OS)

Genitourinary (OS)

Musculoskeletal (OS)

Integumentary (OS)

Neurological (OS)

Psychiatric (OS)

Endocrine (OS)

Hematologic/Lymphatic (OS)

Allergic/Immunologic (OS)

## Past, Family, and Social History (PFSH)

### Past

Contains relevant information about past illness, injury, or treatment, including

- Major illnesses/injuries
- Operations
- Hospitalizations
- Allergies
- Immunizations
- Dietary status
- Current medications

### Family History

Health status or cause of death of family members

- Parents
- Siblings
- Children

Family history items related to CC

- Hereditary diseases

**Social History**
Review of past and current activities

- Marital status

- Employment

- Occupational history

- Use of drugs/alcohol/tobacco

- Educational activities

- Sexual history

- Other relevant or contributory factors

### Four History Levels

1. Problem Focused (PF)

2. Expanded Problem Focused (EPF)

3. Detailed (D)

4. Comprehensive (C)

**Problem-Focused History**
CC

Brief HPI

No ROS

No PFSH

**Expanded Problem-Focused History**
CC

Brief HPI

Problem focused ROS

No PFSH

**Detailed History**
CC

Extended HPI

Problem pertinent ROS, extended to include a limited number of additional systems

Pertinent PFSH directly related to problem

**Comprehensive History**
CC

Extended HPI

Complete ROS directly related to CC, plus review of 10+ systems

Complete PFSH

Summary of elements required for each level of history (Figure 3-2)

**History Elements**

**Chief Complaint (CC)**
Reason for the encounter in the patient's words

**History of Present Illness (HPI)**
Location
Quality
Severity
Duration*
Timing
Context
Modifying factors
Associated signs and symptoms

**Review of Systems (ROS)**
Constitutional symptoms (fever, weight loss, etc.)
Ophthalmologic (eyes)
Otolaryngologic (ears, nose, mouth, throat)
Cardiovascular
Respiratory
Gastrointestinal
Genitourinary
Musculoskeletal
Integumentary (skin and/or breast)
Neurologic
Psychiatric
Endocrine
Hematologic/Lymphatic
Allergic/Immunologic

**Past, Family, and/or Social History (PFSH)**
Past major illnesses, operations, injuries, and treatments
Family medical history for heredity and risk
Social activities, both past and current

**Elements Required for Each Level of History**

| | | Problem Focused | Expanded Problem Focused | Detailed | Comprehensive |
|---|---|---|---|---|---|
| **History** | HPI | Brief 1-3 | Brief 1-3 | Extended 4+ | Extended 4+ |
| | ROS | None | Problem-pertinent 1 | Extended 2-9 | Complete 10+ |
| | PFSH | None | None | Pertinent 1 | Complete 2-3 |

*Duration is not listed in the CPT E/M Guidelines, but is listed in the DGs.

Figure **3-2** History elements required for each level of history.

## Four Examination Levels (Objective)

### Problem-Focused Examination (1995 Documentation Guidelines [DG])
Limited examination of affected body area or organ system

### Expanded Problem-Focused Examination (1995 DG)
Limited examination of affected body area or organ system

Other related body area(s) or organ system(s)

### Detailed Examination (1995 DG)
Extended examination of affected body area(s) and other symptomatic or related organ system(s)

**Examination Elements**

*General (OS)*
Constitutional

*Body Areas (BA)*
Head (including the face)
Neck
Chest (including breasts and axillae)
Abdomen
Genitalia, groin, buttocks
Back
Each extremity

*Organ System (OS)*
Ophthalmologic (eyes)
Otolaryngologic (ears, nose, mouth, throat)
Cardiovascular
Respiratory
Gastrointestinal
Genitourinary
Musculoskeletal
Integumentary
Neurologic
Psychiatric
Hematologic/Lymphatic/Immunologic

**Elements Required for Each Level of Examination**

| | Problem Focused | Expanded Problem Focused | Detailed | Comprehensive |
|---|---|---|---|---|
| **Examination** | Limited to affected BA or OS | Limited to affected BA or OS and other related OS(s) | Extended of affected BA(s) and other related OS(s) | General multi-system (OSs only) |

Figure **3-3** Examination elements required for each level of examination.

## Comprehensive Examination (1995 DG)

Eight or more organ systems

Summary of elements required for each level of examination (Figure 3-3)

## Medical Decision Making Complexity (MDM)

### Management Options

Based on number of possible diagnoses

Levels: Minimal, limited, multiple, or extensive

### Data Reviewed

Laboratory, radiology; any test/procedure results are documented along with the data reviewed and the identity of the reviewer in medical record

- "Hemoglobin within normal limits."

- "Chest x-ray, negative."

Old medical records (data) from others may be requested and reviewed

Levels: Minimal, limited, moderate, or extensive

## Risks

Risks of morbidity (poor outcome), complications, or mortality (death) associated with problem, diagnostic procedure

Other diseases or factors (co-morbidities)

- Diabetes

- Extreme age

Urgency relates to risks

- Myocardial infarction

- Ruptured appendix

Levels: Minimal, low, moderate, or high

See Figure 3-4, CMS Table of Risk

## Four Levels of MDM Complexity

### 1. Straightforward MDM

Number of diagnoses or management options: Minimal

Amount or complexity of data: Minimal/None

Risk of complications or death: Minimal

### 2. Low-complexity MDM

Number of diagnoses or management options: Limited

Amount or complexity of data: Limited

Risk of complications or death: Low

### 3. Moderate-Complexity MDM

Number of diagnoses or management options: Multiple

Amount or complexity of data: Moderate

Risk of complications or death: Moderate

### 4. High-Complexity MDM

Number of diagnoses or management options: Extensive

Amount or complexity of data: Extensive

Risk of complications or death: High

Summary of elements required for each level of MDM (Figure 3-5)

The diagnosis or management options, amount or complexity of data, and risk are totaled to arrive at the level of MDM

- Only two of three categories must meet or exceed each other in any level to assign the MDM

***Example:*** Moderate complexity for diagnosis or management options and moderate complexity of amount or complexity of data, but only a low risk would be assigned a moderate level MDM

***Example:*** Low risk of death, moderate diagnosis or management options, and high amount or complexity of data: Assign the moderate level of MDM

**TABLE OF RISK**
(Total = highest risk in any one category)

| Level of risk | Presenting problem(s) | Diagnostic procedure(s) ordered | Management options selected |
|---|---|---|---|
| *Minimal* | • One self-limited or minor problem, e.g., cold, insect bite, tinea corpus | • Laboratory tests requiring venipuncture<br>• Chest x-rays<br>• EKG/EEG<br>• Urinalysis<br>• Ultrasound, e.g., echocardiography<br>• KOH prep | • Rest<br>• Gargles<br>• Elastic bandages<br>• Superficial dressings |
| *Low* | • Two or more self-limited or minor problems<br>• One stable chronic illness, e.g., well controlled hypertension or non–insulin-dependent diabetes, cataract, BPH<br>• Acute uncomplicated illness or injury, e.g., cystitis, allergic rhinitis, simple sprain | • Physiologic tests not under stress, e.g., pulmonary function tests<br>• Non-cardiovascular imaging studies with contrast, e.g., barium enema<br>• Superficial needle biopsies<br>• Clinical laboratory tests requiring arterial puncture<br>• Skin biopsies | • Over-the-counter drugs<br>• Minor surgery with no identified risk factors<br>• Physical therapy<br>• IV fluids without additives |
| *Moderate* | • One or more chronic illnesses with mild exacerbation, progression, or side effects of treatment<br>• Two or more stable chronic illnesses<br>• Undiagnosed new problem with uncertain prognosis, e.g., lump in breast<br>• Acute illness with systemic symptoms, e.g., pyelonephritis, pneumonitis, colitis<br>• Acute complicated injury, e.g., head injury with brief loss of consciousness | • Physiologic tests under stress, e.g., cardiac stress test, fetal contraction stress test<br>• Diagnostic endoscopies with no identified risk factors<br>• Deep needle or incisional biopsy<br>• Cardiovascular imaging studies with contrast and no identified risk factors, e.g., arteriogram, cardiac catheterization<br>• Obtain fluid from body cavity, e.g., lumbar puncture, thoracentesis, culdocentesis | • Minor surgery with identified risk factors<br>• Elective major surgery (open, percutaneous, or endoscopic) with no identified risk factors<br>• Prescription drug management<br>• Therapeutic nuclear medicine<br>• IV fluids with additives<br>• Closed treatment of fracture or dislocation without manipulation |
| *High* | • One or more chronic illnesses with severe exacerbation, progression, or side effects of treatment<br>• Acute or chronic illnesses or injuries that pose a threat to life or bodily function, e.g., multiple trauma, acute MI, pulmonary embolus, severe respiratory distress, progressive severe rheumatoid arthritis<br>• Psychiatric illness with potential threat to self or others<br>• Peritonitis<br>• Acute renal failure<br>• An abrupt change in neurologic status, e.g., seizure, TIA, weakness, or sensory loss | • Cardiovascular imaging studies with contrast with identified risk factors<br>• Cardiac electrophysiological tests<br>• Diagnostic endoscopies with identified risk factors<br>• Discography | • Elective major surgery (open, percutaneous, or endoscopic) with identified risk factors<br>• Emergency major surgery (open, percutaneous or endoscopic)<br>• Parenteral controlled substances<br>• Drug therapy requiring intensive monitoring for toxicity<br>• Decision not to resuscitate or to de-escalate care because of poor prognosis |

Figure **3-4** Centers for Medicare and Medicaid Services (CMS) Table of Risk. (Courtesy U.S. Department of Health and Human Services, Centers for Medicare and Medicaid Services.)

**Medical Decision-Making Elements**

*Number of Diagnoses or Management Options*
Minimal
Limited
Multiple
Extensive

*Amount or Complexity of Data to Review*
Minimal/None
Limited
Moderate
Extensive

*Risk of Complications or Death If Condition Goes Untreated*
Minimal
Low
Moderate
High

**Elements Required for Each Level of Medical Decision Making**

|  | Straightforward | Low | Moderate | High |
|---|---|---|---|---|
| **Number of diagnoses or management options** | Minimal | Limited | Multiple | Extensive |
| **Amount or complexity of data to review** | Minimal/None | Limited | Moderate | Extensive |
| **Risk** | Minimal | Low | Moderate | High |

Figure **3-5** Elements required for each level of medical decision making.

## Contributory Factors

### Counseling

Provided to patient or family members (synopsis must be stated in medical record)

Discussion of diagnosis, test results, impressions, recommendations, prognosis, risks/benefits of treatment options or lack thereof, and risk factor reduction

### Coordination of Care
Work done on behalf of patient by physician to provide care

### Nature of Presenting Problem
Type of problem patient presents to physician with or reason for encounter

## Levels of Presenting Problem

### Minimal Presenting Problem
May not require a physician

*Example:* A dressing change or removal of an uncomplicated suture

### Self-limiting or Minor Presenting Problem
Self-limiting problems are minor and with a good outcome and no complications predicted

*Example:* Sore throat or a slightly irritated skin tag

### Low-Severity Presenting Problem

Without treatment, low risk

*Example:* A middle-aged, healthy male with an upper respiratory infection

### Moderate-Severity Presenting Problem

Without treatment, moderate risk

*Example:* An elderly male with bacterial pneumonia

### High-Severity Presenting Problem

Without treatment, high risk

*Example:* An elderly male in very poor health with diabetic ketoacidosis

### Time

Direct or face-to-face: Physician or NPP (nonphysician practitioner) and patient together

*Example:* Clinic visit or at bedside in hospital

Calculated for code assignment beginning and ending times documented in medical record

Unit/Floor: Time spent by physician on patient's floor or unit, also at patient's bedside

*Example:* Reviewing patient records or at chart desk and then with patient

---

Over 50% of the total time should include counseling and/or coordination of care, and the documentation must reflect the total time of the visit and the time spent counseling and/or in coordination of care to qualify to assign the code based on time.

---

### Use of E/M Code

Codes are grouped by type of service and place of service

- Consultation

- Office visit

- Hospital admission

Different codes are required for various levels of service assignment

New patient (99201-99205) services to new patient in office or other outpatient setting

### Selection of Level of E/M Services

For the following categories/subcategories, all three of the key components must meet or exceed the level stated in the code description:

- Office or Other Outpatient Services, New Patient

- Hospital Observation Services

- Initial Hospital Care

- Office Consultation

- Inpatient Consultation
- Emergency Department Services
- Initial Nursing Facility Care
- Other Nursing Facility Services
- Domiciliary, Rest Home (e.g., Boarding Home), or Custodial Care Services, New Patient
- Home Services, New Patient

For the following categories/subcategories, two of the three key components must meet or exceed the level stated in the code description:

- Office or Other Outpatient Services, Established Patient
- Subsequent Hospital Care
- Subsequent Nursing Facility Care
- Domiciliary, Rest Home (e.g., Boarding Home), Established Patient
- Home Services, Established Patient

### New Patient (99201-99205)
All new patients must be seen by physician

### Established Patient (99211-99215)
99211 may not require a physician's presence

No such code in New Patient category; all new patients are seen by physician

### Hospital Observation Status (99217-99220, 99224-99226, 99234-99236)
Not officially admitted to "inpatient status"

Patient not ill enough to admit but is too ill not to be monitored or discharged

Read notes at beginning of subsection

Observation services are not codes for "inpatient" services

Observation admission can be reported only for first day of service

*When patient admitted on observation status and discharged on same day:*

- Use code from 99234-99236 (Observation or Inpatient Care Services category including admission and discharge)

*Patient in hospital overnight for observation but less than 48 hours:*

- **First day:** 99218-99220 (Initial Observation Care)
- **Second day:** 99217 (Observation Care Discharge Services)

*If observation stay longer than 48 hours:*

- **First day:** 99218-99220 (Initial Observation Care)
- **Second day:** 99224-99226 (Subsequent Observation Care)
- **Third day:** 99217 (Observation Care Discharge Services)

### Initial Observation Care

- Beginning of observation care service
- Does not require a specific hospital unit; can be a regular bed on a floor or in emergency department (ED)
- Status specified as "observation"

E/M services immediately prior to admission bundled into observation service

*Example:* Office visit prior to observation, bundled into observation service

### Hospital Inpatient Services (99221-99239)
Officially admitted to a hospital setting

Total (all day and night)

Partial (all day and no night, all night and no day, or a variation)

• Time in and out must be specified in medical record

### Types of Physician Status
**Attending:** Primary or admitting physician

**Consultant:** Physician whose opinion and advice requested by attending physician

**Referring:** Physician requesting a consultation from another physician regarding a patient's health status

### Types of Care
Concurrent care given to patient by more than one physician each of different specialties

*Example:* Pulmonologist and cardiologist both treating patient for different conditions at same time

### Three Types of Hospital Inpatient Services
#### Initial Hospital Care (99221-99223)
First service includes admission

Initial paperwork

Initial treatment plans and orders

Used only once for each admission

• Only one admission by the attending or admitting physician billable per hospitalization

#### Subsequent Hospital Care (99231-99233)
After initial service

Physician reviews patient's progress using documentation, information received from nursing staff, examination of patient

• May be reported by multiple physicians of different specialties managing different conditions (concurrent care); only one per day per physician per specialty

#### Hospital Discharge Services (99238, 99239)
Final day of hospital stay when patient in hospital more than 1 day

Documentation indicates final patient status

Time based

• Total time

• Does not need to be continuous time

Beginning and ending time or total time spent must be documented to assign the extended discharge code or use lowest level code

## Final Status of Patient
**Summary of stay (Discharge)**
Condition (final examination)

Medications

Plan for return (follow-up care) to physician

How hospital stay progressed

Discharged destination (to home, nursing facility, etc.)

Only attending physician can use discharge code (only one discharge per admission)

Code based on time spent in service

Beginning and ending time or total time spent must be documented to assign the extended discharge code or must use lowest level code

## Consultation Services (99241-99255)
One physician or appropriate source requests another physician's opinion or advice

Either inpatient or outpatient; outpatient consultations include those provided in ED

Outpatient consultations (99241-99245)

Inpatient consultations (99251-99255)

Effective January 1, 2010, CMS no longer recognizes CPT consultation codes (ranges 99241-99245, and 99251-99255) for inpatient facility and office/outpatient settings where consultation codes were previously billed for services in various settings.

Consultation services reported with

- New patient office/outpatient (99201-99205)

- Established patient office/outpatient (99212-99215)

- Initial hospital codes (99221-99223)

## Third-Party-Payer Consultations
Request consult for

- Past medical treatment

- Current condition

- Payers may request prior to approving procedure

- Report services with -32, mandated services

## Emergency Department Services (99281-99288)
No distinction between new and established patients

Must be open 24 hours a day to qualify as ED (ER)

ED services often require additional codes from Critical Care Services

- Typically billed by ED physicians

Other Emergency Services (99288)

## Critical Care Services (99291, 99292)
*Example:* Vital organ failure

Critical care services are provided to patients over 71 months of age in life-threatening (critically ill/injured) situations

Time-based codes

- Total time under 30 minutes reported with appropriate E/M code (e.g., ED)

**Critical Care Services (99291, 99292)**
Time must be documented in medical record to select from this code range; does not need to be continuous

- Over 71 months of age

99291 and 99292 used to report total length of time a physician spends caring for critically ill patient

99291: 30-74 minutes

99292: Each additional 30 minutes

## Nursing Facility Services (99304-99318)
Non-hospital settings with professional staff

- Provide continuous health care services to patients who are not acutely ill

Formerly known as Skilled Nursing Facility (SNF), Intermediate Care Facility (ICF), and Long-Term Care Facility (LTCF)

Various levels of nursing facility services

**Initial Nursing Facility Assessment (99304-99306)**
Provided at time of patient's initial admission/readmission

**Subsequent Nursing Facility Care codes (99307-99310)**
99307 stable, recovering, or improving

99308 not responding or minor complication

99309 significant complication or new problem

99310 significant new problem requiring immediate physician attention

**Nursing Facility Discharge Services (99315, 99316)**
For final discharge service

Time-based

- Total time, does not need to be continuous

Other Nursing Facility Services (99318)

Annual Nursing Facility Assessment

## Domiciliary, Rest Home, or Custodial Care Services (99324-99337)
Health care services are not available on site

Types of services provided are lodging, meals, supervision, personal care, leisure activities

Residents cannot live independently

Codes for either new or established patients

**Domiciliary, Rest Home, or Home Care Plan Oversight Services (99339, 99340)**
Read notes at beginning of subsection

Reports individual physician supervision of patient in home or domiciliary rest home

Services not face-to-face

Time-based

99339 15-29 minutes

99340 30 minutes or more

Reported once per 30-day period

## Home Services (99341-99350)
Care provided in patient's home

Services based on key components and contributory factors

Codes for new or established patients

## Prolonged Services (99354-99359)
Time codes for direct and non-direct contact

Report time beyond the usual E/M service

- Must be documented in medical record

Codes for first 30-74 minutes and each additional 30 minutes thereafter

If less than 30 minutes, do not report service as prolonged

## Physician Standby Services (99360)
Physician not caring for other patient(s) to use these codes

Physician standing by only for that patient, if needed

Standby requested by another physician

- Must be documented in medical record

Report in 30-minute increments

Less than 30 minutes—do not report

Can report for subsequent 30 minutes only if a full 30 minutes

Carriers have strict policies regarding reimbursement for this service

### Case Management Services (99363-99368)
Anticoagulant Management Services, 99363 and 99364

- Anticoagulants such as warfarin
  - Thins the blood
- By physician or another qualified health care professional
- Provided in an outpatient setting
  - 60 days or more
  - 60 days or less is not reported

### Medical Team Conferences (99366-99368)
Codes for with or without face-to-face patient/family contact

- Minimum of 3 health care professionals, different specialties/disciplines participate in team
- Each member must have performed face-to-face evaluation in past 60 days
- Documentation must reflect member's contribution of information and treatment recommendation
- Not reported for organization or facility contracted services

Time-based

Begins and ends at start and conclusion of review

### Care Plan Oversight Services (99374-99380)
Used to report physician supervision of patient care in home health agency, hospice, domiciliary, or equivalent environment

Patient not present

Codes are time-based

- 15-29 minutes

- 30 minutes or more

- Must be documented in medical record

Reported once for each 30-day period

### Preventive Medicine Services (99381-99429)
Used to report services when patient is not currently ill

*Example:* Annual checkup

Codes divided by new or established and age

If significant problem is encountered during preventive examination

- E/M code also reported, append modifier -25

### Counseling Risk Factor Reduction and Behavior Change Intervention (99401-99429)
Patient is seen specifically to promote health and/or wellness

*Example:* Diet, exercise program

Patient without symptoms or an established diagnosis to use these codes

Codes based on

- Time

- Individual or group

- Physician review of assessment data

### Non-Face-to-Face Physician Services (99441-99444)
Physician E/M services using telephone/Internet

- 99441-99443 telephone E/M services

  Established patient, family member of the patient, or a guardian

- 99444 online E/M services

  Established patient, family member of the patient, or a guardian

### Special E/M Services (99450-99456)
- 99450 is reported for services provided for insurance or disability assessments

Involves no treatment; any treatment provided would be coded separately

99455-99456 reports work related or medical disability evaluation

Codes divided

- 99455: Assessment by treating physician
- 99456: Assessment by nontreating physician

## Newborn Care (99460-99465)

Initial and subsequent care in/other than hospital or birthing center

For normal newborn infant

Per day, for E/M services

99463, initial hospital/birthing center when admission and discharge is same day

### Delivery/Birthing Room Attendance and Resucitation Services (99464-99465)

99464, attendance at delivery

Documented request by attending in medical record

Provides initial stabilization

99465, resuscitation and ventilation

### Inpatient Neonatal Intensive Care Services and Pediatric and Neonatal Critical Care Services Subsection (99466-99480)

Pediatric Critical Care Patient Transport

99466, 99467

First 30-74 minutes

Each additional 30 minutes

Reports interfacility transport

Face-to-face service

Critically ill or injured patient

24 months or younger

### Inpatient Neonatal and Pediatric Critical Care

99468-99476

Divided by

Initial day

Subsequent day

Divided by age

Neonatal (Age 28 days or younger)

Pediatric (29 days-24 months)

Pediatric (2-5 years)

### Initial and Continuing Intensive Care Services

99477-99480

Hospital Care

99477 for neonate 28 days of age or younger

99478-99480 divided by birth weight

very low birth weight (VLBW) ≤1500 grams (≤3.3 pounds)

low birth weight (LBW) 1500-2500 grams (3.3-5.5 pounds)

normal birth weight 2501-5000 grams (5.51-11.01 pounds)

Subdivided on day

Initial

Subsequent

## Other Evaluation and Management Services (99499)

- 99499 reports unlisted E/M services

  Accompanied by a special report

# ■ ANESTHESIA SECTION (00100-01999)

## Anesthesiologist

Doctor of medicine specializing in anesthesia

Usually outside practices, e.g., Anesthesia Associates, Inc., or Pain Clinic, Ltd.

Professional services reported separately

## CRNA

Certified Registered Nurse Anesthetist

## Uses of Anesthesia

Manage unconscious patients, life functions, and resuscitation

## Analgesia

Relieve pain

## Some Methods of Anesthesia

**Endotracheal:** Through mouth (general anesthesia)

**Local:** Application to area (injection or topical)

**Epidural:** Between vertebral spaces—injection into epidural space

**Regional:** Field or nerve block

**MAC:** Monitored anesthesia care (service provided by an anesthesiologist or CRNA)

  Patient is monitored, and if necessary, sedation (including general anesthesia) may be provided

**Spinal:** Anesthesia applied to the spinal cord area, outside the dura mater

**General:** State of unconsciousness accomplished through drug administration or by inhalation

## Patient-Controlled Analgesia (PCA)

Patient self-administers drug

Used to relieve chronic pain or temporarily for severe pain following surgery

## Moderate (Conscious) Sedation

Codes in Medicine Section of CPT

99143-99145 used when surgeon administers sedation

99148-99150 used when another physician administers sedation

• No anesthesia personnel are present

Decreased level of consciousness

Not reported by physician if provided in nonfacility setting

## Anesthesia Formula

(B + T + M) × conversion factor = Anesthesia payment

### B is for Base Units

Published in *Relative Value Guide (RVG)* by American Society of Anesthesiologists

National unit values for anesthesia services based on complexity of service

### T Is for Time

Patient record indicates time, e.g., 60 minutes

Usually, 15 minutes = 1 unit

   *Example:* 60 minutes = 4 units

Some payers may indicate 1 unit = 1 minute

Begins: Anesthesiologist begins to prepare patient for induction—preoperative

Continues throughout procedure—intraoperative

Ends: Patient no longer under care of anesthesiologist—postoperative

### M Is for Modifying Unit

Additional units based on physical status of patient (see modifiers that follow)

### Physical Status Modifiers, P1-P6

Located in Anesthesia Guidelines

Not reported to Medicare

Help to show complexity of service

- P1 Normal healthy
- P2 Mild systemic disease
- P3 Severe systemic disease
- P4 Severe systemic disease is constant threat to life
- P5 Not expected to survive without the operation
- P6 Clinically brain dead

### Qualifying Circumstances Codes (99100-99140)

Anesthesia services provided under difficult circumstances

Located in both Anesthesia Guidelines and Medicine section

Listed in addition to primary anesthesia code

More than one may be reported

### Summing Up Formula

Base units (from *RVG*) based on CPT codes

Time units (usually 15 min is a unit)

- Total time ÷ 15 = time units

Modifiers [Qualifying Circumstances (99100-99140) and/or Physical Status (P1-P6)]

### Conversion Factors

CMS anesthesia conversion factors

Sum of money allocated by payer, per unit for payment of anesthesia services

### Anesthesia for Multiple Surgical Procedures

Once anesthetized, length of time, not number of procedures performed during session

Report highest relative value guide (RVG) valued CPT code

   *Example:* Two procedures during same session

- One, 10 base units; the other, 5 base units
- Report only 10 base units and combined time for all procedures

## Anesthesia Modifiers

Anesthesia code reported twice

- Once for anesthesiologist
- Once for CRNA

Each reports service on separate claim form

- One claim anesthesiologist's service
- One claim CRNA's service

Anesthesia modifiers report supervision/direction circumstances

- AA, anesthesia services performed personally by anesthesiologist
- AD, medical supervision >4 concurrent procedures
- QK, medical direction of 2-4 concurrent procedures
- QX, CRNA service with medical direction
- QY, medical direction of 1 CRNA
- QZ, CRNA service without medical

Anesthesia modifier always precedes the physical status modifier

# ■ CPT/HCPCS LEVEL I MODIFIERS (-22 to -99)

Alters CPT or HCPCS code

Full list, CPT, Appendix A

- Two separate lists
  - One for physician use
  - One for hospital outpatient use

**Modifier Functions**

Altered (i.e., increased or reduced service)

Bilateral

Multiple

Only portions of service (i.e., professional service only)

More than one surgeon

## -22 Increased Procedural Service

Indicates services significantly greater than usual

Accompanied by written report and supportive documentation

## -23 Unusual Anesthesia

Use of general anesthesia where local or regional is norm

> *Example:* Highly agitated senile patient

Used only with anesthesia codes

Written report with submission of modifier

## -24 Unrelated E/M Services by Same Physician During a Postoperative Period

Service not related to surgery

If E/M provided during postoperative global period, no payment considered without -24

## -25 Significant, Separately Identifiable E/M Service, by Same Physician on the Same Day of the Procedure or Other Service

Documentation must support service

> *Example:* Patient seen for sinus congestion, physician performs H&P, prescribes decongestant, notes and removes lesion on back

> Code: Procedure + E/M-25

## -26 Professional Component

Professional component (physician, -26)

Technical component (technician + equipment, -TC)

## -32 Mandated Service

Mandated by payer, workers' comp, or official body or court of law

Not request of patient, patient's family, or another physician

> **Example:** Workers' Compensation requests examination of person currently receiving disability benefits

## -33 Preventive Services

New in 2012 CPT

Patient Protection and Affordable Care Act (PPACA)

- Requires coverage without cost to patient

United States Preventive Services Task Force (USPSTF)

- Grades preventive services
- Example: Grade A: Substantial; Grade B: Moderate

## -47 Anesthesia by Surgeon

Surgeon administers regional or general anesthesia

Physician acts as both surgeon and anesthesiologist

Used only with Surgery codes

## -50 Bilateral Procedure

Organs that are bilateral

> **Example:** Procedure on kidneys

Caution: Some codes describe bilateral procedures

Typically not used on Integumentary System codes

## -51 Multiple Procedure—Three Types

Same procedure, different sites

Multiple operation(s), same operative session

Procedure performed multiple times

- List most resource-intense procedure first, then descending order of resource intensity
- Next, other procedure(s) + -51 (unless code is -51 exempt or add-on code)
  > Usual procedure payment: 1st 100%, 2nd 50%, 3rd 25%-50%, depending on payer

## -52 Reduced Services

Service reduced or not performed to the extent described in code description

There is no other code that accurately reflects the service actually provided

Physician directed reduction

Documentation substantiates reduction

Not to be used for patient unable to pay

Submit regular charge amount, payer will adjust

## -53 Discontinued Procedure

Surgical/diagnostic procedures

Procedure started then stopped due to patient's condition

Does not apply to presurgical discontinuance

Submit regular charge, payer will adjust

DO NOT USE -53

- When patient cancels scheduled procedure
- With E/M codes
- With time-based code

## -54 Surgical Care Only

Physician provides only procedure (intraoperative); other physician performs preoperative and postoperative service

Documented patient transfer must be in record

Some payers require copy of transfer order

## -55 Postoperative Management Only

Physician provides only the care after hospital discharge; report surgical code + modifier -55

If transferred while patient hospitalized, report postoperative management with subsequent hospital codes 99231-99233

Documentation of transfer in medical record

## -56 Preoperative Management Only

Physician provided only preoperative care; report surgical code + modifier -56

Not acceptable for Medicare

Usual reimbursement for portions, surgical package

- 10% preoperative
- 70% intraoperative
- 20% postoperative

Each payer determines reimbursement for portions

## -57 Decision for Surgery Used With

E/M, 99201-99499

Medicine, 92002, 92004, 92012 and 92014 ophthalmologic services

Medicare: Only for preoperative period of major surgery (day before or day of)

## -58 Staged/Related Procedure or Service by Same Physician During Postoperative Period

Subsequent procedure planned at time of initial surgery

- During postoperative period of previous surgery in series

  ***Example:*** Multiple skin grafts completed in several sessions

- Do not use when code describes total sessions

  ***Example:*** 67208 destruction of lesion of retina, one or more sessions

- More extensive than original procedure or

- For therapy following diagnostic procedure (e.g., breast biopsy and subsequent mastectomy)

## -59 Distinct Procedural Service

Used to report non-E/M services not normally reported together

Different session or encounter

Different procedure

Different site

Separate incision, excision, lesion, injury

***Example:*** Physician removes several lesions from patient's leg; also notes a suspicious lesion on torso and biopsies it

- Excision code for lesion removal + biopsy code for torso lesion with -59

- Indicates biopsy as distinct procedure, not part of lesion removal

## -62 Two Surgeons

Both function as cosurgeons (equals)

Usually of different specialties

Each reports same code + -62

Each dictates operative/procedure note for their portion

Total reimbursement = 125%; each physician = $62\frac{1}{2}\%$

## -63 Procedure Performed on Infants Less Than 4 kg

Kilogram = 2.2 pounds (4 kg = 8.8 lb)

Small size increases complexity

Use with all Surgery section codes except Integumentary System or directed otherwise (63700)

## -66 Surgical Team

Team: Several physicians with various specialties plus technicians and other support personnel

Very complex procedures

Payers may increase payment up to 50%

- Each physician's service must be documented in the medical record

## -76 Repeat Procedure/Service by Same Physician or Other Qualified Health Care Professional

Note: "Same Physician"

Used to indicate necessary service

> *Example:* X-rays before and after fracture repair

## -77 Repeat Procedure/Service by Another Physician or Other Qualified Health Care Professional

Note: "Another Physician"

Performed by one physician, repeated by another physician

Submitted with written report to establish medical necessity and identity of performing physician

## -78 Unplanned Return to Operating/Procedure Room by the Same Physician or Other Qualified Health Care Professional Following Initial Procedure for a Related Procedure During Postoperative Period

For complication of first procedure

> *Example:* Patient had outpatient procedure in morning; was returned to operating room in afternoon with severe hemorrhage

Indicates not typographical error

- Medical record must specifically document need for service provided

## -79 Unrelated Procedure or Service by Same Physician During Postoperative Period

> *Example:* Several days after discharge for procedure, patient returns for unrelated problem

Diagnosis code would also be different

## -80 Assistant Surgeon

Reimbursed at 15% to 30%

Payers identify procedures for which they reimburse assistant at surgery

## -81 Minimum Assistant Surgeon

Services at a level less than that described in -80

Reimbursed at 10% if services reported with the modifier are recognized by payer

## -82 Assistant Surgeon

Teaching hospitals

- Have residents who assist as part of education

- Must demonstrate no qualified resident available to use -82
  - Unavailability must be documented in written report

## -90 Reference (Outside) Laboratory

Physician has business relationship with outside lab

Physician pays lab

Physician bills payer for lab services

## -91 Repeat Clinical Diagnostic Laboratory Test

Repeat same laboratory tests on same day for multiple test results

- e.g., serial troponin levels for acute MI confirmation

Not tests rerun to confirm or negate original test results

Not assigned for malfunction of equipment, loss of specimen, or technician error

## -92 Alternative Laboratory Platform Testing

Used to report a laboratory test using portable instrument or kit

Usually single use

86701-86703 HIV testing

## -99 Multiple Modifiers

Used when service needs more than one modifier but payer allows for only one modifier with each code

The new CMS-1500 allows for multiple modifiers (Figure 3-6)

### HCPCS Level II Modifiers

### Examples of HCPCS Anatomical Modifiers

-LT  Left side

-RT  Right side

-E1  Upper left, eyelid

-E2  Lower left, eyelid

-E3  Upper right, eyelid

-E4  Lower right, eyelid

| 24. A. | DATE(S) OF SERVICE | | | | | B. PLACE OF SERVICE | C. EMG | D. PROCEDURES, SERVICES, OR SUPPLIES (Explain Unusual Circumstances) | |
|---|---|---|---|---|---|---|---|---|---|
| | From | | | To | | | | CPT/HCPCS | MODIFIER |
| | MM | DD | YY | MM | DD | YY | | | |
| 1 | | | | | | | | 19306 | ↗ |

Figure **3-6** CMS-1500 (08-05) allows for multiple placement of modifiers. (Courtesy U.S. Department of Health and Human Services, Centers for Medicare and Medicaid Services.)

-FA   Left hand, thumb

-F1   Left hand, second digit

-F2   Left hand, third digit

-F3   Left hand, fourth digit

-F4   Left hand, fifth digit

-F5   Right hand, thumb

-F6   Right hand, second digit

-F7   Right hand, third digit

-F8   Right hand, fourth digit

-F9   Right hand, fifth digit

-TA   Left foot, great toe

-T1   Left foot, second digit

-T2   Left foot, third digit

-T3   Left foot, fourth digit

-T4   Left foot, fifth digit

-T5   Right foot, great toe

-T6   Right foot, second digit

-T7   Right foot, third digit

-T8   Right foot, fourth digit

-T9   Right foot, fifth digit

-LC   Left circumflex coronary artery

-LD   Left anterior descending coronary artery

-RC   Right coronary artery

Anatomical modifiers are not used with skin procedures

> **Example:** Removal of skin tags, any area

Exception is with codes that indicate feet, hands, fingers, legs, arms, and eyelids

# ■ SURGERY SECTION (10021-69990)

Largest CPT Section

## Section Format

Divided by subspecialty, e.g., Integumentary, Cardiovascular

## Notes and Guidelines

Throughout section

Information varied and extensive

"Must" reading

Subsection notes apply to entire subsection

Figure **3-7** Parenthetical information in the CPT manual.

Subheading notes apply to entire subheading

Category notes apply to entire category

Parenthetical information (Figure 3-7)

## Unlisted Procedure Codes

Used only when more specific code not found in Category I or Category III

Written report accompanies submission

Each unlisted code service paid on case-by-case basis

## Separate Procedures

"(Separate procedure)" follows code description

Usually minor surgical procedure

Incidental to more major procedure:

- Breast biopsy before radical mastectomy would not be reported unless results of biopsy resulted in mastectomy, modifier -59 appended to biopsy code

- Appendectomy performed incidentally when other abdominal surgery is performed

Separate procedures reported when

- Only procedure performed

- With another procedure

  - On different site

  - Unrelated to major procedure

## Major Guideline of Surgical Packages

Usually include

- Preoperative (before, preop)

- E/M service subsequent to decision for surgery but prior to surgery date

- Intraoperative (during, intraop)

- Postoperative (after—also known as global period, postop)

  - Post-anesthesia recovery (PAR)

  - Follow-up office visits

- Local/topical anesthesia and digital block

To report these bundled services separately is "unbundling"

Remember to use modifiers during global period for unrelated E/M, return to OR, etc.

### Supplies

Supplies that are beyond those typically included in the procedure are reported separately

> ***Example:*** Report surgical tray with

- 99070 CPT, Medicine section
- A4550 HCPCS

### Special Report

Submitting an unlisted service or one that is unusual, variable, or new may require a special report, as listed in Guidelines

Demonstrates medical necessity/appropriateness of service

Contains pertinent information describing service in terms of

- Nature
- Extent
- Need for procedure
- Time
- Effort
- Equipment necessary

May also include complexity of symptoms, final diagnosis, physical findings, procedures, concurrent problems, and follow-up care

## GENERAL SUBSECTION (10021, 10022)

Fine needle aspirations with or without (w/wo) imaging guidance

Pathology 88172 and 88177 are for evaluation of aspirate

## INTEGUMENTARY SYSTEM SUBSECTION (10040-19499)

Often used in all specialties of medicine

Not just surgeons or dermatologists; wide range of physicians

Subheadings of Integumentary Subsection

- Skin, Subcutaneous, and Accessory Structures
- Nails
- Pilonidal Cyst
- Introduction
- Repair (Closure)
- Destruction
- Breast

## Skin, Subcutaneous and Accessory Structures (10040-11646)

### Incision and Drainage (10040-10180)

I&D of abscess, carbuncle, boil, cyst, infection, hematoma, pilonidal cyst

- Lancing (cutting of skin)

- Aspiration (removal by puncturing lesion with a needle and withdrawing fluid)

Gauze or tube may be inserted for continued drainage

Pilonidal cyst

- Also known as a pilonidal abscess

- May be incised and drained (10080, 10081) or excised (11770-11772)

### Excision—Debridement (11000-11047)

Dead tissue cut away and washed away with sterile saline

**11000, 11001** Eczematous or infected skin

**11004-11006** Debridement of infected area based on location and depth of necrotizing tissue (subcutaneous tissue, muscle, and fascia)

**+11008** Removal of prosthetic material or mesh from abdominal wall

**11010-11012** Foreign material with open fracture or dislocation

- Skin, subcutaneous tissue, muscle fascia, muscle, and bone

**11042-11044** Subcutaneous tissue, muscle, bone

- Debridement partial thickness based on 20 square centimeters or less

**11045-11047** Based on each additional 20 square centimeters

### Paring or Cutting (11055-11057)

Removal by scraping or peeling (e.g., removal of corn or callus)

Codes indicate number: 1, 2-4, 4+

### Biopsy (11100, 11101)

Skin, subcutaneous tissue, or mucous membrane biopsy

Not all of lesion removed

- All lesion removed = excision

Do not use modifier -51

Codes indicate number: 1 or each additional

Tissue removed during excision, shaving, etc., and submitted to pathology is NOT reported separately as a biopsy

- Rather, it is included in the code for the excision

### Skin Tag Removal (11200, 11201)

Benign lesions

Removed with scissors, blade, chemicals, electrosurgery, etc.

Do not use -51

- Codes indicate number: Up to and including 15 lesions and each additional 10 lesions or part thereof

### Shaving of Lesions (11300-11313)

Removed by transverse incision or sliced horizontally

Based on

- Size (e.g., 1.1-2.0 cm)
- Location (e.g., arm, hand, nose)

Does not require suture closure

- Report most extensive lesion first with no modifier, then least extensive lesions with modifier -51

### Benign/Malignant Lesions (11400-11646)

Codes divided: Benign or malignant

Physician assesses lesion as benign or malignant

Codes include local anesthesia and simple closure

Report each excised lesion separately

Lesion size

- Taken from physician's notes
- Includes greatest diameter plus narrowest margins of two sides (Figure 3-8)

  ***Example:*** A benign lesion measuring 0.5 cm at widest point is removed with 0.5-cm margin at narrowest point (each side, 0.5 + 0.5 = 1.0 cm). Reported as 1.5-cm lesion excision (11402)

  - Do not take size from pathology report—storage solution shrinks tissue
  - Margins (healthy tissue) are also taken for comparison with unhealthy tissue
  - Re-excisions following initial excision of malignant lesion coded as excision of malignant lesion

All excised tissue pathologically examined

Codes 11400-11646 report excision of lesion

Destroyed lesions have no pathology samples

  ***Example:*** Laser or chemical

Lesion closure

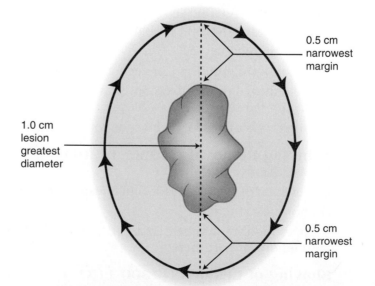

Figure **3-8** Calculating the size of a lesion.

- Simple or subcutaneous closure included in removal
- Reported separately
  - Layered or intermediate, 12031-12057 (Repair—Intermediate)
  - Complex, 13100-13153 (Repair—Complex)

## Nails (11719-11765)

Includes toes and fingers

Types of services

- Trimming, debridement, removal, biopsy, repair

## Pilonidal Cyst (11770-11772)

Codes divided by

- Simple
- Extensive
- Complicated

## Introduction (11900-11983)

Types of services

- Lesion injections (therapeutic or diagnostic), tattooing, tissue expansion, contraceptive insertion/removal, hormone implantation services, and insertion/removal of non-biodegradable drug delivery implant

## Repair (Closure) (12001-13160)

### Repair Factors in Wound Repair

As types of wounds vary, types of wound repair also vary

Length, complexity (simple, intermediate, complex), and site must be documented

- Length measured in centimeters
- Measured prior to closure

### Types of Wound Repair

**Simple.** Superficial, epidermis, dermis, or subcutaneous tissue

- One-layer closure
- Dermabond closure
- Medicare report Dermabond closure with G0168

**Intermediate.** Layered closure of deeper layers of subcutaneous tissue and superficial fascia with skin closure

- Single-layer closure can be coded as intermediate if extensive debridement required

**Complex.** Greater than layered; may include multiple layers of tissue and fascia or extensive debridement

> *Example:* Scar revision, complicated debridement, extensive undermining, stents, extensive retention sutures

### Included in Wound Repair Codes

Simple ligation of vessels in an open wound

Simple exploration of nerves, blood vessels, and exposed tendons

Normal debridement

- Additional codes for debridement can be used when
  - Gross contamination requires prolonged cleaning
  - Appreciable amounts of devitalized/contaminated tissue are removed to expose healthy tissue
  - Debridement is provided without immediate primary closure

### Grouping of Wound Repair
Add together lengths by
- **Complexity** of Wound
  - Simple, intermediate, complex
- **Location** of Wound
  - e.g., face, ears, eyelids, nose, lips

1 inch = 2.54 cm

> *Example:* **Same complexity, same codes description location:** Intermediate repairs of 2.9-cm laceration of leg and 1.1-cm laceration of buttocks. 2.9 + 1.1 = 4.0 cm (12032)

> *Example:* **Different complexity:** Intermediate repair of 2.9-cm laceration of leg and simple repair of 1.1-cm laceration of buttocks. 2.9-cm intermediate repair (12032) and 1.1-cm simple repair (12001)

> *Example:* **Same complexity, different code description locations:** Intermediate repair of 2.9-cm laceration of leg and intermediate repair of 1.1-cm laceration of nose. 2.9-cm intermediate repair of leg (12032) and 1.1-cm intermediate repair of nose (12051)

### Do Not Group Wound Repairs That Are
Different complexities

> *Example:* Simple repair and complex repair

Different locations as stated in the code description

> *Example:* Simple repairs of scalp (12001) and nose (12011)

## Adjacent Tissue Transfer, Flaps, and Grafts (14000-15776)

### Information Needed to Code Graft
Type of graft—adjacent, free, flap, etc.

Donor site (from)

Recipient site (to)

Any repair to donor site

Size of graft

### Adjacent Tissue Transfer/Rearrangement (14000-14350)
Includes lesion excision and/or repair (e.g., Z-plasty, W-plasty, V-plasty, Y-plasty, rotation flap, advancement flap)

Codes based on size and location of graft

Primary defect results from excision of lesion

Secondary defect results from formation of flap

To select code, add the size of the primary and secondary defects together

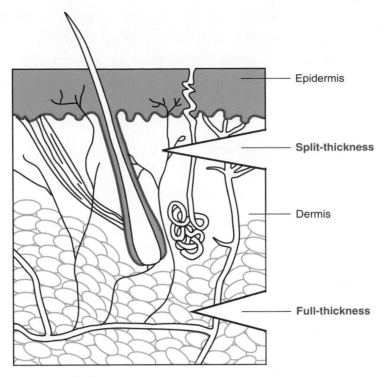

Figure **3-9** Split-thickness and full-thickness skin grafts.

## Skin Replacement Surgery and Skin Substitutes (15002-15278)

15002-15005 Site preparation based on size and site

15040 Harvest for tissue culture

15050-15278 Graft codes by type and size

**Split-thickness:** Epidermis and some dermis (Figure 3-9)

**Full-thickness:** Epidermis and all dermis

### Skin Replacement Surgery (15002-15278)

- Surgical Preparation (15002-15005)
- Autografts/Tissue Cultured Autografts (15040-15261)
- Skin Substitute Grafts (15271-15278)

**Allograft:** Donor graft

**Xenograft:** Nonhuman donor

### Flaps (15570-15776)

Some skin left attached to blood supply

- Keeps flap viable

Donor site may be far from recipient site

Flaps may be in stages

Codes divided by location and size

Formation of flap (15570-15576)

- Based on recipient location: Trunk, scalp, nose, etc.

Transfer of flap (15650): Previously placed flap released from donor site

- Also known as walking or walk up of flap

Muscle, Myocutaneous, or Fasciocutaneous Flaps (15732-15738)

- Based on recipient location; head and neck, trunk, upper or lower extremity

- Repairs made with

  - Muscle

  - Muscle and skin

  - Fascia and skin

- Flaps rotated from donor to recipient site

- Includes closure donor site unless skin graft or local flaps are necessary

### Other Procedures (15780-15879)

Many cosmetic procedures including:

- Dermabrasion

- Chemical peel

- Blepharoplasty

- Rhytidectomy

- Excessive skin excision

### Pressure (Decubitus) Ulcers (15920-15999)

Excision and various closures

- Primary, skin flap, muscle, etc.

Many codes "with ostectomy"

- Bone removal

Locations

- Coccygeal (end of spine)

- Sacral (between hips)

- Ischial (lower hip)

- Trochanteric (outer hip)

Site preparation only: 15936, 15937, 15946, 15956 or 15958

- Defect repair of donor site reported separately

### Burns Local Treatment (16000-16036)

Codes for small, medium, and large

Must calculate percentage of body burned using Rule of Nines for adults (Figure 3-10)

- <5% small

- 5% to 10% medium

- >10% large

Lund-Browder for children (Figure 3-11)

- Proportions of children differ from adults

- Heads are larger

Often require multiple debridements and redressing

Figure **3-10** The Rule of Nines is used to calculate burn area on an adult.

**Anterior**                    **Posterior**

Relative percentage of body surface areas (% BSA) affected by growth

|  | 0 yr | 1 yr | 5 yr | 10 yr | 15 yr |
|---|---|---|---|---|---|
| a – ½ of head | 9½ | 8½ | 6½ | 5½ | 4½ |
| b – ½ of 1 thigh | 2¾ | 3¼ | 4 | 4¼ | 4½ |
| c – ½ of lower leg | 2½ | 2½ | 2¾ | 3 | 3¼ |

Figure **3-11** Lund-Browder chart for estimating the extent of burns on children.

Based on

- Initial treatment of 1st-degree burn (16000)
- Size

Report percent of burn and depth

### Destruction (17000-17286)
Ablation (destruction) of tissue

- Laser, electrosurgery, cryosurgery, chemosurgery, etc.
- Benign/premalignant or malignant tissue
- Malignant tissue is based on location and size of lesion
- Benign/premalignant is based on the number of lesions removed/destroyed or size (sq cm)

### Mohs Micrographic Surgery (17311-17315)
Surgeon acts as pathologist and surgeon

Removes one layer of lesion at a time

Continues until no malignant cells remain

Based on stages and number of specimens per stage indicated in medical record

### Other Procedures (17340-17999)
Treatment of acne

- Cryotherapy
- Chemical exfoliation
- Electrolysis
- Unlisted procedures

### Breast Procedures (19000-19499)
Divided based on procedure

- Incision
- Excision
- Introduction
- Mastectomy procedures
- Repair/Reconstruction

Use excision of lesion codes if entire lesion is removed during incisional biopsy

Use additional code for placement of radiological marker

Mastectomies based on extent of procedure

- Wide excision
- Removal of neoplasm, capsule, and surrounding margins
- Radical
- Wide excision and anatomical structure surrounding neoplasm
    ***Example:*** Muscle or fascia
- Conservative partial mastectomy in which lesion is removed with adequate margins (19301)
- Axillary dissection and partial mastectomy, 19302
- Radical and modified radical 19305, 19306, and 19307 based on extent

Confirm whether pectoral muscles, axillary, or internal lymph nodes were removed

19307 most common and includes breast and axillary lymph node removal

Code removal of lymph nodes separately unless included in code description

Bilateral procedures, use -50

## Biopsy/Removal of Lesion

Incisional biopsy: Incision made into lesion and small portion of lesion removed

Excisional biopsy: Entire lesion removed

Open incisional biopsy most complex (19101)

Percutaneous needle core biopsy without imaging guidance (19100)

- Same procedure with imaging guidance is 19102

Automated vacuum assisted or rotating biopsy device described in 19103 is the use of advanced breast biopsy instrumentation

- Image guidance performed by physician reported separately
- Complete, simple removal of a mass is reported with 19120

Lesion may be preoperatively marked by placing thin wire (radiologic marker) down to lesion

- Wire placement reported separately (19290)
- Additional wires reported with 19291
- Metallic localization clips may be placed during biopsy operative session so the site can be located later, if necessary
- Placement of clip reported with 19295, once for each clip placed
- Image guidance performed by physician reported separately

# MUSCULOSKELETAL SYSTEM SUBSECTION (20005-29999)

Subsection divided: Anatomic site, then service (e.g., excision)

Used extensively by orthopedic surgeons

- Many codes commonly used by variety of physicians

Extensive notes

Most common

- Fracture and dislocation treatments
- "General" subheading
- Arthroscopic procedures
- Casting and strapping

Eponyms are "things" named after "people"

> ***Example:*** Barr procedure is a tendon transfer of the lower leg (27690-27692), and Mitchell, Chevron or concentric type procedure is a complex metatarsal osteotomy (bunion correction) (28296)

- Procedures are often referred to with eponyms
- Check the index of the CPT manual for directions to eponym codes

## Fracture Treatment

Type of treatment depends on type and severity of fracture

Diagnosis codes must support the procedure codes and document the medical necessity

**Open:** Surgically opened to view or remotely opened to place nail across fracture site

- Open reduction with internal fixation is ORIF

**Closed:** Not surgically opened

**Percutaneous:** Insertion of devices through skin or a remote site

- Percutaneous fracture treatment neither open nor closed

Treatment terms should not be confused with **types** of fractures:

- Open fracture: Fractured bone penetrates skin

- Closed fracture: Fractured bone does not penetrate skin

### Traction

- Application of force to align bone

- Force applied by internal device (e.g., wire, pin) inserted into bone (skeletal fixation)

- Application of force by means of adhesion to skin (skin traction)

### Manipulation

Use of force to return bone back to normal alignment by manual manipulation (reduction) or temporary traction

Codes often divided based on whether manipulation was or was not used

### Dislocation

Bone displaced from normal joint position

Treatment: Return bone to normal joint location

### Subheading "General"

Begins "Incision" (20005)

Depth: Difference between Integumentary and Musculoskeletal incision codes

Musculoskeletal used when underlying bone or muscle is involved or procedure is deep subcutaneous

## Wound Exploration (20100-20103)

Traumatic penetrating wounds

Divided by wound location

Includes

- Enlargement

- Debridement

- Foreign body(ies) removal

- Ligation

- Repair of tissue and muscle

Use additional code for repair of major structures or blood vessels

Not used for integumentary repairs

- Unless the repair requires extension, enlargement, or exploration

## Excision (20150-20251)

Biopsies for bone and muscle

Divided by

- Type of biopsy (bone/muscle)
- Depth
- Some by method

Can be percutaneous needle or excisional

Does not include tumor excision, which is coded separately

Biopsy with excision: Code only excision

## Introduction or Removal (20500-20697)

Codes for

- Injections
- Aspirations
- Insertions
- Applications
- Removals
- Adjustments

Therapeutic sinus tract injection procedures

- Not nasal sinus
- Abscess or cyst with passage (sinus tract) to skin
- Antibiotic injected with use of radiographic guidance

Removal of foreign bodies lodged in muscle or tendon sheath

Integumentary removal codes for removal from skin

Injection into

- Tendon sheath
- Tendon origin
- Ligament
- Ganglion cyst
- Trigger points

Placement of needles or catheters into muscle and/or soft tissue

- For interstitial radioelement application

Arthrocentesis: Injection "and/or" aspiration of a joint

- Both aspiration and injection reported with one code (20600-20610)
- Codes based on joint size: Small, intermediate, major
- Do not unbundle and report aspiration/injection with two codes

### External Fixation

(20690-20697)

Device that holds bone in place

- Application, adjustment, removal under anesthesia

Code fracture treatment and external fixation device (EFD)

- Unless treatment and fixation both included in fracture care code description
- Adjustment to (20693) and removal of (20694 [under anesthesia]) EFD are coded separately

## Replantation (20802-20838)

Used to report reattachment of amputated limb

Code by body area

## Grafts (or Implants) (20900-20938)

### Autogenous Grafts

Used to report harvesting through separate incision of

- Bone
- Cartilage
- Tendon
- Fascia lata
- Tissue

Fascia lata grafts: From upper lateral thigh where fascia is thickest

Some codes include obtaining grafting material (not coded separately)

Some grafts are add-on codes for spine surgery only (20930-20938)

## Other Procedures (20950-20999)

Monitoring interstitial fluid pressure (interstitial for compartment syndrome, etc.)

- Pressure increases when blood supply decreases due to increased accumulation of fluids

Bone grafts identified by donor site

Free osseocutaneous flaps: Bone grafts

- Taken along with skin and tissue overlying bone

Electrical stimulation

- Used to speed bone healing
- Placement of stimulators externally or internally
- Ultrasound also used externally

## Soft Tissue Tumors

New in 2010, codes to identify excision of soft tissue and subfascial (intramuscular) tumors

- Subcutaneous soft tissue tumors: Below skin but above deep fascia
- Fascial or subfascial soft tissue tumors: Within or below deep fascia (not bone)
- Soft tissue tumors: May involve resection from one or more layer (i.e., subcutaneous, subfascial)

  *Example:* 21011-21016 to report subcutaneous, subfascial, and soft tissue tumors

## Arthrodesis

Fixation of joint (arthro = joint, desis = fusion)

- Bony structures of joint fused together to form one solid bone
- Fixation with pins, wires, rods, etc. to hold the joint immobile

Often performed with other procedure such as fracture repair

• Arthrodesis of the spine is also called spinal fusion

## Subsequent Subheadings

After General subheading, divided by anatomic location

• Anatomic subheadings divided by type procedure

*Example:* Subheading "Head" divided by procedure

• Incision

• Excision

• Manipulation

• Head prosthesis

• Introduction or Removal

• Repair, Revision, and/or Reconstruction

• Fracture and/or Dislocation

• Other Procedures

• Fracture and/or Dislocation

## Spine and Spinal Instrumentation

Insertion of spinal instrumentation reported in addition to arthrodesis (fusion)

Many add-on codes reported in addition to definitive procedure

Spine (Vertebral Column), 22100-22899, divided by repair location (Figure 3-12)

• Cervical (C1-C7)

C1 = Atlas

C2 = Axis

• Thoracic (T1-T12)

• Lumbar (L1-L5)

• Sacral (S1-S5)

Coccyx (tailbone)

Vertebral segment: Single complete vertebral bone with articular processes and laminae

Vertebral interspace: Non-bony compartment between two vertebral bodies which contains the disc

Single level = two vertebrae and the disc that separates them

Percutaneous vertebroplasty

• Use of polymethylmethacrylate injected into the vertebral space

• Polymethylmethacrylate is a type of bone cement/glue like silicone but not silicone

• Adheres bone fragments together

• Fills vertebral body defects

### Types of spinal instrumentation

**Segmental:** Devices at each end of repair area + at least one other attachment

**Nonsegmental:** Devices at each end of defect only

**Approach:** Pay special attention to the approach used to perform the surgery

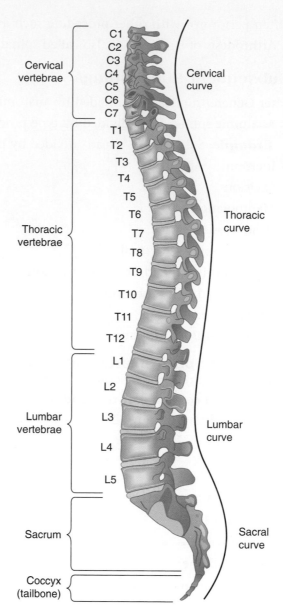

Figure **3-12** The spinal cord is part of central nervous system (CNS) and extends from the brain to the lower back.

- Several different approaches to spine: Most common are anterior (front) and posterior (back)

- Most spinal instrumentation codes divided based on approach

### Casting and Strapping (29000-29799)
Replacement procedure or initial placement to stabilize without additional restorative treatment

   ***Example:*** Application of wrist splint or cast for wrist sprain

Initial fracture treatment includes placement and removal of first cast

- Subsequent cast applications coded separately

- Payers have strict individual reimbursement policies for subsequent casting

Application not coded when part of surgical procedure

   *Example:* Application of wrist splint or cast for wrist sprain

Initial fracture treatment includes placement and removal of first cast

Elastic bandage application is not billed separately

Removal bundled into surgical procedure

Supplies reported separately

### Endoscopy/Arthroscopy (29800-29999)
Surgical arthroscopy always includes diagnostic arthroscopy

Codes divided by joint

- Subdivided by procedure

Be aware of subterms and bundled procedures within code descriptions

**Note:** Parenthetical information following codes indicates codes to use if procedure was an open procedure

## RESPIRATORY SYSTEM SUBSECTION (30000-32999)

Anatomic site arrangement

- Nose
- Larynx

Further subdivided by procedure

- Incision
- Excision

## Endoscopy

Endoscopy in all subheadings except Nose

Each preceded by "Notes"

### Endoscopy Rule One
Code full extent of endoscopic procedure performed

   *Example:* Procedure begins at mouth and ends at bronchial tube

- Bronchial tube = full extent

### Endoscopy Rule Two
Code correct approach

   *Example:* For removal:

- Interior lung lesion via endoscope inserted through mouth
- Exterior lung lesion via endoscope inserted through skin into chest

Incorrect approach = incorrect code = incorrect or no reimbursement

### Endoscopy Rule Three
Diagnostic always included in surgical

*Examples:*

- Diagnostic bronchial endoscopy begins
- Identified foreign body
- Removed foreign body (surgical endoscopy)

## Multiple Procedures

Frequent in respiratory coding

- **Watch for bundled services**

Sequence primary procedure first, no modifier

Sequence secondary procedures next, with -51

Bilateral procedures often performed, use -50

Format for reporting chosen by payer

> *Example:* Nasal lavage

- 31000 × 2
- 31000 and 31000-50
- 31000-50
- 31000-RT and 31000-LT

## Nose (30000-30999)

Used extensively by otorhinolaryngologists (ear, nose, and throat [ENT] specialists)

Also used by wide variety of physicians in other specialties

Approach to nose

- External approach, use Integumentary System
- Internal approach, use Respiratory System

## Incision (30000-30020)

Bundled into Incision codes are drain or gauze insertion and removal

Supplies reported separately

## Excision (30100-30160)

Contains intranasal biopsy codes

Polyp excision, coded by complexity

- Excision includes any method of destruction, even laser
- Use -50 (bilateral) for both sides

Turbinate excision and resection

- Three turbinates: Superior, middle, inferior
- Excision of inferior turbinate, 30130
- Excision of superior or middle turbinate, 30999
- Submucous resection of inferior turbinate, 30140
- Submucous resection of superior or middle turbinate, 30999

### Introduction (30200-30220)
Common procedures

**Example:** Injections to shrink nasal tissue or displacement therapy (saline flushes) to remove mucus

- Displacement therapy performed through nose

### Removal of Foreign Body (30300-30320)
Distinguished by the site of removal, whether at office or hospital (requires general anesthesia)

### Repair (30400-30630)
Many plastic procedures

- Rhinoplasty (reshaping nose internal and/or external)

- Septoplasty (rearrangement or repair of nasal septum)

### Destruction (30801-30802)
Use of ablation (removing by cutting)

Used for removal of excess nasal mucosa or to reduce turbinate inflammation

Based on intramural or superficial extent of destruction

- **Intramural:** Deeper mucosa
- **Superficial:** Outer layer of mucosa

### Other Procedures (30901-30999)
Control of nasal hemorrhage

- Packing
- Ligation
- Cauterization
- The packing may be anterior or posterior

### Accessory Sinuses (31000-31299)
Subheadings include:

Incision (31000-31090)

Excision (31200-31230)

Endoscopy (31231-31297)

Other Procedures (31299)

Codes for lavage (washing) of sinuses

- Cannula (hollow tube) placed into sinus
- Sterile saline solution flushed through

Procedures may involve multiple codes when multiple locations are accessed

**Example:** 31020, Sinusotomy, maxillary, can be coded with 31050 sinusotomy, sphenoid, and 31070 sinusotomy, frontal

Use -50 (bilateral) for both sides

Maxillary sinusotomy may use an external and intranasal approach to creating passage between sinus and nose

- Used to clear blocked or infected sinus
- Intranasal sinusotomy, 31020
- External sinusotomy, radical (such as Caldwell-Luc)

  Access through mouth

  Incision above eyetooth

  Sinus is cleaned

  New opening created or old opening enlarged

Repair of fractures occurring during procedure may be coded separately if not included in code description

### Larynx (31300-31599)

### Excision (31300-31420)

Laryngotomy: Open surgical procedure to expose larynx

- For removal procedure (e.g., tumor)

May be confused with Trachea/Bronchi codes for tracheostomy used to establish airflow

### Introduction (31500-31502)

Used to establish, maintain, and protect air flow

Endotracheal intubation, establishment of airway

Based on planned (ventilation support) or emergency procedure

### Endoscopy (31505-31579)

Uses terms *indirect* and *direct*

- **Indirect:** Tongue depressor with mirror used to view larynx
- **Direct:** Endoscopy passed into larynx; physician directly views vocal cords

### Repair (31580-31590)

Several plastic procedures and fracture repairs

Laryngoplasty procedures based on purpose

Fracture code is open reduction code

### Trachea and Bronchi (31600-31899)

### Incision (31600-31614)

Most codes: Tracheostomy divided by

- Planned (ventilation support), based on age
- Emergency

Divided by type

- Transtracheal or cricothyroid (location of incision)

### Endoscopy (31615-31656)

Bronchoscope may be inserted into nose or mouth

Rigid endoscopy performed under general anesthesia

Flexible endoscopy usually performed under local or moderate (conscious) sedation

### Introduction (31715-31730)

Catheterization

Instillation

Injection

Aspiration

Tracheal tube placement

Some include inhaled gas as contrast material

### Excision, Repair (31750-31830)

Repairs of trachea and bronchi

## Lungs and Pleura (32035-32999)

### Incision (32035-32225)

**Thoracotomy.** Surgical opening of chest to expose to view.

Used for

- Biopsy
- Cyst
- Foreign body removal
- Cardiac massage, etc.

### Excision/Removal (32310-32540)

Biopsy codes in both Excision and Incision categories

- Excisional biopsy with percutaneous needle
- Incisional biopsy with chest open

Also services of pleurectomy, pneumocentesis, and lung removal

- **Segmentectomy:** 1 segment
- **Lobectomy:** 1 lobe
- **Bilobectomy:** 2 lobes
- **Total Pneumonectomy:** 1 lung

**Thoracentesis.** Needle inserted into pleural space for aspiration (withdrawal) of fluid and/or air (32421, 32422)

### Introduction and Removal (32550-32553)

- Insertion of indwelling tunneled pleural catheter (removal 32552)
- Tube thoracostomy
- Placement of interstitial device(s) for radiation therapy guidance

### Destruction (32560-32562)

- Chemical pleurodesis
- Fibrinolysis, initial day, subsequent day

## CARDIOVASCULAR SYSTEM SUBSECTION (33010-37799)

CV coding may require codes from

- **Radiology:** Diagnostic studies

- **Medicine:** Nonsurgical and percutaneous
- **Surgery:** Open and percutaneous

Both Medicine and Surgery sections contain invasive procedures

## Cardiology Coding Terminology

**Invasive:** Enters body

- Incision

    *Example:* Opening chest for removal (e.g., tumor on heart)

- Percutaneous

    • Placement of catheter into artery or vein through the skin by means of wire threaded through needle and catheter slid over wire

    *Example:* PTCA (percutaneous transluminal coronary angioplasty) procedure

Percutaneous—wire threaded through needle placed through skin into vessel and catheter placed over wire

- Cut down—small nick made into vessel under direct vision and catheter inserted

    *Example:* Catheter inserted into femoral or brachial artery

Common catheters are:

- Broviac
- Hickman
- HydroCath
- Arrow multi-lumen
- Groshong
- Dual-lumen
- Triple-lumen

**Noninvasive:** Procedures that do not break skin

*Example:* Electrocardiogram

**Electrophysiology (EP):** Study of electrical system of heart

*Example:* Study of irregular heartbeat (arrhythmia)

- EP studies are in Medicine section, 93600-93662
- Electrophysiologic Operative Procedures are in Surgery section, 33250-33266

**Nuclear Cardiology:** Diagnostic and treatment specialty; uses radioactive substances to diagnose cardiac conditions

*Example:* Myocardial perfusion and cardiac blood pooling imaging studies

## ■ Cardiovascular in Surgery Section

### Codes for Procedures

Heart/Pericardium (33010-33999)

- Pacemakers, valve disorders

Arteries/Veins (34001-37799)

### Heart/Pericardium (33010-33999)

Both percutaneous and open surgical

- Cardiologists often use percutaneous intervention; cardiovascular or thoracic surgeons often use open surgical procedures

Extensive notes throughout

Frequent changes with medical advances

Examples of categories of Heart/Pericardium subheading

- Pericardium
- Cardiac Tumor
- Pacemaker or Pacing Cardioverter-Defibrillator

Examples of services

- Pericardiocentesis: Percutaneous withdrawal of fluid from pericardial space (pericarditis) (33010-33011)
- Cardiac Tumor: Open surgical procedure for removal of tumor on heart (33130)

### Pacemakers or Pacing Cardioverter-Defibrillators (33202-33249)

Devices that assist heart in electrical function

- Differentiate between temporary and permanent devices
- Differentiate between one-chamber (one lead) and dual-chamber (two leads) devices

Divided by where pacer placed, approach, and type of service

Patient record indicates revision or replacement

- Pacemaker pulse generator is also called a battery
- Pacemaker leads are also called electrodes

Usual follow-up 90 days (global period)

#### Placed

Atrium (single chamber)

- Pulse generator and one or more electrodes in atrium (single-chamber pacemaker)

Ventricle (single chamber)

- Pulse generator and one or more electrodes in ventricle (single-chamber pacemaker)

Both (dual chamber)

- Pulse generator and one electrode in right ventricle and one electrode in right atrium

Biventricular, right ventricle, right atrium, and coronary sinus

- Pulse generator and one electrode in right ventricle, one electrode(s) may be placed in right atrium, and one electrode in the coronary sinus over the left ventricle

#### Approach

**Epicardial:** Open procedure to place electrodes on heart

**Transvenous:** Through vein to place in heart

#### Type of service

Initial placement or replacement of all or part of device

Number of leads placed is important in code selection

### Electrophysiologic Operative Procedures (33250-33266)

Surgeon repairs defect causing abnormal rhythm

Chest opened to full view

- Cardiopulmonary (CP) bypass usually used

Endoscopy procedure

- Without cardiopulmonary bypass

Codes based on reason for procedure and if CP bypass used

### Patient-Activated Event Recorder (33282-33284)

Also known as cardiac event recorder or loop recorder

Internal surgical implantation required

Divided based on whether device is being implanted or removed

## Cardiac Valves (33400-33496)

Divided by valve

- Aortic

- Mitral

- Tricuspid

- Pulmonary

Subdivided by whether replacement, repair, or resection is completed (all done with bypass machine)

Code descriptions are all similar, requiring careful reading

### Coronary Artery Bypass Graft (CABG)

CABG performed for bypassing coronary arteries severely obstructed as in atherosclerosis or arteriosclerosis

Determine what was used in repair

- Vein (33510-33516)

- Artery (33533-33536)

- Both artery and vein (33517-33523 and 33533-33536)

Based on number of bypass grafts performed and if combined venous and arterial grafts are used

> *Example:* Three venous grafts

## Venous Grafting Only for Coronary Artery Bypass (33510-33516)

Based on number of grafts being replaced

## Combined Arterial-Venous Grafting (33517-33530)

Divided based on number of grafts and if procedure initial or reoperation

Procuring saphenous vein included, unless performed endoscopically

These codes are never used alone

- Arterial-Venous codes (33517-33523) report only **venous** graft portion of procedure

- Always used with Arterial Grafting codes (33533-33536)

> *Example:* 3 vein grafts and 2 arterial grafts = 33519 and 33534

Open procurement of saphenous vein is included in procedure (not coded separately)

Code harvesting of saphenous vein graft separately when endoscopic video-assisted procurement is performed (33508)

Code harvesting separately for upper extremity or femoral vein

## Arterial Grafting for Coronary Artery Bypass (33533-33536)

Divided based on number of grafts

Obtaining artery for grafting included in codes, except

- Procuring upper-extremity artery (e.g., radial artery), coded separately (35600)

Several codes (33542-33548) for myocardial resection, repair of ventricular septal defect (VSD), and ventricular restoration

## Endovascular Repair of Descending Thoracic Aorta (33880-33891)

Placement of an endovascular aortic prosthesis for repair of descending thoracic aorta

- Less invasive than traditional approach of chest or abdominal incision

Synthetic aortic prosthesis placed via catheter

- Report fluoroscopic guidance separately 75956-75959

  Fluoroscopic guidance codes include diagnostic imaging prior to placement and intraprocedurally

Stent-graft (endoprosthesis) is deployed to reinforce weakened area

## Arteries and Veins Subheading (34001-37799)

Only for noncoronary vessels

- Divided based on whether artery or vein involved

  *Example:* Different codes for embolectomy, depending on artery or vein

Catheters placed into vessels for monitoring, removal, repair

Nonselective or selective catheter placement

- Nonselective: Direct placement without further manipulation
- Selective: Place and then manipulate into further order(s)

Catheter placement example

- Nonselective: 36000 Introduction of needle into vein
- Selective: 36012 Placement of catheter into second-order venous system

### Vascular Families Are Like a Tree

First-order (main) branch (tree trunk)

Second-order branch (tree limb)

Third-order branch (tree branch)

Brachiocephalic vascular family (Figure 3-13)

- Report farthest extent of catheter placement in a vascular family; labor intensity is increased with the extent of catheter placement

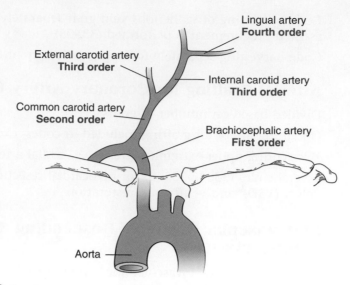

Figure **3-13** Brachiocephalic vascular family with first-, second-, third-, and fourth-order vessels.

## Embolectomy and Thrombectomy (34001-34490)
**Embolus:** Dislodged thrombus

**Thrombus:** Mass of material in vessel located in place of formation

• May be removed by dissection or balloon

**Balloon:** Threaded into vessel, inflated under mass, pulled out with mass

• Codes are divided by site of incision and whether artery or vein

## Venous Reconstruction (34501-34530)
Types of repairs
• Valve of the femoral vein

• Vena cava

• Saphenopopliteal vein anastomosis

Aneurysm
Aneurysm: Weakened arterial wall causing a bulge or ballooning

Repair by removal, bypass, or coil placement

Endovascular repair (34800-34900) from inside vessel

Direct (35001-35152) from outside vessel

## Endovascular Repair of Abdominal Aortic Aneurysm (34800-34834)
Fluoroscopic guidance: Use Radiology 75952 or 75953

Includes access, catheter manipulation, balloon angioplasty, stent placement, site closure

Reported separately: Introduction of guideline and catheters

Other procedures performed at same time coded separately

### Endovascular Repair of Iliac Aneurysm (34900)

Extensive notes preceding codes—"must" reading

Uses fluoroscopic guidance report: Radiology 75954

Includes introduction, positioning, and deployment of graft, stent and balloon angioplasty

Reported separately: Introduction of guidewire and catheters

### Repair Arteriovenous Fistula (35180-35190)

Abnormal passage from artery or vein

Divided based on fistula type

- Congenital
- Acquired/traumatic
- By site

Repair methods

- Autogenous graft—fistula created artery to vein
- Non-auto fistula—biocompatible tube connecting artery to vein

### Angioplasty (35450-35476)

Divided as open or percutaneous and by vessel

- **Transluminal:** By way of vessel
- **Transluminal Angioplasty:** Catheter passed into vessel and a balloon is inflated to crush/flatten fatty deposits in vessel
  - Placement of eluding or noneluding stents coded in addition to catheter placement

### Noncoronary Bypass Grafts (35500-35671)

Divided by

- Vein
- In-Situ Vein (veins repaired in their original place)
- Other Than Vein

Code by type of graft and vessels being used to bypass

>   *Example:* 35506 Bypass graft, with vein; carotid-subclavian

- Graft attached to carotid and to subclavian, bypassing defect of subclavian

Procurement of saphenous vein graft is included and not reported separately

Harvesting of upper-extremity vein (35500) or femoropopliteal vein (35572) is reported separately

### Vascular Injection Procedures (36000-36598)

Divided into

- Intravenous
- Intra-arterial—Intra-aortic
- Venous
- Central venous access procedures

Used for many procedures, including

- Local anesthesia
- Introduction of needle
- Injection of contrast material

- Preinjection and postinjection care related to injection procedure
  ***Example:*** Injection of opaque substance for venography (radiography of vein)

## Central Venous Access (CVA) Procedures

Long term use for medication/chemotherapy administration and short-term use for monitoring

Approach

- Central: jugular, subclavian, or femoral vein
- Peripheral: basilic or cephalic vein

Categories

1. Insertion
2. Repair
3. Replacement, partial or complete
4. Removal
5. Other central venous access procedure
6. Guidance for vascular access

### Insertion (36555-36571)

Insertion of newly established venous access

- Tunneled under skin (e.g., Hickman, Broviac, Groshong)
- Nontunneled (e.g., Hohn catheter, triple lumen, PICC)
- Central (e.g., subclavian, internal jugular, femoral, inferior vena cava)
- Peripheral (basilic or cephalic vein)

Codes divided by tunneled/non-tunneled, with/without port, central/peripheral, and age

### Repair (36575-36576)

Repair of malfunction without replacement with or without subcutaneous port or pump

Repair of central venous access device

No differentiation between age of patient or central/peripheral insertion

### Replacement (Partial or Complete) (36578-36585)

Partial (36578) is replacement of catheter only

Complete (36580-36585) is replacement through same venous access site

Differentiated by tunneled/non-tunneled, central/peripheral, and with or without subcutaneous port or pump

### Removal (36589, 36590)

To be used for tunneled catheter

Removal of non-tunneled catheter is not reported separately

### Other Central Venous Access Procedures (36591-36598)

Collection of blood specimen

Declotting of catheter or access device by thrombolytic agent

Mechanical removal of obstructive material from around catheter or within lumen

### Guidance for Vascular Access

77001, Fluoroscopic guidance for central venous access device placement, replacement, or removal

- Reported in addition to primary procedure

76937, Ultrasound guidance for vascular access

- Reported in addition to primary procedure

## Transcatheter Procedures (37184-37216)

Arterial mechanical thrombectomy (37184-37186)

- Removal of thrombus by means of mechanical device

   From artery or arterial bypass graft

Venous mechanical thrombectomy (37187-37188)

- Removal of a thrombus by means of a mechanical device

   From vein

Arterial and venous mechanical thrombectomy may be performed as primary procedure or add-on

- Include

   Introduction of device into thrombus

   Thrombus removal

   Injection of thrombolytic drug(s), if used

   Fluoroscopic and contrast guidance

   Follow-up angiography

- Report separately

   Diagnostic angiography

   Catheter placement(s)

   Diagnostic studies

   Pharmacologic thrombolytic infusion before or after (37201, 75896, 75898)

   Other interventions

## Other Procedures (37191-37216)

- Used to report a variety of transcatheter procedures

   ***Example:*** Transcatheter biopsy, therapy, infusion for thrombolysis or antispasmotic treatment of a vessel, retrieval of foreign object, occlusion or embolization, and intravascular stents

Endovascular Revascularization (Open or Percutaneous, Transcatheter) (37220-37235)

## ■ Cardiovascular in Medicine Section

Services can be

- Invasive or noninvasive
- Diagnostic or therapeutic

Subheadings

- Therapeutic Services
- Cardiography
- Echocardiography

- Cardiac Catheterization
- Intracardiac Electrophysiologic (EP) Procedures/Studies
- Peripheral Arterial Disease Rehabilitation
- Other Vascular Studies

### Therapeutic Services (92950-92998)
Types of services

- Cardioversion
- Infusions
- Thrombolysis
- Catheter placement

Codes divided by

- Method (e.g., balloon, blade)
- Location (e.g., aortic or mitral valve)
- Number (e.g., single or multiple vessels)

### Intracoronary Brachytherapy (92974)
Uses radioactive substances to destroy re-stenosis of coronary vessel

Patients have had stent placed in coronary vessel

Add-on code

Includes moderate sedation

Stent "re-stenosis" (re-formation of plaque)

Cardiologist: Places guidewire and catheter

Radiation oncologist: Places radioactive elements

### Cardiography (93000-93278)
Types of services

- Stress tests
- Holter monitor
- Electrocardiogram

Separate codes for components of study, such as

- 93000 global
- 93005 tracing only
- 93010 interpretation and report only

**Note:** Coding structure eliminates use of modifiers -26 or -TC

### Implantable and Wearable Cardiac Device Evaluations (93279-93299)
Diagnostic medical procedures for cardiac rhythm devices

- Devices are internal or external
- In-person or remote assessments

Codes divided by

- Type of Service

Implantation

Interrogation

Programming

- Device

  Implantable cardioverter-defibrillator

  Loop recorder

- Number of leads or chambers

- Monitoring period must exceed 10 days

Implantation procedures (93279-93292)

- Reported once per procedure

Interrogation device evaluation of implantable cardioverter-defibrillator (ICD) (93293-93296)

  - ICDs may act as defibrillator or pacemaker

- Report interrogation or monitoring once per 90-day period

Interrogation device evaluation implantable cardiovascular monitor system (93297-93299)

- Report interrogation or monitoring once per 30-day period

### Echocardiography (93303-93352)
**Noninvasive diagnostic procedure.** Ultrasound detects presence of cardiac or vascular disease

Codes divided by

- Approach

- Extent of study (e.g., limited, complete)

- Service provided (e.g., probe only, interpretation and report)

### Cardiac Catheterization (93451-93568)
Used to identify valve disorders, abnormal blood flow

Many bundled services in catheterization codes

  ***Examples:***
  - Introduction
  - Positioning/Repositioning of catheter
  - Pressure readings inside heart or vessels
  - Blood samples
  - Rest/Exercise studies
  - Final evaluation and report
  - Many codes are -51 exempt
  - Many codes include moderate (conscious) sedation

**Three components of coding cardiac catheterization**
1. Placement of catheter
2. Injection
3. Imaging supervision, interpretation, and report

Most codes have all three components in the code

- Example: 93456 includes catheterization, injection, imaging

Some codes require multiple codes

- Example: 93531 reports catheterization for congenital cardiac anomalies, injection code (93563/93564) must be added

### Intracardiac Electrophysiologic Procedures/Studies (93600-93662)

Services to diagnose and treat conditions of electrical system of heart

- Arrhythmic induction
- Mapping
- Ablation

**EP system of heart**

Electrical conduction system

Electrical recording codes divided based on location of recording device

> *Example:* Bundle of His or right ventricle

Pacing: Temporary pacing to stabilize beating of heart

> *Example:* Intraventricular or intra-arterial pacing

### Peripheral Arterial Disease (PAD) Rehabilitation (93668)

Rehabilitation sessions: 45-60 minutes

Use of motorized treadmill/track/bicycle to build patient's CV function

Supervised by exercise physiologist or nurse

If E/M is provided by physician, service is reported separately

### Noninvasive Physiologic Studies and Procedures (93701-93790)

Category contains codes for services such as

- **Plethysmography:** Recordings of changes in size of body part when blood passes through it
- **Electronic Analysis:** Checks electronic function of devices, such as pacemakers
- **Ambulatory Blood Pressure Monitoring:** Outpatient basis over 24-hour period
- **Thermograms:** Visual recordings of body temperature

## ■ Cardiovascular in Radiology Section

Radiology section, Heart (75557-75574) and Aorta/Arteries (75600-75791) subsections

Prior to 1992, Radiology section contained codes for entire CV procedures

Major revision to CV radiology codes 1992

Divided complete procedures into two components: technical and professional

> *Example:* Angiography

- Technical component angiography—remains in Radiology section
- Professional component injection—moved to Surgery section

Complete angiography requires radiology code and surgery code

Reflects common practice of cardiologist's performing injection and radiologist's performing angiography

### Contrast Material

Often radiologic procedures use contrast material to improve image

Many codes have contrast material bundled into service

- "With contrast" or "with or without contrast"

Only injected contrast qualifies as with contrast

Contrast not included in description but used in procedure: Code contrast material and injection separately

- Specify site where service is received to differentiate between global, technical, and professional components of the procedure

Non-hospital-based (not employed by hospital) physician usually performs procedure in hospital outpatient department: Use -26 for professional component only

---

### A COMPONENT CODING EXAMPLE

Two physicians (cardiologist and radiologist from same facility) perform angiography of third-order brachio-cephalic artery with contrast

- Cardiologist places catheter (36217), Surgery section
- Radiologist performs angiography (75658), Radiology section
- Supply of contrast material (99070), Medicine section

---

## HEMIC AND LYMPHATIC SYSTEM SUBSECTION (38100-38999)

### Divisions

- Spleen

- General

- Lymph Nodes and Lymphatic Channels

### Spleen Subheading (38100-38200)

Spleen easily ruptured, causing massive and potentially lethal hemorrhage

Excision:

- Splenectomy: Total or partial/open or laparoscopic

Often done as part of more major procedure

- Bundled into major procedure

- Repair

- Laparoscopy

### General (38204-38242)

#### Bone Marrow
Codes divided based on

- Preservation

- Preparation

- Purification

- Aspiration

- Biopsy

- Harvesting

- Transplantation

### Stem Cells

Immature blood cells originating in bone marrow

Used in treatment of leukemia

**Types of stem cells**

*Allogenic:* Same species

*Autologous:* Patient's own

## Lymph Nodes and Lymphatic Channels Subheading (38300-38999)

Two types of lymphadenectomies:

1. **Limited:** Pelvic and para-aortic lymph nodes only for neoplasm staging
2. **Radical:** Aortic and/or splenic lymph nodes and surrounding tissue for neoplasm staging

Often bundled into more major procedure (e.g., prostatectomy)

Do not unbundle and report lymphadenectomy separately

# MEDIASTINUM SUBSECTION (39000-39499)

Incision codes for foreign body removal, biopsy, or drainage

Excision codes for removal of cyst or tumor

## Diaphragm (39501-39599)

Only two categories: Repair and Other Procedures

Includes hernia and laceration repairs

# DIGESTIVE SYSTEM SUBSECTION (40490-49999)

Divided by anatomic site from mouth to anus + organs that aid digestive process

> *Example:* Liver and gallbladder

Many bundled procedures

## Endoscopy

Diagnostic procedure always bundled into surgical endoscopic

Code to furthest extent of procedure

### Endoscopy Terminology

Notes define specific terminology

Code descriptions are specific regarding

- Technique and depth of scope

  Esophagoscopy: Esophagus only

  Esophagogastroscopy: Esophagus and past diaphragm

  Esophagogastroduodenoscopy: Esophagus and beyond pyloric channel

- Proctosigmoidoscopy: Rectum and sigmoid colon (6-25 cm)

- Sigmoidoscopy: Entire rectum, sigmoid colon, and may include part of descending colon (26-60 cm)

- Colonoscopy: Entire colon, rectum to cecum, and may include terminal ileum (greater than 60 cm)

## Laparoscopy and Endoscopy

Some subheadings have both laparoscopy (outside) and endoscopy (inside) procedures

> *Example:* Subheading Esophagus

- Endoscopy views inside

- Laparoscopy—scope inserted through umbilicus; views from outside

## Hemorrhoidectomy and Fistulectomy Codes (46221-46320)

Divided by

- Location
  - Internal
  - External
- Complexity
  - Simple: No repair procedure involved
  - Complex: Includes repair procedure and fissurectomy
- Anatomy
  - Subcutaneous: No muscle involvement
  - Submuscular: sphincter muscle
- Complex fistulectomy involves excision/incision of multiple fistulas

## Hernia Codes (49491-49659)

Divided by

- Type of hernia

  > *Example:* Inguinal, femoral

- Initial or subsequent repair
- Age of patient determines code choice
- Clinical presentation
  - **Strangulated:** Blood supply cut off
  - **Incarcerated:** Cannot be returned to cavity (not reducible)

Additional code is used for implantation of mesh or prosthesis

- Laparoscopy surgical procedures

## URINARY SYSTEM SUBSECTION (50010-53899)

Anatomic division

- Kidney
- Ureters
- Bladder
- Urethra

Further divided by procedure

- Incision

- Excision

- Introduction

- Repair

- Laparoscopy

- Endoscopy

## Kidney Subheading (50010-50593)

Endoscopy codes are for procedure done through previously established stoma or incision

Caution: Codes may be unilateral or bilateral

### Introduction Category (50382-50398)
Codes divided by renal pelvis catheter procedures or other introduction procedures

Renal pelvis catheters further divided; internally dwelling or externally accessible

Catheters for drainage and injections and for radiography

Aspirations

Insertion of guidewires

Tube changes

Usually reported with radiology component

## Ureter Subheading (50600-50980)

Caution: Codes may be unilateral or bilateral

Divided by type of procedure

- Incision

- Excision

- Introduction

- Repair

- Laparoscopy

- Endoscopy

## Bladder Subheading (51020-52700)

Includes codes for

- Incision

- Removal

- Excision

- Introduction

- Urodynamics

- Repair

- Laparoscopy
- Endoscopy
- Cystoscopy
- Urethroscopy
- Cystourethroscopy
- Transurethral surgery

Many bundled codes

> *Example:* Urethral dilation is included with insertion of cystoscope

Read all descriptions carefully

### Urodynamics (51725-51798)

Procedures relate to motion and flow of urine

Used to diagnose urine flow obstructions

Bundled: All usual, necessary instruments, equipment, supplies, and technical assistance

### Vesical Neck and Prostate (52400-52700)

Contains codes for transurethral resection of the prostate (TURP)

> *Example:* 52601 reports a complete transurethral electrosurgical resection of the prostate and includes vasectomy, meatotomy, cystourethroscopy, urethral calibration and/or dilation, internal urethrotomy, and control of any postoperative bleeding

Other approaches are reported with 55801-55845

> *Example:* 55801 reports a removal of the prostate gland (prostatectomy) through an incision in the perineum and includes vasectomy, meatotomy, urethral calibration and/or dilation, internal urethrotomy, and control of any postoperative bleeding

## MALE GENITAL SYSTEM SUBSECTION (54000-55899)

Penis

Testis

Epididymis

Tunica Vaginalis

Scrotum

Vas Deferens

Spermatic Cord

Seminal Vesicles

Prostate

### Biopsy Codes

Located in anatomical subheading to which the codes refer

> *Example:* Biopsy codes in subheadings

- Epididymis (Excision)

*Example:* 54800, needle biopsy of epididymis

- Testis (Excision)

*Example:* 54500, needle biopsy of testis

### Penis (54000-54450)

Incision codes (54000-54015) differ from Integumentary System codes

- Penis incision codes used for deeper structures

### Destruction (54050-54065)

Codes divided by

- Extent: Simple or extensive

- Method of destruction, e.g., chemical, cryosurgery

Extensive destruction can be by any method

### Excision (54100-54164)

Commonly used codes biopsy and circumcision

### Introduction (54200-54250)

Many procedures for corpora cavernosa (spongy bodies of penis)

- Injection procedures for Peyronie disease (toughening of corpora cavernosa)

- Treatments for erectile dysfunction (ED)

### Repair (54300-54440)

Many plastic repairs

Some repairs are staged (more than one stage)

- Stage indicated in code description

## REPRODUCTIVE SYSTEM PROCEDURES (55920)

Code 55920 reports the placement of catheters/needles into pelvic organs/genitalia

- For subsequent interstitial radioelement application

## INTERSEX SURGERY SUBSECTION (55970-55980)

Only 2 codes within subsection

1. Male to female

2. Female to male

Complicated procedures completed over extended period of time

Performed by multiple physicians with extensive specialized training

## FEMALE GENITAL SYSTEM SUBSECTION (56405-58999)

Anatomic division: From vulva to ovaries

- Many bundled services

### Vulva, Perineum, and Introitus (56405-56821)

Skene's gland coded with Urinary System, Incision or Excision codes

- Group of small mucous glands, lower end of urethra

  - Paraurethral duct

## Incision (56405-56442)
**I&D of abscess.** Vulva, perineal area, or Bartholin's gland

## Marsupialization (56440)
Cyst incised

Drained

Edges sutured to sides to keep cyst open, creating a pouchlike repair

## Destruction (56501, 56515)
Lesions destroyed by variety of methods

- Destruction = Eradication (not to be confused with excision; excision is removal)

Divided by simple or extensive destruction

- Complexity based on physician's judgment

- Stated in medical record

Destruction has no pathology report

## Excision (56605-56740)
Biopsy includes

- Local anesthetic

- Biopsy

- Simple closure

Code based on number of lesions biopsied

Place number of lesions on CMS-1500 in Block 24-G (see Figure 3-1)

**Vulvectomy.** Surgical removal of portion of vulva (56620-56640)

Based on extent and size of area removed

*Extent*

- Simple: Skin and superficial subcutaneous tissues

- Radical: Skin and deep subcutaneous tissues

*Size*

- Partial: <80% vulvar area

- Complete: >80% vulvar area

Extent and size indicated in operative report

## Repair (56800-56810)
Includes plastic repair

Read notes following category

- If repair procedure for wound of genitalia, use Integumentary System code

### Endoscopy (56820-56821)
By means of a colposcope with or without biopsy

### Vagina (57000-57426)

Codes divided based on service, e.g., incision, excision

### Introduction (57150-57180)
Includes vaginal irrigation, insertion of devices, diaphragm, cervical caps

Report device inserted separately

- 99070 or HCPCS National Level II codes, such as A4261 (cervical cap)

### Repair (57200-57335)
For nonobstetric repairs

- Obstetric repairs, use Maternity Care and Delivery codes

### Manipulation (57400-57415)
**Dilation:** Speculum inserted into vagina, which is enlarged by dilator

### Endoscopy/Laparoscopy (57420-57426)
Colposcopy codes based on purpose

- e.g., biopsy, diagnostic

Includes code for laparoscopic approach for repair of paravaginal defect

### Cervix Uteri (57452-57800)

Cervix uteri, narrow lower end of uterus

Services include endoscopy, excision, repair, manipulation

### Excision (57500-57558)
Conization codes

**Conization:** Removal of cone of tissue from cervix

LEEP (loop electrocautery excision procedure) technology may be used for conizations or loop electrode biopsies

### Corpus Uteri (58100-58579)

Many complex procedures

- Often very similar wording in code descriptions

- Requires careful reading and specific documentation in the medical record

### Excision (58100-58294)
Dilation and curettage (D&C, 58120) of uterus

- After dilation, curette scrapes uterus

- Coded according to circumstances: Obstetrical or nonobstetrical

Do not report postpartum hemorrhage service with 58120

- Report 59160—Maternity and Delivery code

Many hysterectomy codes

- Based on approach (vaginal, abdominal) and extent (uterus, fallopian tubes, etc.)

Often secondary procedures performed with hysterectomy

Do not code secondary, related minor procedures separately

### Introduction (58300-58356)
Common procedures

- e.g., insertion of an IUD

Report supply of device separately

Specialized services

- e.g., artificial insemination procedures

Used to report physician component of service

Component coding

- Necessary with catheter procedures for hysterosonography
- Notes following codes indicate radiology guidance component codes

### Laparoscopy/Hysteroscopy (58541-58579)
Laparoscopic approach for:

- Removal of myomas
- Radical hysterectomy
- Supracervical and laparoscopic vaginal hysterectomies

Codes divided by tissue removed and weight

- Hysteroscopy codes divided on procedure performed (e.g., lysis of uterine adhesions, endometrial ablation)

### Oviduct/Ovary (58600-58770)

**Oviduct.** Fallopian tube
Incision category contains tubal ligations

- When during same hospitalization (but not at same session as delivery), is coded separately

### Laparoscopy (58660-58679)
Through abdominal wall

Codes in the laparoscopy and hysteroscopy section are divided by procedure performed (e.g., lysis of adhesions, removal adnexal structures)

*Caution:* If only diagnostic laparoscopy

- Do not report Female Genital System codes
- Report 49320, Digestive System

Many codes can be reported separately with appropriate modifiers

> ***Example:*** 58660 Laparoscopy, surgical, with lysis of adhesions, can be coded with any of the indented codes that follow 58660 (58661, 58662, 58670-58673)

## Ovary (58800-58960)

Two categories only: Incision and Excision

**Incision:** Primarily for drainage of cysts and abscesses

• Divided by surgical approach

**Excision:** Biopsy, wedge resection, and oophorectomy

## In Vitro Fertilization (58970-58976)

Specialized codes used by physicians trained in fertilization procedures

• Codes divided by type of procedure and method used

# MATERNITY CARE AND DELIVERY SUBSECTION (59000-59899)

Divided by service

• Antepartum and Fetal Invasive Services

   Amniocentesis

   Fetal non-stress test

   Fetal monitoring during labor

• Type of delivery

   Vaginal delivery

   C-section

   Delivery after previous C-section

• Abortion

## Gestation

**Fetal gestation:** Approximately 266 days (40 weeks)

**EDD:** Estimated Date of Delivery

• 280 days from last menstrual period (LMP)

### Trimesters

First, LMP to week 12

Second, weeks 13-27

Third, week 28 to EDD

## Global Package and Delivery

Uncomplicated maternity care includes

• Antepartum care = Before delivery

• Delivery

• Postpartum care = After delivery

## Antepartum Care Includes

Initial and subsequent H&P (history and physical)

Blood pressures

Weight

Routine urinalysis

Fetal heart tones

Monthly visits to 28 weeks

Twice-a-month visits, weeks 29 to 36

Weekly visits from week 37 to delivery

Listed in notes preceding 59000

- Services not related to antepartum care are reported separately

  *Example:* Pregnant female with complaint of suspicious mole on left shoulder

  - Visits OB/GYN physician, who provides antepartum care

  - Service regarding mole, not antepartum care, requires good documentation in the maternity record and a specific diagnosis relative to the treatment provided

## Delivery Includes
Admission to hospital with admitting H&P

Management of uncomplicated labor

Vaginal or cesarean section delivery

- Complications coded separately

- Listed in notes preceding 59000

## Postpartum Care Includes
Normal follow-up care for 6 weeks after delivery

- Hospital visits, office visits

- Listed in notes preceding 59000

## Antepartum and Fetal Invasive Services (59000-59076)
**Amniocentesis:** Insertion of needle into pregnant uterus, withdrawal of fluid (59000, 59001)

- Ultrasound guidance with 59000 (76946)

- Ultrasound guidance included with 59001

- Component coding often part of services in subheading

**Fetal services:** Include stress tests, blood sampling, monitoring, and therapeutic procedures

## Excision (59100-59160)
**Postpartum curettage:** Removes remaining pieces of placenta or clotted blood (59160)

**Nonobstetric curettage:** 58120 (Corpus Uteri, Excision)

## Introduction (59200)
**Insertion of cervical dilator:** Used to prepare and soften the cervix for an abortive procedure or delivery (for abortive procedure, see 59855)

Cervical ripening agents may be introduced to prepare cervix

- Is a separate procedure and not reported when part of more major procedure

### Repair (59300-59350)
Only for repairs during pregnancy

Repairs done as a result of delivery or during pregnancy

Episiotomy or vaginal repair by other than attending

Suture closure (cerclage) of cervix or repair of uterus (hysterorrhaphy)

### Routine Global Obstetric Care
Includes delivery, antepartum, and postpartum care

59400, Vaginal delivery

59510, Cesarean delivery

59610, Vaginal delivery after previous cesarean delivery (VBAC)

59618, Cesarean delivery following attempted vaginal delivery after previous cesarean delivery

**Note:** Take care when assigning diagnosis codes for normal versus complicated delivery. ICD-9-CM states specific guidelines for a normal delivery.

### Episiotomies and Use of Forceps
Included in delivery

Not reported separately

### Physician Provides Only Portion of Global Routine Care, Delivery
59409, Vaginal delivery only

59514, Cesarean delivery only

59612, Vaginal delivery only, after previous cesarean delivery

59620, Cesarean delivery only, following attempted vaginal delivery after previous cesarean delivery

## Delivery of Twins

Payers differ on reporting format

- -22 (Unusual Procedural Services)
- -51 (Multiple Procedures)

## Abortion Services (59812-59857)

**Spontaneous:** Happens naturally (for a complete spontaneous abortion, report with a code from the E/M section)

**Incomplete:** Requires medical intervention

**Induced:** Intentional termination of pregnancy

**Missed:** Fetus dies naturally but does not abort during first 22 weeks of gestation

**Septic:** Abortion with infection

**Medical intervention**

- Dilation and curettage or evacuation (suction removal)
- Intra-amniotic injections (saline or urea)
- Vaginal suppositories (prostaglandin)

## ENDOCRINE SYSTEM SUBSECTION (60000-60699)

Nine glands in endocrine system; only four included in subsection

1. Thyroid
2. Parathyroid
3. Thymus
4. Adrenal

**Pituitary and Pineal.** *See* Nervous System subsection

**Pancreas.** Digestive System

**Ovaries and Testes.** Respective genital systems

Divided into two subheadings

- Thyroid Gland
- Parathyroid, Thymus, Adrenal Glands, Pancreas, and Carotid Body

**Carotid Body.** Refers to area adjacent to the bifurcation of the carotid artery

Can be site of tumors

### Thyroid Gland, Excision Category (60100-60281)

- **Lobectomy:** Partial or subtotal (something less than total)
- **Thyroidectomy:** Total (all)

Thyroid, 1 gland with 2 lobes

## NERVOUS SYSTEM SUBSECTION (61000-64999)

Divided anatomically

- Skull, Meninges, and Brain
- Spine and Spinal Cord
- Extracranial Nerves, Peripheral Nerves, and Autonomic Nervous System

### Skull, Meninges, and Brain (61000-62258)

**Categories**

Injection, Drainage, or Aspiration

Twist Drills, Burr Hole(s), or Trephine

**Conditions that Require Openings Into Brain to**

Relieve pressure

Insert monitoring devices

Place tubing

Inject contrast material

### Craniectomy or Craniotomy (61304-61576)

Craniectomy involves removal of portion of skull, at operative site, performed emergently to prevent herniation of brain into the brainstem

Craniotomy—bone flap is replaced after surgery

Codes divided by site and condition for which procedure is performed

### Surgery of Skull Base (61580-61619)

**Skull base:** Area at base of cranium

- Lesion removal from this area very complex

### Surgery of Skull Base Terminology

Approach procedure used to gain exposure of lesion

Definitive procedure is what is done to lesion

Repair/reconstruction procedure reported separately only if extensive repair

### Surgery of Skull Base (61580-61619)

Approach procedure and definitive procedure coded separately

   *Example:* Removal of an intradural lesion using middle cranial fossa approach

- 61590 approach procedure, middle cranial fossa and

- 61608 definitive procedure of intradural resection of lesion

### Cerebrospinal Fluid (CSF) Shunt (62180-62258)

Used to drain fluid

Codes describe

- Placement of devices

- Reprogramming

- Replacement

- Removal of shunting devices

## Spine and Spinal Cord (62263-63746)

Codes divided by condition and approach

Often used are

- Unilateral or bilateral procedures (-50)

- Multiple procedures (-51)

- Radiologic supervision and fluoroscopic guidance reported separately

Includes codes for

- Spinal or steroid anesthetic injections 62310-62319

- Intrathecal or epidural catheter placement/implantation 62350-62355

**Introduction/Injection of Anesthetic Agent (Nerve Block), Diagnostic or Therapeutic Category (64400-64530)**

Includes codes for

- Nerve blocks 64400-64530

  - Bundled when used as anesthesia for procedure

- Paravertebral facet joint injections 64490-64495

- Epidural injections 64479-64484

  - Used to provide pain relief

  - As compared with an epidural catheter placement used for anesthetic purposes

## EYE AND OCULAR ADNEXA SUBSECTION (65091-68899)

Terminology extremely important

- Code descriptions often vary only slightly

Understanding of eye anatomy is necessary for proper coding in this subsection

Codes divided anatomically, e.g.,

- Eyeball

- Anterior segment

- Posterior segment

- Ocular adnexa

- Conjunctiva

Some codes specifically for previous surgery

> *Example:* Insertion of ocular implant, secondary (65130)

Much bundling

> *Example:* Subheading Posterior Segment, Prophylaxis category notes indicate:

- "The following descriptors (67141, 67145) are intended to include all sessions in defined treatment period."

## Cataracts

Method used depends on type of cataract and surgeon preference

> Nuclear cataract: Most common, center of lens (nucleus), due to aging process

> Cortical cataract: Forms in lens of cortex and extends outward; frequent in diabetics

> Subcapsular cataract: Forms at back of lens

Removal and lens replacement (66830-66986)

- Extracapsular cataract extraction (ECCE)

  Removes hard nucleus in one piece

  Removes soft cortex in multiple pieces

  Posterior capsule is left in place, supporting IOL implant

- Intracapsular cataract extraction (ICCE) is total removal

Removes lens and capsule in one piece

- Phacoemulsification

Small incision into eye and introduction of probe

High-frequency waves fragment cataract (extracapsular); then suctioned out

Lens placed through same small incision

### Eyelids (67700-67999)
Blepharotomy (67700)

- Incision into eyelid for drainage of abscess

Blepharoplasty

- Repair of eyelid

- Codes in Integumentary System (15820-15823)

- Codes in Eye and Ocular Adnexa (67916, 67917, 67923, 67924)

- These codes are strictly for entropion and ectropion repair

Selection of code depends on technique used to repair eyelid

- Blepharoplasty codes with specific techniques, 67901-67908

## AUDITORY SYSTEM SUBSECTION (69000-69979)

Codes divided by

- External Ear (69000-69399)

- Middle Ear (69400-69799)

- Inner Ear (69801-69949)

- Temporal Bone, Middle Fossa Approach (69950-69979)

Understanding of ear anatomy is necessary for proper coding in this subsection

External, middle, and inner ear further divided by procedure

- Incision
- Excision
- Removal
- Repair

Myringotomy and tympanostomy

- Eustachian tube connects middle ear to back of throat for drainage

- Fluid collects in middle ear when tube does not function properly

- Prevents air from entering middle ear and pressure builds

- Surgical intervention

Myringotomy (incision into tympanic membrane)

Tympanostomy (placement of PE [pressure equalization] tube)

## OPERATING MICROSCOPE SUBSECTION (+69990)

Employed with procedures using microsurgical techniques

Code in addition to primary procedure performed

Do not report separately when primary procedure description includes microsurgical techniques

*Example:* 15758 Free fascial flap with microvascular anastomosis

Note that following 15758 is the statement:

- "(Do not report code 69990 in addition to code 15758)" indicating to the coder not to report the use of the operating microscope separately

Do not report 69990 when magnifying loupes are used

# ■ RADIOLOGY SECTION (70010-79999)

**Radiology:** Branch of medicine that uses radiant energy to diagnose and treat patients

**Specialist in radiology:** Radiologist (doctor of medicine)

## Radiology Subsections

1. Diagnostic Radiology
2. Diagnostic Ultrasound
3. Radiologic Guidance
4. Breast Mammography
5. Bone/Joint Studies
6. Radiation Oncology
7. Nuclear Medicine

## Procedures

Fluoroscopy views inside of body, projects onto television screen

Live images by which physician can view function, structure, and defects or anomalies within an organ

*Example:* 71034 chest x-ray with fluoroscopy

### Magnetic Resonance Imaging (MRI)

*Example:* 72148 MRI of spinal canal

### Tomography or Computed Axial Tomography (CAT or CT Scan)

*Example:* 70450 tomographic scan of head or brain

### Planes of Body (Figure 3-14)

### Position and Projection

Position = method of positioning patients for examination

Projection path = pathway traveled by x-ray beam

### Component Coding

Three component terms

1. Professional

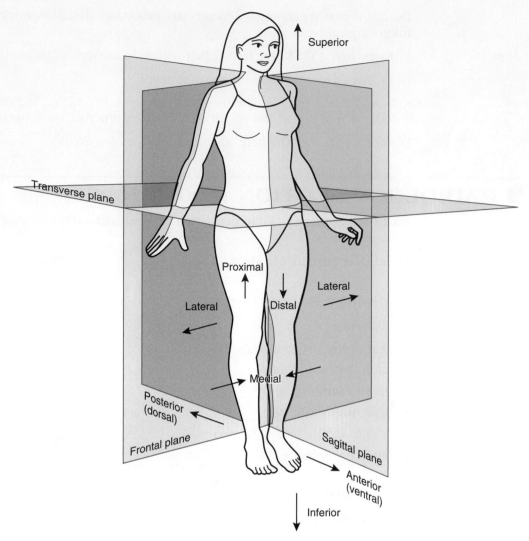

Figure **3-14** Planes of the body.

2. Technical

3. Global

## Professional Component
Physician portion of service, includes

• Supervision of technician

• Interpretation of results, including written report

## Technical Component
• Technologist's services

• Equipment, film, and supplies

## Global Procedure
Both professional and technical portions of radiology service

## Component Modifiers
If only professional component of radiology service provided: -26 to code

If only technical component provided: -TC to code

- -TC HCPCS modifier used with CPT and HCPCS codes

If both professional and technical components of radiology service are provided by physician who owns equipment and facility, pays technician and supplies (global), no modifier is needed

> *Example:* Chest x-ray

- Professional component: 71030-26 (supervision and final report)
- Technical component: 71030-TC (technician, supplies, equipment)
- Global procedure: 71030 (both professional and technical)

Third-party payers usually reimburse

- 40% professional component
- 60% technical component
- 100% global procedure

## Contrast Material

Statement "with contrast" implies injection service included in code

Oral or rectal contrast does not qualify for "with contrast"

Notes indicate codes for components

> *Example:* 75801, Lymphangiography; see 38790 (Injection procedure)

## Interventional Radiologist

Combination radiologist and surgeon

Provides total procedure for cystography with contrast

- Report 74430, x-ray portion
- 51600 for injection procedure
- Plus code for supply of contrast material (e.g., 99070)

## DIAGNOSTIC RADIOLOGY SUBSECTION (70010-76499)

Most standard radiographic procedures

Codes often divided by whether contrast material used

Codes further divided by number of views

> *Example:* 71030, Chest x-ray, complete, minimum of 4 views

Used to:

- Diagnose disease
- Monitor disease process—progression or remission
- Therapeutic procedures (guidance)

## Diagnostic Procedures Include

X-ray

Computerized axial tomography (CAT or CT scan)

Magnetic resonance imaging (MRI)

Angiography

### Computed Axial Tomography (CAT or CT)
X-ray image taken in sections

Computer reconstructs and enhances image

### Magnetic Resonance Imaging (MRI)
Uses magnetic fields to produce an image displayed on computer screen

Codes of same area (e.g., spine) divided by whether or not contrast material used

### Angiography
Used to view vessel obstructions

Dye injected into vessel

Radiologist uses angiography to diagnose vascular conditions

> ***Example:***
>
> • Malformation
>
> • Stroke (cerebrovascular accident, CVA)
>
> • Myocardial infarction (MI)

---

**Remember**
• If fewer than total number of views specified in code provided: Report -52, Reduced Service

---

## DIAGNOSTIC ULTRASOUND SUBSECTION (76506-76999)

Uses high-frequency sound waves to image anatomic structures

Nine subheadings of Diagnostic Ultrasound

Primarily based on anatomy

### A-mode (A = Amplitude)
Technique used to map structure outline in one-dimensional image

### M-mode (M = Motion)
Technique used to display one-dimensional movement of structure

### B-scan (B = Brightness)
Technique used to display two-dimensional movement of tissues and organs

Known as gray scale ultrasound

### Real-Time Scan
Technique used to display both structure and motion with time of organ and tissues in a two-dimensional image

### Extent of Study
Codes often divided on extent of study

*Example:* Extent of scan as follows

- **Complete:** Scans entire body or body region
- **Limited:** Scans part of body, e.g., one organ
- **Follow-up/repeat:** Limited study of part of body that was scanned previously

### Three Locations for Ultrasound Services

**76506-76999:** Radiology codes for diagnostic ultrasound services

**93880-93990:** Medicine codes for non-invasive vascular studies

**93303-93352:** Medicine codes for echocardiography

## RADIOLOGIC GUIDANCE SUBSECTION (77001-77032)

Guidance

- Fluoroscopic
- Computed tomography
- Magnetic resonance
- Other

## BREAST MAMMOGRAPHY SUBSECTION (77051-77059)

*Example:* Computer-aided detection and screening

Some codes specified unilateral/bilateral

## BONE/JOINT STUDIES SUBSECTION (77071-77084)

*Example:* Bone density, bone mineral density, and joint survey

## RADIATION ONCOLOGY SUBSECTION (77261-77799)

Therapeutic use of radiation

Codes both professional and technical services

Subheadings divided based on treatment

Initial consultation, prior to decision to treat, reported with E/M consultation code

- **Outpatient:** 99241-99245
- **Inpatient:** 99251-99255

No reimbursement through CMS for consultation codes

### Clinical Treatment Planning—Professional Component (77261-77299)

Includes

- Interpretation of special testing
- Tumor localization

- Determination of treatment volume
- Choice of treatment method
- Determination of number of treatment ports
- Selection of treatment devices
- Other necessary procedures

Clinical Treatment Planning consists of

- Planning
- Simulation

### Three Levels of Planning (77261-77263, 77299)
1. **Simple:** One treatment area, one port, or one set of parallel ports
2. **Intermediate:** Three or more ports, two separate treatment areas, multiple blocking
3. **Complex:** Complex blocking, custom shielding blocks, tangential ports, special wedges, 3+ treatment areas, special beams

### Simulation (77280-77295)

Determining placement of treatment areas/ports for radiation treatment

Does not include administration of radiation

### Definitions of Simulation
1. **Simple:** 1 treatment area with 1 port or pair of ports
2. **Intermediate:** 3+ ports, 2 separate treatment areas, multiple blocking
3. **Complex:** Tangential ports, 3+ treatment areas, complex blocking
4. **Computer-generated 3-D** reconstruction of volume of tumor and critical structures

### Medical Radiation, Physics, Dosimetry, Treatment Devices, and Special Services (77300-77370)

Decision making services of physicians
- Treatment types
- Dose calculation and placement (dosimetry)
- Development of treatment device

### Stereotactic Radiation Treatment Delivery (77371-77373)

Delivers large radiation dose to specific tumor sites
- Computer(s) map location
- Radiation delivered to one or more sites

### Radiation Treatment Delivery (77401-77423, 77520-77525)

Technical component of actual delivery of radiation

## Information Needed to Code Radiation Treatment Delivery

Amount of radiation delivered

Type of radiation—electron (most common), neutron, or proton

Number of

- Areas treated (single, two, three or more)
- Ports involved (single, three or more, tangential)
- Blocks used (none, multiple, custom)

## Reporting Radiation Treatment Management (77427-77499)

Professional (physician) portion of services, including

- Review port films
- Review dosimetry, dose delivery, treatment parameters
- Treatment set-up
- Patient examination for medical E/M

Report in units of five fractions, unless last 3-4 fractions are at the end of the treatment; then you can count the last 3-4 as an additional fraction

## Clinical Brachytherapy (77750-77799)

Placement of radioactive material into or around site of tumor

- Intracavitary (within body cavity)
- Interstitial (within tissues)

### Source

Radioactive element delivers radiation dose over time

> **Example:** Seeds, ribbons, or capsules

- **Ribbons:** Seeds embedded on tape and inserted into tissue
- Tape is cut to desired length, thereby controlling amount of radiation

## Clinical Brachytherapy Codes Divided Based on

Number of sources applied

- Simple 1-4
- Intermediate 5-10
- Complex 11+

# NUCLEAR MEDICINE SUBSECTION (78000-79999)

Placement of radioactive material into body and measurement of emissions

Used for both diagnosis and treatment

Codes divided primarily on organ system

- Except "Therapeutic," which is for radiopharmaceutical therapies

# ■ PATHOLOGY AND LABORATORY SECTION (80047-89398)

- Organ or Disease-Oriented Panels
- Drug Testing
- Therapeutic Drug Assays
- Evocative/Suppression Testing
- Consultation (Clinical Pathology)
- Urinalysis
- Chemistry
- Hematology and Coagulation
- Immunology
- Transfusion Medicine
- Microbiology
- Anatomic Pathology
- Cytopathology
- Cytogenetic Studies
- Surgical Pathology
- In Vivo (Transcutaneous) Laboratory Procedures
- Other Procedures
- Reproductive Medicine Procedures

## Pathology and Laboratory

Codes for laboratory test only

Specimen collection coded separately

*Example:* Venous blood draw reported 36415 (Surgery section)

## Facility Indicators

Allow additional tests without physician written order

*Example:* Urinalysis positive for bacteria, built-in indicator for culture

### Pathology/Laboratory Caution

Report second or subsequent tests without -51, multiple procedures

## Organ or Disease Oriented Panels (80047-80076)

Groups of tests often ordered together

*Examples:*

- Basic Metabolic Panel
- General Health Panel
- Electrolyte Panel

### Rules of Panels

All tests must have been conducted

Do not use -52, Reduced Service

Additional tests, over those in panel, reported separately

If all tests in panel not done

- List each test separately

- Do not use panel code

## Drug Testing (80100-80104)

Identifies presence or absence of drug—qualitative analysis

Confirmation conducted to double-check results of positive drug test (80102)

Chromatography procedure in which multiple drugs identified (80100)

- Some machines identify all drugs present in 1 procedure

- Others require 2+ procedures to identify 2+ drugs

Code the number of procedures, not number of drugs tested for

> *Example:*
> - 2 procedures to identify 3 drugs = 80100 × 2
> - 1 procedure to identify 3 drugs = 80100

Does not identify amount of drug present

- Only presence or absence

Other than chromatographic method, each procedure, 80104

## Therapeutic Drug Assays (80150-80299)

Reports the presence and amount (quantitative)

Material examined can be from any source

Drugs listed by generic names

> *Example:* Amitriptyline, generic name for brand name Elavil

## Evocative/Suppression Testing (80400-80440)

Measures stimulating (evocative) or suppressing agents

Codes report only technical component of service

Additional services reported

- Supplies and/or drugs used in testing (99070 or HCPCS code)

E/M code reported for physician monitoring of test

### Consultations (Clinical Pathology) (80500, 80502)

At request of physician

Additional information about specimen

Consultant prepares written report

**Levels**

Limited without review of medical record

Comprehensive with review of medical record

## More Consultation Codes (88321-88334)

Surgical Pathology

Used when pathologist either

- Reviews slides, material, or reports

- Provides consultation during surgery

Reported by number of specimens

## Urinalysis (81000-81099)

### Tests on Urine

Method of test

- e.g., tablet, reagent, or dipstick

Reason for test

- e.g., pregnancy

Constituents being tested for

- e.g., bilirubin, glucose

### Equipment Used

Automated or nonautomated

With or without microscope

## Molecular Pathology Procedures (81200-81406)

- 81200-81383 are Tier 1 procedures that report molecular assay

  - More common gene specific procedures

  - Example, breast cancer gene—81211 (BRCA1 or BRCA2)

- 81400-81406 are Tier 2 procedures to report less commonly performed analyses

## Chemistry (82000-84999)

Specific tests on any bodily substances

- Urine

- Blood

- Breath

- Feces

- Sputum

Most are for quantitative (amount of) screenings only

Few report qualitative (presence of) screenings

Samples from different sources reported separately, e.g., blood, feces

Samples taken different times of day reported separately

## Hematology and Coagulation (85002-85999)

Laboratory procedures on blood

> *Example:*

- Complete blood count (CBC)
- White blood cell count (WBC)

Codes divided based on method of

- Blood draw
- Test being conducted

## Immunology (86000-86849)

Identifying immune system conditions caused by antibodies and antigens

> *Example:* Hepatitis C antibody screening

## Tissue Typing (86805-86849)

Compatibility test on tissue

- Match donor to recipient
- Measure/monitor cytotoxic reactions

## Transfusion Medicine (86850-86999)

Blood bank codes

Tests performed on blood or blood products

Identifies

- Collection
- Processing
- Typing

## Microbiology (87001-87999)

### Study of Microorganisms
Identification of organism

Sensitivities of organism to antibiotics

---

**Microbiology Caution:** Many code descriptions are similar to those in Immunology (86000-86849), with only difference being **technique** used

---

## Anatomic Pathology (88000-88099)

Postmortem examinations

- Autopsies

Reports only physician service

Codes divided on extent of exam and type of examination—gross versus gross and microscopic

> *Example:* Gross examination without central nervous system (88000)

## Cytopathology (88104-88199)

Identifies cellular changes

Common laboratory procedures, e.g., Pap smear

Codes divided by

- Type of procedure
- Technique used

## Cytogenetic Studies (88230-88299)

Branch of genetics concerned with cellular abnormalities and pathologic conditions

> *Example:* Chromosomes

## Surgical Pathology (88300-88399)

### Pathology Terminology

Specimen sample of tissue of suspect area

- Basis of reporting determined by number of labeled specimens

Block: Frozen piece of specimen

Section is a slice of frozen block

### Evaluation of Specimens to Determine Disease Pathology

All tissue removed during procedures undergoes pathology evaluation

Operative report usually coded after pathology report received

Pathology reports usually coded with operative report

Unit of measure (88300-88309), specimen

- 2 separately identifiable anus tags, each examined, 88304 × 2
- 1 anus tag examined in 2 different areas of tag, 88304

### Types of Pathologic Examination

**Microscopic:** With microscope

**Gross:** Without microscope

- 88300, only gross exam code
- Other codes are gross and microscopic

### Six levels of surgical pathology

Based on specimen examined (e.g., breast, prostate, lung) and reason for evaluation (e.g., radical procedure for suspected carcinoma)

Levels divided on complexity of examination

> *Example:*
>
> 88305, Colon, Biopsy
>
> 88307, Colon, Segmental Resection, Other than for Tumor
>
> 88309, Colon, Total Resection

### Level I

- Specimen can be accurately diagnosed without microscopic examination

**Level II**
- Gross and microscopic examination is performed on the specimen

**Levels III, IV, V, and VI**
- Include gross and microscopic examination and additional ascending levels of physician work (increasing difficulty)

Based upon method of or need for removal

Same anatomical site can be listed in each level

Additional service codes 88311-88399 are not included in codes 88300-88309

> *Example:* Special stains (88312)

---

# ■ MEDICINE SECTION (90281-99607)

Most procedures noninvasive (not entering body)

Contains invasive procedures

> *Example:* 92973, Percutaneous thrombectomy

Many specialized tests

> *Example:* Audiology and biofeedback

Special lightning bolt icon (⚡)

- Indicates substances pending FDA (Food and Drug Administration) approval

## Immunizations

Often used

Two types of immunizations

- Active and passive

Correct coding includes

- Supply injected
- Administration of injection

### Active—Bacteria or Virus
Bacteria that cause disease made nontoxic (toxoid)

- Injected to build immunity

Small dose active virus injected (vaccine)

- Injected to build immunity

> *Example:* Poliovirus

### Passive Immunization
Does not cause immune response

Contains antibodies against certain diseases—immune globulins

### Immune Globulins (90281-90399)

Identifies immune globulin product

> *Example:* Botulism antitoxin

Report administration separately

### Immune Globulin Codes Divided by

**Type**
e.g., rabies, hepatitis B

**Method**
e.g., intramuscular, intravenous, subcutaneous

**Dose**
e.g., full dose, minidose

## Immunization Administration (90460-90474)

Administration (giving of substance)

- Reported in addition to substance given

- 90460, 90461 Patients through age 18 when counseled regarding immunization

- 90471-90474 Patients over 18

- 90471, +90472 = Percutaneous, intradermal, subcutaneous, or intramuscular injection

- 90473, +90474 = Oral or intranasal

### Methods of Administration

- Percutaneous

- Intradermal

- Subcutaneous

- Intramuscular

- Intranasal

- Oral

### Report Administration for Each Dose—Single or Combination

*Example:* 10-year-old patient receives 3 separate injections

- 90471 administration tetanus

- 90472 administration rubella

- 90472 administration diphtheria

**OR depending on payer:**

- 90471 administration tetanus

- 90472 × 2 administration rubella and diphtheria

### Vaccines, Toxoids (Vaccine Product Codes) (90476-90749)

Many codes age-specific

*Example:* 90658, influenza vaccine, for ages 3 and over

Codes for products for single diseases

*Example:* 90703, tetanus

Codes for combination diseases

*Example:* 90701, diphtheria, tetanus, and whole cell pertussis (DTP)

Some vaccines given on schedule

*Example:* 90634, 2-dose hepatitis A vaccine

- 1st dose, 1st visit

- 2nd dose, 2nd visit

### Caution: There Are Multiple Diphtheria Codes

- 90696-90702, 90719-90723 diphtheria and diphtheria with other substances

*Example:* 90719, diphtheria for IM use

*Example:* 90698, diphtheria, tetanus toxoids, and acellular pertussis (synthetic form of pertussis) (DTaP), *Haemophilus influenza* Type B (HiB), and inactivated poliovirus (IPV) for IM use

---

**Remember**

Third-party payers do not usually require modifier -51 used with Vaccine/Toxoid codes

Rather, depending on payer:

- List each code multiple times or
- Use times (×) symbol and indicate number

---

**Important Reporting Rule.** If vaccine administered during an office visit that was not related to the E/M

- Report E/M service (with modifier -25) + Vaccine + administration

Office visit for vaccine only: Code only vaccine and the administration (no E/M service)

### Routine Vaccinations

Influenza

### Substance (vaccine) 90655-90668

### Administration for patients age 19 years and over

- G0008 HCPCS National Level II for Medicare patients

- 90471/90472

Pneumococcal

### Substance (vaccine) 90732

### Administration

- G0009 HCPCS National Level II for Medicare

- 90471/90472 administration

## Psychiatry (90801-90899)

Psychiatric treatment at same time as E/M service, report

- One code for psychotherapy with E/M

Time major billing factor

- Record indicates session time

Many services provided in partial hospital settings

• Patient in hospital during day, returns home for evenings and weekends

### Codes Divided Based on

Interactive or insight-oriented psychotherapy

Inpatient or outpatient

With or without E/M service

Individual or group

## Biofeedback (90901, 90911)

Used to help patients gain control over body processes

> *Example:* Elevated BP (blood pressure) or manage chronic pain

Patient training in biofeedback by professional

• Continues on own

Services often part psychophysiologic (mind/body) therapy

## Dialysis (90935-90999)

Cleanses blood

• Temporary (non-ESRD [end-stage renal disease])

• Permanent (ESRD)

Two parts to report ESRD dialysis services

• Physician service

• Hemodialysis procedure

### Hemodialysis Service (90935-90940)

Hemodialysis is the procedure

Used for ESRD and non-ESRD

Billed per day for inpatients receiving hemodialysis and also for outpatient non-ESRD

Includes all physician E/M services related to procedure

• Use modifier -25 if separate E/M service provided

### Miscellaneous Dialysis Procedures (90945-90947)

Describes other dialysis procedures

> *Example:* Peritoneal dialysis in which toxins are passively absorbed into dialysis fluid

#### Peritoneal Dialysis (90945-90947)

Services billed on per-day basis for inpatient ESRD patients

### ESRD Physician Services (90951-90970)

Include

• Establishment of dialyzing cycle

- Physician services
- E/M outpatient dialysis visits
- Telephone calls
- Patient management during dialysis

**Reported per month: 90951-90966**
Month is defined as 30 days

Less than full month of service 90967-90970 per day

Codes divided by age and number of encounters

Codes are used to report outpatient dialysis services for ESRD patients

## Other Diagnosis Procedures (90989-90999)
Patients can receive training in self-dialysis (90989, 90993)

Codes divided by complete or partial training program

## Gastroenterology (91010-91299)

For tests and treatments of esophagus, stomach, and intestine

Codes usually reported with E/M or consultation service code

- **Caution:** Many bundled services

## Ophthalmology (92002-92499)

Contains E/M "eye" codes

Definitions for new and established patients same as for E/M section

Codes are for bilateral services

- If only one eye, use modifier -52 (reduced service)

## Special Ophthalmologic Services (92015-92287)

For special evaluations of visual system

Goes beyond those usually provided in evaluation

May be reported in addition to basic visual service

## Special Otorhinolaryngologic Services (92502-92700)

Special treatments and diagnostic services

   *Example:* Nasal function tests (rhinomanometry) or audiometric tests

All hearing tests bilateral unless one ear indicated in description

## Cardiovascular in Medicine Section

Services can be

- Invasive or noninvasive
- Diagnostic or therapeutic

Subheadings

- Therapeutic Services
- Cardiography
- Echocardiography
- Cardiac Catheterization
- Intracardiac Electrophysiologic (EP) Procedures/Studies
- Peripheral Arterial Disease Rehabilitation
- Other Vascular Studies

## Noninvasive Vascular Diagnostic Studies (93880-93990)

Vascular codes for procedures on noncoronary veins and arteries

Include

- Patient care
- Supervision and interpretation (S&I)
- Copy of results

## Pulmonary (94002-94799)

For ventilation management therapies and diagnostic tests

Includes procedure and interpretation of test results

- Additional E/M service reported separately

## Allergy and Clinical Immunology (95004-95199)

Divided into two subheadings

1. Allergy Testing (95004-95075)
2. Allergen Immunotherapy (95115-95199)

### Allergy Testing (95004-95075)

Sensitivity testing using various types of tests

   ***Example:*** Percutaneous, intracutaneous, inhalation

Tests use numerous substances

   ***Example:*** Extracts, venoms, biologics, and foods

Type and number of tests based on physician's judgment

**Coding allergy testing**

Medical record will indicate

- Number of tests
- Type of test
- Method testing

**Allergen Immunotherapy (95115-95199)**

Codes divided into three types of services:

1. Injection only

2. Prescription and injection

3. Provision of antigen (substance) only

Physician service bundled into immunotherapy codes

If separate E/M service provided, report separately

## Neurology and Neuromuscular Procedures (95800-96020)

Contains codes to report tests, such as

- Sleep tests
- Muscle tests (electromyography)
- Range-of-motion measurements
- Electroencephalogram (EEG)
- Electromyography (EMG)
- Analysis and programming of neurostimulators
- Motion analysis
- Functional brain mapping

Many bundled services

Services usually provided in addition to E/M service

## Medical Genetics and Genetic Counseling Services (96040)

Trained genetic counselors assess risk of genetic defects in offspring

Includes

- Pedigree construction
- Obtaining structured genetic history
- Analysis of risk
- Counseling

## Central Nervous System (CNS) Assessments/Tests (96101-96125)

Used to report

- Psychological tests
- Speech/Language assessments
- Developmental progress assessments
- Thinking/Reasoning examinations

Standardized cognitive performance testing

Codes based on per-hour basis

- Includes written report of results

### Health and Behavior Assessment/Intervention (96150-96155)

- Identify psychological behavior, emotional, cognitive, or social factors important to treatment or management of physical health problems

### Hydration, Therapeutic, Prophylactic, Diagnostic Injections and Infusions, and Chemotherapy and Other Highly Complex Drug or Highly Complex Biologic Agent Administration (96360-96549)

**Infusion:** Therapeutic procedure to introduce fluid into body

**Hydration:** Infusion for purpose of rehydration; includes prepackaged fluid

**Injection:** Subcutaneous (Sub-Q), intramuscular (IM), intra-arterial (IA), and intravenous (IV)

Codes report the physician work related to the infusion, hydration, or injection

- Affirmation of treatment plan

- Direct supervision of staff

- Significant, separately identifiable E/M is reported with -25

Codes include

- Local anesthesia

- Intravenous start

- Access to indwelling intravenous catheter or port

- Flush at conclusion

- Standard tubing, syringes, and supplies

Multiple drug administrations in same session are reported separately

Use only one initial code to report multiple infusions or injections or combinations

> For the physician, assign initial code based on primary reason for encounter

> The secondary infusion/injection is reported with a subsequent or concurrent code, unless the protocol requires two separate IV sites

> > **Example:** If three different agents were administered in the same session, report one initial code and two additional sequential codes

> Determination of initial code is based on primary reason for encounter

Some codes are time based, so medical documentation must indicate time infusion begins and ends

Time is defined as the actual time used to administer the drug/substance

### Hydration (96360, 96361)

IV infusion for hydration and includes prepackaged fluid/electrolytes

- 96360 IV infusion for hydration up to 1 hour

- 96361 IV infusion for hydration, each additional hour

- Report for hydration intervals greater than 30 minutes beyond 1 hour
- Start infusion time over if a different bag is started
- Do not report hydration codes when the fluid is used to administer a drug (incidental hydration)
- Do not report hydration codes for infusion of <30 minutes

## Therapeutic, Prophylactic, and Diagnostic Injections and Infusions (Excludes Chemotherapy and Other Highly Complex Drug or Highly Complex Biologic Agent Administration) (96365-96379)

Types of drug administration

- Therapeutic
- Prophylactic
- Diagnostic

Codes divided by administration method

- Subcutaneous
- Intramuscular
- Intra-arterial
- Intravenous push

A push is defined as when a health care professional is needed to administer the drug/substance and monitor the patient or an infusion that takes 15 minutes or less to administer

Also report the substance administered

96365-96368 report therapeutic, prophylactic, or diagnostic IV infusions, other than hydration and chemotherapy

- Typically require direct physician supervision
- Special consideration for preparing, dosing, or disposing
- Trained staff who administer infusion
- Monitoring of vital signs during infusion

## Chemotherapy Administration (96401-96549)

Represents only preparation and administration of chemotherapy

- If separate E/M service provided, report E/M code + -25

Report all drugs/substances separately

Codes are not limited to patients with diagnosis of cancer

Codes also include infusion of antineoplastic agents, monoclonal antibody agents, and biological response modifiers for treatment of noncancer diagnoses

Chemical can be administered (injected) into

- Lesion
- Vein

- Tissue

- Muscle

- Artery

- Cavity

- Nerve

Intravenously injected chemicals: Two methods of delivery of chemical

1. IV push quickly delivers substance/medication into vein (15 minutes or less)

2. IV infusion delivers over longer period of time

Codes often divided by time the infusion/injection procedure takes

> **Example:** 96413 chemotherapy administration, intravenous, infusion up to 1 hour

Report the initial code that represents the main reason why the patient was being treated, even though it might not be the first drug/substance infused

> **Example:** Patient received 1 hour of hydration first, then 2 hours of chemotherapy intravenously. Code the initial chemotherapy infusion 96413 for the first hour of chemo, 96415 for the second hour, then code 96360 for the hydration

Special supplies (e.g., special needles) reported separately using 99070 or HCPCS National Level II code

Report any intra-arterial catheter placement with 36620-36640

Injections with chemotherapy

- Report separately any analgesic or antiemetic (for vomiting)

- Given before or after chemotherapy

---

Use code J0881 to report injection of darbepoetin alfa and J0885 to report injection of epoetin alfa

---

## Photodynamic Therapy (96567-96571)

Used in addition to bronchoscopy or endoscopy codes

Injected agent remains in cancerous cells longer than normal cells

- After agent dissipates from normal cells, patient exposed to laser light

- Agent absorbs light

- Light produces oxygen and cancer cells destroyed

## Special Dermatologic Procedures (96900-96999)

Usually specialized procedures provided on consultation basis

- Separate E/M consultation code would then be appropriate

Treatment of skin conditions:

**Actinotherapy**—with ultraviolet light

**Photochemotherapy**—with light-sensitive chemicals and light rays

## Physical Medicine & Rehabilitation (97001-97799)

Used by physicians and therapists to report a variety of services

### Treatments

Traction

Modalities

Electrical stimulation (used to help heal fractures)

Therapeutic procedures

Gait training

Functional activities

### Patient Training

Codes often have time components

> *Example:* 97761 reports prosthetic training, extremity, each 15 minutes

## Active Wound Care Management (97597-97606)

### Debridement

Debridement without anesthesia with removal of devitalized tissue by different techniques, such as water pressure, sharp selective debridement with scissors, scalpel, and forceps

97597 and 97598 include total surface area of all wounds

Codes based on centimeters treated

Nonselective debridement (97602): Healthy tissue removed along with necrotic tissue, with wet-to-moist dressings, enzymatic or abrasive methods

Negative pressure wound therapy (NPWT) (97605, 97606)

- Vacuuming of drainage and tissue from wound
  - Then negative pressure draws the edges of the wound together
- Application of topical medications/ointments
- Assessment of wound
- Directions to patient on continued care of wound
- Each code for ongoing care reported on per-session basis

## Osteopathic and Chiropractic Services (98925-98943)

Both inpatient and outpatient settings

Physician services bundled into codes

Codes divided by body area

## Education and Training for Patient Self-Management (98960-98962)

- Use of standardized curriculum for education to individual or group for management of illness

### Non–Face-to-Face Nonphysician Services (98966-98969)

Reports nonphysician E/M services using telephone/Internet

Established patient, family member of the patient, or a guardian

98966-98968 telephone E/M services

98969 online E/M services

To report physician services, see 99441-99443

### Special Services, Procedures, and Reports (99000-99091)

Handling and conveyance of laboratory specimens

- 99000-99002

Postoperative follow-up visits included in surgical package

- 99024

Office visits after posted hours or in locations other than office

- 99050-99060

Supplies and materials

- 99070

Hospital mandated on-call services

- 99026, 99027

### Moderate (Conscious) Sedation (99143-99150)

Type of sedation in which the patient can respond to verbal commands

- Appendix G of the CPT manual contains summary of codes that include moderate (conscious) sedation

The bullseye symbol ⊙ indicates these codes in the CPT manual

Do not report sedation services with codes marked with bullseye when sedation is provided by same physician performing procedure

- Second physician provides sedation, report with 99148-99150

Included in service is:

- Patient assessment
- IV establishment
- Administration of agent
- Maintenance of sedation
- Monitoring of vital signs
- Recovery

Codes divided based on patient age (under 5 and 5 and over) and time (30 minutes and each 15 minutes over)

# ◼ HCPCS CODING

> Developed by Centers for Medicare and Medicaid Services (CMS)
>
> • Formerly HCFA
>
> HCPCS developed, 1983
> CPT did not contain all codes necessary for Medicare services reporting

## One of Two Levels of Codes

1. Level I, CPT

2. Level II, HCPCS, also known as national codes

## Phased Out Level III, Local Codes

Developed by Medicare and other carriers for use at local level

Varied by locale

Discontinued October 2002 due to HIPAA code set regulations

Some codes incorporated into HCPCS Level I and Level II

## Level II, National Codes

Codes for wide variety of providers

- Physicians

- Dentists

- Orthodontists

Codes for wide variety of services

- Specific drugs

- Durable medical equipment (DME)

- Ambulance services

Code book published every January, but codes are added and deleted throughout the year and providers are notified through carrier bulletins

## Format

Begins with letter, followed by four digits

> *Example:* E0605, vaporizer, room type

Each letter represents group codes

> *Example:* "J" codes used to report drugs, J0585, onabotulinumtoxina, 1 unit

## Temporary Codes

Certain letters indicate temporary codes

> *Example:* K0552, Supplies for external drug infusion pump

- K codes are temporary codes

### HCPCS National Level II Index

Directs coder to specific codes

Do not code directly from index

Reference main portion of text before assigning code

Alphabetical order

### Table of Drugs

Listed by generic name, not brand name

# ■ AN OVERVIEW OF THE ICD-9-CM

## INTRODUCTION

Morbidity (illness)

Mortality (death)

CM = Clinical Modification

Provides continuity of data

World Health Organization's (WHO) ICD-9 used globally; many countries already use ICD-10

1977: United States develops ICD-9 version

• Has more code subsets

• Data collapse back to ICD-9 for uniformity of data

## Medicare

Medicare Catastrophic Act of 1988

Required use of ICD-9-CM codes for outpatient claims

Act abolished but codes still used

## Uses of ICD-9-CM

Facilities track patient use through codes

Fiscal entities track health care costs

Research

• Health care quality

• Future needs

• Newer cancer center built if patient use warrants

## ICD-9-CM on Insurance Forms

Diagnoses establish medical necessity

Services and diagnoses must correlate

CMS-1500 in Block 21 and 24E (Figure 3-15)

**Office visit:** Croup, 464.4, Block 21, 1; 1 placed in Block 24E, Line 1

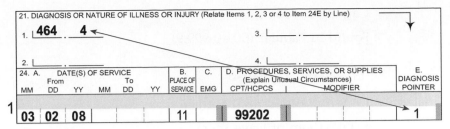

Figure **3-15** Diagnosis code and service must correlate.

---

**Ethics**

Documentation must support diagnosis and match procedures or service performed

**Example:**
- Services provided
- Diagnosis justifies services

If in doubt, check it out; don't make assumptions

**Your Job:** Translate documentation into ICD-9-CM codes

---

## FORMAT OF ICD-9-CM

Volume 1, Diseases, Tabular

Volume 2, Diseases, Index

### Volume 1, Diseases, Tabular

Contains code numbers

001.0-999.9 Diagnosis codes describe condition

V & E codes = supplemental information

### Volume 2, Diseases, Index

Appears first in book

Refers coder to code numbers in Volume 1

Never code directly from Index!

## ICD-9-CM CONVENTIONS

Symbols, abbreviations, punctuation, and notations

NEC: Not elsewhere classifiable

- No more-specific code exists

NOS: Not otherwise specified

- Unspecified in documentation

### [ ] Brackets

Enclose synonyms, alternative wording, or explanatory phrases

Helpful, additional information

Can affect code

Found in Tabular (001.0-999.9)

## ( ) Parentheses

Contain nonessential modifiers

• Take them or leave them

Found in Tabular and Index

Do not affect code assignment

## Colon & Brace

: **Colon:** Tabular, completes statement with one or more modifiers

} **Brace:** Tabular, modifying statements to right of brace

## Lozenge, Section Mark, & Bold Type

□ **Lozenge:** Can indicate code unique to ICD-9-CM

§ **Section mark:** Can be footnote indicator

**Bold type:** Codes and code titles in Tabular, Volume 1

## Italicized Type

All excludes notes

Codes NOT used as principal diagnosis

## Slanted Brackets [ ]

Enclose manifestations of underlying condition

Code underlying condition first

## Includes, Excludes, Use Additional Code

**Includes notes:** In chapter, section, or category

**Excludes notes:** Conditions are coded elsewhere

**Use Additional Code:** Assignment of other code(s) is necessary

## And/With

**And:** Means and/or

**With:** One condition with (in addition to) another condition

## Code, If Applicable, Any Causal Condition First

May be first-listed diagnosis if no causal condition applicable or known

>  ***Example:*** 707.10, Ulcer of lower limb, except decubitus; states
>  • Chronic venous hypertension with ulcer (459.31)

If ulcer caused by chronic venous hypertension

- **First:** 459.31 chronic venous hypertension
- **Second:** 707.10 ulcer of lower limb

## VOLUME 2, INDEX

Nonessential Modifiers: Have no effect on code selection

Enclosed in parentheses

Clarify diagnosis

> ***Example:*** Ileus (adynamic) (bowel) . . .

### Terms

Main terms (bold typeface)

- Subterms
- Indented two spaces to right
- Not bold

### Cross References

Directs you: *see, see also*

- "*see*" directs you to specific term, must be referenced

  > ***Example:*** Panotitis—*see* Otitis media

- "*see also*" directs you to another term for more information, may also be referenced

  > ***Example:*** Perivaginitis (*see also* Vaginitis)

- "*see* category" Volume 1, Tabular, specific information about use of code

  > ***Example:*** Mesencephalitis (*see also* Encephalitis) 323.9; late effect—*see* category 326

### Notes

Define terms

Give further coding instructions

> ***Example:*** Index: "Melanoma"

> **Note:** "Except where otherwise indicated . . ."

Mandatory fifth digits also appear as notes (one reason to never code from Index)

### Eponyms

Disease or syndrome named for person

> ***Example:*** Arnold-Chiari (*see also* Spina bifida)

### Etiology and Manifestation of Disease

**Etiology** = cause of disease

**Manifestation** = symptom

**Combination codes** = etiology and manifestation in one code

## Neoplasm

In Volume 2, Index, locate Neoplasm Table under the alphabetic entry "N"

## SECTIONS

Section 1, Index to Diseases and Injuries

Section 2, Table of Drugs and Chemicals

Section 3, Index to External Causes of Injuries and Poisonings (E Codes)

### Section 1, Index to Diseases

Largest part of Volume 2—Index

First step in coding, locate main term in Index

Subterms indented two spaces to right

May have more than one subterm

### Section 2, Table of Drugs and Chemicals

Located after the Index to Diseases

Contains classification of drugs and substances to identify poisoning and adverse effects

- Adverse effect occurs when substance is taken correctly but patient has a negative reaction to substance

  Condition E-code for drug found under therapeutic column

- Poisoning occurs when substance is incorrectly taken

  ***Example:*** Amoxicillin prescribed for bronchitis causes rash (adverse effect). Rather than one tablet of prescribed amoxicillin, patient takes 4 tablets and nausea results (poisoning)

Drug name placed alphabetically on left under heading "Substance" (Figure 3-16)

First column: "Poisoning" code for substance involved if not related to an adverse effect

E codes identify how poisoning occurred

  ***Example:*** If alkaline antiseptic solution poisoning occurred by accident, E858.7

- Accidental poisoning by alkaline antiseptic solution: 976.6 (substance) and E858.7 (how it occurred)

- Identify agent condition E code for occurrence

- Code any resulting condition (e.g., coma)

### Headings
*Accident:* Unintentional

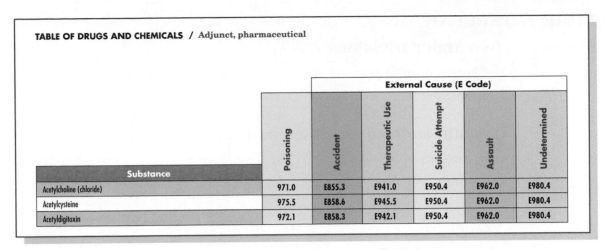

**TABLE OF DRUGS AND CHEMICALS** / **Adjunct, pharmaceutical**

| Substance | Poisoning | External Cause (E Code) | | | | |
|---|---|---|---|---|---|---|
| | | Accident | Therapeutic Use | Suicide Attempt | Assault | Undetermined |
| Acetylcholine (chloride) | 971.0 | E855.3 | E941.0 | E950.4 | E962.0 | E980.4 |
| Acetylcysteine | 975.5 | E858.6 | E945.5 | E950.4 | E962.0 | E980.4 |
| Acetyldigitoxin | 972.1 | E858.3 | E942.1 | E950.4 | E962.0 | E980.4 |

Figure **3-16** Section 2, Table of Drugs and Chemicals. (Modified from Buck CJ: *2012 ICD-9-CM, Volumes 1, 2, and 3, Professional Edition*, St. Louis, 2012, Saunders.)

*Therapeutic:* Correct dosage, correctly administered, with adverse effects

*Suicide attempt:* Self-inflicted

*Assault:* Intentionally inflicted by another person

*Undetermined:* Unknown cause

## Section 3, E Codes

Index to External Causes of Injuries and Poisonings

Provides additional information about the nature of the injury/poisoning and locality

Never principal (inpatient), sole, or primary (outpatient) diagnosis

Separate Index to External Causes

- Alphabetical, main terms in bold
- Subterms are indented 2 spaces to right under main term

## A Word of Caution about the Index

Some words in Index do not appear in Tabular—saves space

Exact word may not be in code description in Tabular

- Usually found in Index
- Must locate the term in the Index, then locate in Tabular
- Additional coding instructions found in Tabular

## VOLUME 1, TABULAR

### Two Major Divisions

1. Classification of Diseases and Injuries (codes 001.0-999.9)

2. Supplementary Classification (V codes and E codes)

### Classification of Diseases and Injuries

Main portion of ICD-9-CM

Codes from 001.0 to 999.9

Most chapters are body systems

> *Example:*

- Digestive System
- Respiratory System

### Divisions of Classification of Diseases and Injuries

Chapters 1 through 17

- *Section:* A group of related conditions
- *Category:* Represents single disease/condition
- *Subcategory:* More specific
- *Subclassification:* Most specific

---

**Remember**

Assign to highest level of specificity, based on documentation

If 4-digit code exists, do not report 3-digit code

If 5-digit code exists, do not report 4-digit code

---

# ■ USING THE ICD-9-CM

Guidelines developed by Cooperating Parties

- American Hospital Association (AHA)
- American Health Information Management Association (AHIMA)
- Centers for Medicare and Medicaid Services (CMS)
- National Center for Health Statistics (NCHS)

## GENERAL GUIDELINES

Appendix A of this text contains resources to view the *ICD-9-CM Official Guidelines for Coding and Reporting*

You must know and follow the Guidelines when assigning diagnoses codes

- All certification examinations adhere to the Guidelines
- As you review this ICD-9-CM material, locate the information in the Guidelines of your ICD-9-CM
- In this way, you will become familiar with the location of Guidelines content to be able to quickly reference the Guidelines during the examination

Outpatient coders primarily use Sections I and IV

Diagnostic Coding and Reporting Guidelines do NOT cover all situations

- Outpatient coders also use many Section II and III guidelines

## STEPS TO DIAGNOSIS CODING

Identify MAIN term(s) in diagnosis

Locate MAIN term(s) in Index

Review subterms

Follow cross-reference instructions (e.g., *see, see also*)

Verify code(s) in Tabular

- Read Tabular notes

- Code to highest specificity

- Never code from Index!

### Level of Detail in Coding

Assign diagnosis (dx) to highest level of specificity

Do NOT use 3-digit code if there is 4th

Do NOT use 4-digit code if there is 5th

### Acute and Chronic Conditions

Exists alone or together

May be separate or combination codes

If two codes, code acute first

    ***Example:*** acute (577.0) and chronic (577.1) pancreatitis

Combination code: Both acute and chronic condition

- Diarrhea (acute) (chronic) 787.91, Acute and subacute bacterial endocarditis 421.0

- Otitis acute, chronic, and subacute 382.9

### Combination Code

Always use combination code if one exists

    ***Example:*** encephalomyelitis (dx) due to rubella (manifestation), 056.01

### Multiple Coding for Single Condition

Etiology (cause)

Manifestation (symptom)

- Slanted brackets *[ ]*

    ***Example:*** Retinopathy, diabetic 250.5 *[362.01]*

- Must check Tabular notes to assign correct 5th digit for diabetes

- Tabular: 362.0, Diabetic retinopathy, instructs to "Code first diabetes 249.5, 250.5"

# SELECTION OF PRIMARY DIAGNOSIS

Condition for encounter

Documented in medical record

Condition that is responsible for services provided

Also list coexisting condition(s) or comorbidity(ies)

Diagnosis and procedure MUST correlate

- Medical necessity established
- No correlation = no reimbursement

## Codes in Brackets

Never sequence as primary diagnosis

Always sequence in order listed in Index

### *Example:*

- Index lists: Diabetes, gangrene 250.7 *[785.4]*
- 785.4 = gangrene
- Tabular, 785.4 indicates "Code first any associated underlying condition: diabetes (250.7X)..."
- Code first diabetes, then gangrene
- 250.7X = diabetes (X = 5th digit)
- 785.4 = gangrene

## Two or More Interrelated Conditions

When two or more interrelated conditions exist and either could be primary diagnosis, either may be sequenced first

### *Example:* Patient with mitral valve stenosis and coronary artery disease (two interrelated conditions)

- Either can be primary diagnosis and sequenced first
- Resource intensiveness affects choice

# V CODES

Located after 999.9 in Tabular

Two digits before decimal (e.g., V10.10)

Index for V codes, Index to Diseases and Injuries

**Main terms:** contraception, counseling, dialysis, status, examination

## Uses of V Codes

Not sick BUT receives health care (e.g., vaccination)

Services for known disease/injury (e.g., chemotherapy)

A circumstance/problem that influences patient's health BUT NOT current illness/injury

> *Example:* Organ transplant status

> *Example:* Birth status and outcome of delivery (newborn)

Section I.C.18.e. of the *Official Guidelines for Coding and Reporting* contains the V Code Table

- Identifies how V codes are listed (first, first/additional, additional only)

---

**Special Note about "History of"**
Index to Disease, MAIN term "History"
Entries between "family" and "visual loss V19.0" = "Family history of"
Entries before "family" and after "visual loss V19.0" = "Personal history of"

---

## History V Code Categories in Tabular

V10 Personal history of malignant neoplasm

V11 Personal history of mental disorder

V12 Personal history of certain other diseases

V13 Personal history of other diseases

Except: V13.4 Personal history of arthritis, and V13.6 Personal history of congenital malformations. These conditions are life-long so are not true history codes

V14 Personal history of allergy to medicinal agents

V15 Other personal history presenting hazards to health

Except: V15.7 Personal history of contraception

V16 Family history of malignant neoplasm

V17 Family history of certain chronic disabling diseases

V18 Family history of certain other specific conditions

V19 Family history of other conditions

## LATE EFFECTS

Late effect residual of (remaining from) previous illness/injury, e.g., burn that leaves scar

Residual coded first (scar)

Cause (burn) coded second

Late effect codes are not in a separate chapter; rather, throughout Tabular

Reference the term "Late" in the Index

There is no time limit on developing a residual

There may be more than one residual

*Example:* Patient has a stroke (434.91) and develops paralysis on dominant side (hemiparesis, 438.21) and loss of ability to communicate (aphasia, 438.11)

## DIAGNOSTIC CODING AND REPORTING GUIDELINES FOR OUTPATIENT SERVICES

Physician's office

Hospital-based outpatient services

Part of *ICD-9-CM Official Guidelines for Coding and Reporting*, Section IV

### Guideline A

The term *first-listed diagnosis* is used rather than *principal diagnosis*

Outpatient Surgery: Reason for surgery

Observation Stay: Medical condition that occasioned admission

### Guideline B

Use codes 001.0 through V91.99 to code dx, symptoms, conditions, problems, complaints, or other reason(s) for visit

### Guideline C

Documentation should describe patient's condition, using terminology that includes specific diagnoses as well as symptoms, problems, or reasons for encounter

### Guideline D

Selection of codes 001.0 through 999.9 (Chapters 1-17) will frequently be used to describe reason for encounter

### Guideline E

Codes that describe symptoms and signs, as opposed to diagnoses, acceptable for reporting purposes when an established dx has NOT been confirmed by physician

### Guideline F

V codes deal with encounters for circumstances other than disease or injury

*Example:* Well-baby checkup (V20.2)

### Guideline G

Codes have either three, four, or five digits

4th and/or 5th digit codes provide greater specificity

Three-digit code used ONLY if there is NO 4th or 5th digit

Where 4th and/or 5th digits provided, must be assigned

Diagnoses NOT coded to full digits available are invalid

## Guideline H

List first code for dx, condition, problem, or other reason for encounter/visit shown in medical record to be chiefly responsible for services provided

List additional codes that describe any coexisting conditions

## Guideline I

Do NOT code diagnoses documented as probable, suspected, questionable, ruled out, or working diagnoses

Rather, code condition(s) to highest degree of certainty for that encounter/visit, such as symptoms, signs, abnormal test results, or other reason for visit

*Example:* Cough and fever, probably pneumonia

- Code as cough (786.2) and fever (780.6X) (in this order)

## Guideline J

Chronic diseases treated on an ongoing basis may be coded and reported as many times as patient receives treatment and care for condition(s)

## Guideline K

Code all documented conditions that coexist at time of visit, that require or affect patient care, treatment, or management

Do NOT code conditions previously treated, no longer existing

"History of" codes (V10-V19) may be used as secondary codes if

- Impacts current care or treatment

## Guidelines L and M

For patients receiving diagnostic or therapeutic services ONLY

Sequence first

- Diagnosis,
- Condition,
- Problem, or
- Other reason shown in medical record to be chiefly responsible for encounter

Codes for other diagnoses (e.g., chronic conditions)

- May be sequenced as secondary diagnoses

   **Exception:**

Patients receiving chemotherapy (V58.11), radiation therapy (V58.0), or rehabilitation (code depends on type)

- V code first; dx or problem for which service being performed second

## Guideline N

For patients receiving preoperative evaluations ONLY

- Code from category V72.8 (Other specified examinations)

- Assign secondary code for reason for surgery
- Code also any findings related to preoperative evaluation

### Guideline O

Code dx which required ambulatory surgery

If postoperative dx different

- Code postoperative dx

### Guideline P

Code routine prenatal visits with no complications

- V22.0 (Supervision of normal first pregnancy)
- V22.1 (Supervision of other normal pregnancy)
- Do NOT use these codes with pregnancy complication codes

## ICD-9-CM, CHAPTER 1, INFECTIOUS AND PARASITIC DISEASES

Divided based on etiology (cause of disease)

### Many Combination Codes

*Example:* 112.0 candidiasis infection of mouth, which reports both organism and condition with one code

### Multiple Codes

Sequencing must be considered

- UTI due to *Escherichia coli*
- 599.0 (UTI) etiology
- 041.4X *(E. coli)* organism (in this order)

### Human Immunodeficiency Virus

Code HIV or HIV-related illness ONLY if stated as confirmed in diagnostic statement

- 042 HIV or HIV-related illness
- V08 Asymptomatic HIV status
- 795.71 Nonspecific HIV serology

### Previously Diagnosed HIV-Related Illness

Code prior dx HIV-related disease 042 (HIV)

NEVER assign these patients to:

- V08 (Asymptomatic) or
- 795.71 (Nonspecific serologic evidence of HIV)

## HIV Sequencing

Sequence first that reason most responsible for encounter, if HIV (042)

Followed by secondary dx that affects encounter or patient care

## HIV and Pregnancy

This is an exception to HIV sequencing

During pregnancy, childbirth, or puerperium, code

- 647.6X (Other specified infectious and parasitic diseases), followed by 042 (HIV)

Asymptomatic HIV during pregnancy, childbirth, or puerperium

- 647.6X (Other specified infections and parasitic diseases) and

- V08 (Asymptomatic HIV infection status)

- Reporting asymptomatic HIV varies by state

  - Check the state's reporting laws

## Inconclusive Laboratory Test for HIV

795.71 (Inconclusive serologic test for HIV)

- Reporting inconclusive laboratory HIV tests varies by state

  - Check the state's reporting laws

## HIV Screening

Code V73.89 (Screening for other specified viral disease)

- Patient in high-risk group for HIV

- V69.8 (Other problems related to lifestyle)

Patients returning for HIV screening results = V65.44 (HIV counseling)

---

**Caution**

Incorrectly applying these HIV coding rules can cause patient hardship and may be a violation of law

- Insurance claims for patients with HIV usually need patient's written agreement for disclosure

---

## Section I.C.1.b. Septicemia, Systemic Inflammatory Response Syndrome (SIRS), Sepsis, Severe Sepsis, and Septic Shock

Sepsis: Assign systemic infection code as first listed when sepsis is present

- Assign a sepsis code as secondary when sepsis develops during encounter

Septicemia/Sepsis: Usually a 038 septicemia code and a 995.9x SIRS code (in this order)

- Code the organ system dysfunction followed by the SIRS (e.g., 518.81 respiratory failure followed by 995.92)

Septic Shock: Organ dysfunction associated with severe sepsis

- Code underlying systemic infection (e.g., 038.xx) followed by the SIRS code (995.92), followed by septic shock (785.52)

## ICD-9-CM, CHAPTER 2, NEOPLASMS

Two steps for coding neoplasms

- Incorrectly applying these neoplasm codes can also cause patient hardship

### Index

1. Locate histologic type of neoplasm (e.g., sarcoma, melanoma)
   - Review all instructions
2. Locate code identified by body site
   - Usually in Neoplasm Table in Index under "N"
   - Neoplasm Table divided into columns:
     · Malignant (Primary, Secondary, Ca in situ)
     · Benign
     · Uncertain behavior
     · Unspecified

***Example:*** Pathology report confirmed diagnosis stated in operative report of primary malignant neoplasm of the bladder neck. ICD-9-CM Index, Neoplasm Table, bladder, neck, under Primary column, 188.5. Code then referenced in Tabular to ensure accurate assignment.

Treatment directed at malignancy: Neoplasm is principal dx

#### Except for Chemotherapy or Radiotherapy:

- Therapy (treatment) followed by neoplasm code
  · Chemotherapy: V58.11
  · Radiotherapy: V58.0

Surgical removal of neoplasm and subsequent chemotherapy or radiotherapy

- Code malignancy as principal dx

Surgery to determine extent of malignancy

- Code malignancy as principal dx
  - V10, "Personal history of malignant neoplasm" if
    · Neoplasm was previously destroyed
    · No longer being treated

If patient receives treatment for secondary neoplasm (metastasis)

- Secondary neoplasm is documented principal dx
- Even though primary is still present

Patient treated for anemia or dehydration due to neoplasm or therapy code

- Anemia or dehydration followed by neoplasm

Patient admitted to repair complication of surgery for an intestinal malignancy

- Complication principal dx
- Complication is reason for encounter
- Malignancy secondary dx

Patient receiving chemotherapy or radiotherapy post-op removal of neoplasm

- Code: Therapy followed by active neoplasm
- Do NOT report H/O (history of) neoplasm

## ICD-9-CM, CHAPTER 3, ENDOCRINE, NUTRITIONAL, AND METABOLIC DISEASES AND IMMUNITY DISORDERS

### Disorders of Other Endocrine Glands

Diabetes Mellitus 250 coded frequently

Subterms in Index often have two codes

> ***Example:***
>
> - Diabetic iritis 250.5X for diabetes (etiology)
> - *[364.42]* for iritis (manifestation)

5th digit indicates type of diabetes

> 0  type II or unspecified type, not stated as uncontrolled
>
> > Fifth-digit 0 is for use for type II patients, even if the patient requires insulin
>
> 1  type I [juvenile type], not stated as uncontrolled
>
> 2  type II or unspecified type, uncontrolled
>
> > Fifth-digit 2 is for use for type II diabetic patients, even if the patient requires insulin
>
> 3  type I [juvenile type], uncontrolled

V58.67 used in addition to diabetes code to report long-term use of insulin

> If type is not indicated, code type II diabetes
>
> > Patient with type II diabetes can receive insulin for periods when diabetes is uncontrolled
> >
> > Type I diabetic is one who is insulin-dependent

### Other Metabolic and Immunity Disorders Section

Disorders such as gout and dehydration

Disorders often have many names

> ***Example:*** 242.0X Toxic diffuse goiter, also known as
>
> - Basedow's disease
> - Graves' disease
> - Primary thyroid hyperplasia

## ICD-9-CM, CHAPTER 4, DISEASES OF BLOOD AND BLOOD-FORMING ORGANS

Short chapter with 10 sections

Includes anemia, blood disorders, coagulation defects

Often used code, anemia

Many different types of anemia

- Hereditary hemolytic (282)

- Iron deficiency (280)

- Acquired hemolytic (283)

- Aplastic (284)

- Other and Unspecified (285)

Multiple coding often necessary

Identify underlying disease condition

## ICD-9-CM, CHAPTER 5, MENTAL, BEHAVIORAL AND NEURODEVELOPMENTAL DISORDERS

Includes codes for

- Personality disorders

- Stress disorders

- Neuroses

- Psychoses

- Sexual deviation/dysfunction, etc.

5th digit = status of episode

> **Example:** 304.2, cocaine dependence, is assigned the following 5th digits:

- 0 unspecified (episode)

- 1 continuous

- 2 episodic

- 3 in remission

## ICD-9-CM, CHAPTER 6, DISEASES OF NERVOUS SYSTEM AND SENSE ORGANS

Central Nervous System

Peripheral Nervous System

Disorders of Eye

Diseases of Ear

Pain—Category 338

Acute or chronic pain not elsewhere classified due to:

- Trauma
- Neoplasm
- Postoperative
- Psychosocial dysfunction

Principal/Primary diagnosis

- When definitive diagnosis not established
- Pain management is reason for encounter/admission

## ICD-9-CM, CHAPTER 7, DISEASES OF CIRCULATORY SYSTEM

Three types of hypertension

1. Malignant accelerated, severe, poor prognosis
2. Benign continuous, mild (BP elevated) controllable
3. Unspecified NOT indicated as either malignant or benign

Hypertension (401-405)

Hypertension table located in Index of ICD-9-CM

- Under "H," Hypertension
- Codes divided based on type (Malignant, Benign, Unspecified)

### Hypertension, Essential, or NOS

Assign hypertension (arterial, essential, primary, systemic, NOS) to 401

4th digit indicates type

- 0 Malignant
- 1 Benign
- 9 Unspecified

### Hypertension with Heart Disease

#### 402 Category
Certain heart conditions when stated "due to hypertension" or implied ("hypertensive")

Add 4th digit for type

Use additional code to specify type of heart failure (428)

### Hypertensive Chronic Kidney Disease

Cause-and-effect relationship assumed in chronic kidney disease (CKD) with hypertension

Category 403, Hypertensive chronic kidney disease, used when following present:

- Chronic kidney disease (585.X)

5th digit assignment required for stage of CKD

- 0 CKD stage I through IV

- 1 CKD stage V or end stage

Use additional code to identify stage of chronic kidney disease

## Hypertensive Heart and Chronic Kidney Disease

Assign 404 when both hypertensive chronic kidney disease and hypertensive heart disease stated

Assume cause-and-effect relationship

Assign 5th digit for mention kidney stage of chronic disease and/or heart failure

- Use additional code to specify type of heart failure (428)

## Hypertensive Cerebrovascular Disease

Code

- Cerebrovascular disease (430-438)

- Type of hypertension (401-405)

## Hypertensive Retinopathy

Code

- Hypertensive retinopathy (362.11)

- Type of hypertension (401-405)

## Hypertension, Secondary

Hypertension caused by an underlying condition

- Code

  - Underlying condition

  - Type of hypertension (405)

## Hypertension, Transient

Transient hypertension: Temporary elevated BP

Do NOT assign 401-405, Hypertensive Disease

- Hypertension dx is NOT established

- Use

  - 796.2, Elevated blood pressure or

  - 642.3X, Transient hypertension of pregnancy

## Hypertension, Controlled

Hypertension controlled by therapy

- Assign code from 401-405

### Hypertension, Uncontrolled

Untreated or uncontrolled hypertension

- Assign code from 401-405

Documentation must state malignant hypertension to use 404

### Elevated Blood Pressure

Elevated blood pressure coded 796.2

- Elevated BP reading without hypertension is dx

- Hypertension NOT stated, NOT coded to 401

## ICD-9-CM, CHAPTER 8, DISEASES OF RESPIRATORY SYSTEM

Watch for "Use additional code to identify infectious organism"

Some codes indicate specific organism and do not need an additional code

Respiratory failure sequencing

If the respiratory failure is due to an acute condition (such as MI [myocardial infarction]) or acute exacerbation of a chronic condition (such as COPD [chronic obstructive pulmonary disease]), sequence the acute condition first

**Example:** MI (acute condition) and respiratory failure

- Sequence MI first and respiratory failure second

If the respiratory failure (acute condition) is due to a chronic nonrespiratory condition (such as myasthenia gravis), sequence the respiratory failure first

**Example:** Acute respiratory failure (acute) and myasthenia gravis (chronic)

- Sequence acute respiratory failure first and myasthenia gravis second

### Acute Respiratory Infection Section

Frequently used codes, such as

- Common cold (460, acute nasopharyngitis)

- Sore throat (462, acute pharyngitis)

- Acute tonsillitis (463)

- Bronchitis (490-491)

- Acute upper respiratory infection (465, URI)

- Influenza (487, flu)

- Pneumonia (480-486)

## ICD-9-CM, CHAPTER 9, DISEASES OF DIGESTIVE SYSTEM

Mouth to anus + accessory organs

Extensive subcategories

- 574 Cholelithiasis (10 subcategories)

- Each has 5th digit subclassification

Commonly used codes

- Ulcers (531-534)
  - Gastric (531)
  - Duodenal (532)
  - Peptic (533)
  - Gastrojejunal (534)
- Hernias (550-553)

## ICD-9-CM, CHAPTER 10, DISEASES OF GENITOURINARY SYSTEM

Commonly used codes

- Urinary tract infection (599.0)
- Inflammation of prostate (601.X)
- Disorders of female genitalia organs (625-627)

Stages of chronic kidney disease

- Stage I: Blood flow through kidney increases, kidney enlarges (585.1)
- Stage II: (mild) Small amounts of blood protein (albumin) leak into urine (microalbuminuria) (585.2)
- Stage III: (moderate) Albumin and other protein losses increase. Patient may develop high blood pressure and kidney loses ability to filter waste (585.3)
- Stage IV: (severe) Large amounts of urine pass through kidney, blood pressure increases (585.4)
- Stage V: Ability to filter waste nearly stops (585.5)
- End-stage renal failure (585.6)

    When documentation indicates chronic renal disease (CKD) and ESRD, report ESRD

- Unspecified 585.9

Status post kidney transplant, assign V42.0

- Patient may still have CKD

## ICD-9-CM, CHAPTER 11, COMPLICATIONS OF PREGNANCY, CHILDBIRTH, AND THE PUERPERIUM

Extensive multiple coding with many 5th digit assignments and notes

Admission for pregnancy, complication

- Obstetric complication = primary dx

Chapter 11 ICD-9-CM codes take precedence over codes from other chapters

Codes 640-676.9 share same 5th digit subclassification

- Denotes current episode of care
- 0 Unspecified as to episode of care or not applicable
- 1 Delivered, with or without mention of antepartum condition

- 2 Delivered, with mention of postpartum complication
- 3 Antepartum condition or complication
- 4 Postpartum condition or complication

## General Rules

Not all encounters are pregnancy-related

> ***Example:*** Pregnant woman, broken ankle (medial malleolus, open)

- Broken ankle (824.1)
- V22.2 Pregnant state incidental; must be documented in medical record that condition being treated not affecting pregnancy

## Complications of Pregnancy, Childbirth, and Puerperium

Chapter 11 codes (630-679)

Used only on mother's medical record

Not on newborn medical record

## Selection of Primary Diagnosis

Routine prenatal visits, no complications:

- V22.0, Supervision, normal **first** pregnancy or
- V22.1, Supervision, **other** normal pregnancy

Prenatal outpatient visits for high-risk pregnancies:

- V23, Supervision of high-risk pregnancy

## Fifth Digit

All categories EXCEPT 650 (Normal delivery)

Requires 5th digit for

- Antepartum
- Postpartum
- If delivery has occurred

Appropriate 5th digit listed under each code

> ***Example:*** 640.0, Threatened abortion

- 0 unspecified episode
- 1 delivered with or without complication
- 3 antepartum condition or complication

Note that NOT all 5th digits are applicable (640.0, cannot assign 2 or 4)

## Postpartum Period

After delivery +6 weeks

### Abortions

Codes 634-637 require 5th digits

- 0 unspecified

- 1 incomplete; POC (product of conception) NOT expelled

- 2 complete; all POC expelled prior to care

### Abortions with Liveborn Fetus
Attempted abortion results in liveborn fetus

- 644.21 (Early onset of delivery)

- Use V27.X (Outcome of delivery)

- Attempted abortion code also assigned

## ICD-9-CM, CHAPTER 12, DISEASES OF SKIN AND SUBCUTANEOUS TISSUE

### Skin

Epidermis

Dermis

Subcutaneous tissue

Infectious skin/subcutaneous tissue

Scar tissue

### Accessory Organs

Sweat glands

Sebaceous glands

Nails

Hair and hair follicles

Other

### Multiple Codes Often Necessary

> **Example:** Cellulitis due to *Staphylococcus,* report

- Cellulitis 682.X

- Staph 041.X

## ICD-9-CM, CHAPTER 13, DISEASES OF MUSCULOSKELETAL SYSTEM AND CONNECTIVE TISSUE

Bone

Bursa

Cartilage

Fascia

Ligaments

Muscle

Synovia

Tendons

### Chapter 13 Sections

Extensive notes and 5th digits

- Arthropathies (joint disease) and related disorders

- Dorsopathies (curvature of spine)

- Rheumatism, Excluding Back

- Osteopathies, Chondropathies, and Acquired Musculoskeletal Deformities

## ICD-9-CM, CHAPTERS 14 AND 15, CONGENITAL ANOMALIES AND CONDITIONS ORIGINATING IN PERINATAL PERIOD

Congenital Anomalies (abnormalities at birth), 740-759

Conditions Originating in Perinatal Period

- Perinatal period through 28th day following birth

- Codes can be used after 28th day if documented that condition originated during perinatal period

Chapter 17 codes are only for the newborn record; never on the maternal record

Assign V30-V39 as first listed according to type of birth

## ICD-9-CM, CHAPTER 16, SYMPTOMS, SIGNS, AND ILL-DEFINED CONDITIONS

Do NOT code a sign or symptom if

- Definitive dx made (symptoms are part of disease)

Used only if no specific dx made

## ICD-9-CM, CHAPTER 17, INJURY AND POISONING

### Section Examples

Fractures

Dislocations

Sprains and Strains

Intracranial Injury

Internal Injury

Crushing Injury

Foreign Body

Burns

Late Effects

Poisoning

Acute fracture care vs. aftercare

Use aftercare codes after completion of active treatment

- Cast change/removal (V53.7)

- Removal of external/internal devices (V54.0X)

- Medication adjustments

- Follow-up visits following fracture treatment

## E Codes

Provide supplemental information

Never principal diagnosis

### Index and Tabular

E code Index located in Section III

   Directly before the Tabular

   Not in the Index to Disease, Volume 2

E codes are located after the V codes in the Tabular

Identify

- Cause of an injury or poisoning

- Intent (unintentional or intentional)

- Place it occurred

### General E Code Guidelines

Use with any code in Volume 1

Initial encounter

- Use E code

Subsequent encounter

- Use late effects E codes, if appropriate

### Intent

Unknown, Undetermined (E980-E989)

Unspecified, Undetermined (E980-E989)

Questionable, Undetermined (E980-E989)

### Table of Drugs and Chemicals

Alphabetic listing with codes (see Figure 3-16)

Do NOT code directly from Table

Always reference Tabular

#### Two or more substances involved

If two or more substances involved

- Code each unless combination code exists

- Code substance more closely related to principal dx

- Include one code from each category (cause, intent, place)

Interaction of drug(s) and alcohol

- Use poisoning and E codes for both

**Unknown or suspected intent**
Unknown

Unspecified

Questionable

**Undetermined cause**
Intent known, cause unknown, use

- E928.9, Unspecified accident

- E958.9, Suicide and self-inflicted injury by unspecified means

- E968.9, Assault by unspecified means

**Late effects of external cause**
Should be used with late effect of a previous injury/poisoning

Should NOT be used with related current injury code

## Coding of Burns
**Multiple injuries and burns**
Sequence most severe injury first (physician determined)

**Current burns**
Sequence highest-degree burn first

Current burns (940-948) classified by

- Depth (severity)

- Extent (% body surface)

- Agent (if necessary)

**Depth of burn (Fig. 3-17)**
1st degree: Erythema

2nd degree: Blistering

3rd degree: Full-thickness involvement

**Burns classified**
- According to extent of body surface involved

**Category 948**
- 4th digits = % body surface involved

- 5th digits = % body surface involved in 3rd-degree burns

- Rule of Nines applies

**Burn Example:** 3rd-degree burn of abdomen (10%) and 2nd-degree burn of thigh (5%) by hot water

- 942.33 Burn, abdomen, 3rd degree

- 945.26 Burn, thigh, 2nd degree

Figure **3-17** Degree of burns.

- 948.11 15% total burn area and 10% 3rd degree
- E924.0 Burn by hot liquid

**Coding for multiple injuries**
Separate code for each injury

Sequence most serious injury first

**Vessel and nerve damage**
Code primary injury first

- Use additional code if minor nerve damage

Primary injury = nerve damage

- Code nerve damage first

**Multiple fractures**
Same coding principles as multiple injuries

Code multiple fractures by site

Sequenced by severity

**Fractures**
Not indicated as closed or open = closed

Same bone fractured AND dislocated:

- Code fracture ONLY (highest level of injury)

# Coding Challenge

Make sure to check
**evolve**
learning system
**for the latest
content updates**

# EXAMINATIONS

You have three opportunities to practice taking an examination:

- Pre-Examination (before study)

- Post-Examination (after study)

- Final Examination (at the end of your complete program of study)

You should have a current edition of the following texts:

- ICD-9-CM (*International Classification of Diseases,* 9th Edition, Clinical Modification), Volumes 1 and 2

- HCPCS (*Healthcare Common Procedure Coding System*)

- CPT (*Current Procedural Terminology*)

No other reference material is allowed for any of the examinations.

- For the Pre-Examination and Post-Examination, you will need a computer and the three coding references listed above (ICD-9-CM [Vols. 1 and 2], HCPCS, CPT).

- For the Final Examination, you will need paper, pencils, and an eraser, along with the three coding references.

- Each organization's certification examination has different scoring requirements, but as you take the examinations with this text, you should strive for 80% to 90% on the Post-Examination and 70% as a minimum on the Final Examination. AAPC's standard for passing is 70%.

**NOTE:** To enable the learner to calculate an examination score, minimums have been identified as "passing" within this text; however, this may or may not be the percentage identified by the American Academy of Professional Coders as a "passing" grade. It is your responsibility to review all certification information published by the American Academy of Professional Coders as they are the definitive source for information regarding the CPC® certification examination.

**NOTE:** It is expected that the examiner is able to assign key components when reporting evaluation and management services. See updated E/M questions for examples of the new format. All categories of codes (I, II, and III) are potentially on the examination.

## PRE-EXAMINATION AND POST-EXAMINATION

The Pre-Examination contains 150 questions and is located on the companion Evolve website. The purpose of the Pre-Examination is only to assess your beginning level of knowledge and skill—your starting place. Based on your scores, you can tailor your study to target your weakest areas and increase your scores. Take the Pre-Examination before you begin your studies.

Your score will automatically be calculated for you. A passing score for the examinations in this text requires 70%.

The software will calculate and retain your scoring information.

Immediately on completion of your study, you should complete the Post-Examination on Evolve. After you are finished, the program on Evolve will automatically compare your Pre-Examination scores with your Post-Examination scores and will store your results. By comparing the results of the Pre-Examination and the Post-Examination (the same examination will be taken twice), the software illustrates the improvements you have achieved or the areas that you will need to practice more on before taking the Final Examination.

Rationales for each question are available for review after you complete the Post-Examination. Study the questions for which you did not choose the right response. Did you misread the question, did you not know the material well enough to answer correctly, or did you run out of time? Knowing why you missed a question is an important step toward improving your skill level.

Ideally, you should complete each examination in one sitting (5 hours and 40 minutes, or 340 minutes); if time does not allow, spread the examination times over several periods. There are no time extensions during an actual examination setting, and learning how to judge the amount of time you should spend on each question is an important part of this learning experience to prepare you for the real certification examination.

## FINAL EXAMINATION

If you scored well on all areas of the Post-Examination (80% to 90%), you are ready to move on to the Final Examination, located in Unit 4 of the text.

There is an answer sheet on which to place your answers; it is located directly before the examination. Remove your answer sheet from this text, and enter your answer for each of the 150 questions using paper and pencil.

**NOTE:** The real certification examination is currently paper and pencil.

Once you have completed the Final Examination, go to Evolve to enter your answers on the electronic score sheet. The software will then provide you with the answers and compare your scores to illustrate your improvement.

A passing score for the Final Examination is the same as for the Pre/Post-Examination—70%.

If you did not attain a minimum score on each section, you should develop a plan to restudy those particular areas where the examination indicates you are having difficulties. There are rationales for each question in the Final Examination, and you should review that information as well as material in the text. You can take any of the practice examinations again after your additional study.

## FINAL EXAMINATION ANSWER SHEET

**Medical Terminology**
1. Ⓐ Ⓑ Ⓒ Ⓓ
2. Ⓐ Ⓑ Ⓒ Ⓓ
3. Ⓐ Ⓑ Ⓒ Ⓓ
4. Ⓐ Ⓑ Ⓒ Ⓓ
5. Ⓐ Ⓑ Ⓒ Ⓓ
6. Ⓐ Ⓑ Ⓒ Ⓓ
7. Ⓐ Ⓑ Ⓒ Ⓓ
8. Ⓐ Ⓑ Ⓒ Ⓓ

**Anatomy**
9. Ⓐ Ⓑ Ⓒ Ⓓ
10. Ⓐ Ⓑ Ⓒ Ⓓ
11. Ⓐ Ⓑ Ⓒ Ⓓ
12. Ⓐ Ⓑ Ⓒ Ⓓ
13. Ⓐ Ⓑ Ⓒ Ⓓ
14. Ⓐ Ⓑ Ⓒ Ⓓ
15. Ⓐ Ⓑ Ⓒ Ⓓ
16. Ⓐ Ⓑ Ⓒ Ⓓ

**ICD-9-CM**
17. Ⓐ Ⓑ Ⓒ Ⓓ
18. Ⓐ Ⓑ Ⓒ Ⓓ
19. Ⓐ Ⓑ Ⓒ Ⓓ
20. Ⓐ Ⓑ Ⓒ Ⓓ
21. Ⓐ Ⓑ Ⓒ Ⓓ
22. Ⓐ Ⓑ Ⓒ Ⓓ
23. Ⓐ Ⓑ Ⓒ Ⓓ
24. Ⓐ Ⓑ Ⓒ Ⓓ
25. Ⓐ Ⓑ Ⓒ Ⓓ
26. Ⓐ Ⓑ Ⓒ Ⓓ

**HCPCS**
27. Ⓐ Ⓑ Ⓒ Ⓓ
28. Ⓐ Ⓑ Ⓒ Ⓓ
29. Ⓐ Ⓑ Ⓒ Ⓓ
30. Ⓐ Ⓑ Ⓒ Ⓓ
31. Ⓐ Ⓑ Ⓒ Ⓓ

**Practice Management**
32. Ⓐ Ⓑ Ⓒ Ⓓ
33. Ⓐ Ⓑ Ⓒ Ⓓ
34. Ⓐ Ⓑ Ⓒ Ⓓ
35. Ⓐ Ⓑ Ⓒ Ⓓ
36. Ⓐ Ⓑ Ⓒ Ⓓ
37. Ⓐ Ⓑ Ⓒ Ⓓ

**Coding Guidelines**
38. Ⓐ Ⓑ Ⓒ Ⓓ
39. Ⓐ Ⓑ Ⓒ Ⓓ
40. Ⓐ Ⓑ Ⓒ Ⓓ
41. Ⓐ Ⓑ Ⓒ Ⓓ
42. Ⓐ Ⓑ Ⓒ Ⓓ
43. Ⓐ Ⓑ Ⓒ Ⓓ

**10000 Integumentary System**
44. Ⓐ Ⓑ Ⓒ Ⓓ
45. Ⓐ Ⓑ Ⓒ Ⓓ
46. Ⓐ Ⓑ Ⓒ Ⓓ
47. Ⓐ Ⓑ Ⓒ Ⓓ
48. Ⓐ Ⓑ Ⓒ Ⓓ
49. Ⓐ Ⓑ Ⓒ Ⓓ
50. Ⓐ Ⓑ Ⓒ Ⓓ
51. Ⓐ Ⓑ Ⓒ Ⓓ
52. Ⓐ Ⓑ Ⓒ Ⓓ
53. Ⓐ Ⓑ Ⓒ Ⓓ

**20000 Musculoskeletal System**
54. Ⓐ Ⓑ Ⓒ Ⓓ
55. Ⓐ Ⓑ Ⓒ Ⓓ
56. Ⓐ Ⓑ Ⓒ Ⓓ
57. Ⓐ Ⓑ Ⓒ Ⓓ
58. Ⓐ Ⓑ Ⓒ Ⓓ
59. Ⓐ Ⓑ Ⓒ Ⓓ
60. Ⓐ Ⓑ Ⓒ Ⓓ
61. Ⓐ Ⓑ Ⓒ Ⓓ
62. Ⓐ Ⓑ Ⓒ Ⓓ
63. Ⓐ Ⓑ Ⓒ Ⓓ

**30000 Respiratory and Cardiovascular System**
64. Ⓐ Ⓑ Ⓒ Ⓓ
65. Ⓐ Ⓑ Ⓒ Ⓓ
66. Ⓐ Ⓑ Ⓒ Ⓓ
67. Ⓐ Ⓑ Ⓒ Ⓓ
68. Ⓐ Ⓑ Ⓒ Ⓓ
69. Ⓐ Ⓑ Ⓒ Ⓓ
70. Ⓐ Ⓑ Ⓒ Ⓓ
71. Ⓐ Ⓑ Ⓒ Ⓓ
72. Ⓐ Ⓑ Ⓒ Ⓓ
73. Ⓐ Ⓑ Ⓒ Ⓓ

**40000 Digestive System**
74. Ⓐ Ⓑ Ⓒ Ⓓ
75. Ⓐ Ⓑ Ⓒ Ⓓ
76. Ⓐ Ⓑ Ⓒ Ⓓ
77. Ⓐ Ⓑ Ⓒ Ⓓ
78. Ⓐ Ⓑ Ⓒ Ⓓ
79. Ⓐ Ⓑ Ⓒ Ⓓ
80. Ⓐ Ⓑ Ⓒ Ⓓ
81. Ⓐ Ⓑ Ⓒ Ⓓ
82. Ⓐ Ⓑ Ⓒ Ⓓ
83. Ⓐ Ⓑ Ⓒ Ⓓ

**50000 Urinary, Male Genital System, Female Genital System, and Maternity Care and Delivery**
84. Ⓐ Ⓑ Ⓒ Ⓓ
85. Ⓐ Ⓑ Ⓒ Ⓓ
86. Ⓐ Ⓑ Ⓒ Ⓓ
87. Ⓐ Ⓑ Ⓒ Ⓓ
88. Ⓐ Ⓑ Ⓒ Ⓓ
89. Ⓐ Ⓑ Ⓒ Ⓓ
90. Ⓐ Ⓑ Ⓒ Ⓓ
91. Ⓐ Ⓑ Ⓒ Ⓓ
92. Ⓐ Ⓑ Ⓒ Ⓓ
93. Ⓐ Ⓑ Ⓒ Ⓓ

**60000 Endocrine System, Nervous System, Eye and Ocular Adnexa**
94. Ⓐ Ⓑ Ⓒ Ⓓ
95. Ⓐ Ⓑ Ⓒ Ⓓ
96. Ⓐ Ⓑ Ⓒ Ⓓ
97. Ⓐ Ⓑ Ⓒ Ⓓ
98. Ⓐ Ⓑ Ⓒ Ⓓ
99. Ⓐ Ⓑ Ⓒ Ⓓ
100. Ⓐ Ⓑ Ⓒ Ⓓ
101. Ⓐ Ⓑ Ⓒ Ⓓ
102. Ⓐ Ⓑ Ⓒ Ⓓ
103. Ⓐ Ⓑ Ⓒ Ⓓ

**Evaluation and Management (E/M)**
104. Ⓐ Ⓑ Ⓒ Ⓓ
105. Ⓐ Ⓑ Ⓒ Ⓓ
106. Ⓐ Ⓑ Ⓒ Ⓓ
107. Ⓐ Ⓑ Ⓒ Ⓓ
108. Ⓐ Ⓑ Ⓒ Ⓓ
109. Ⓐ Ⓑ Ⓒ Ⓓ
110. Ⓐ Ⓑ Ⓒ Ⓓ
111. Ⓐ Ⓑ Ⓒ Ⓓ
112. Ⓐ Ⓑ Ⓒ Ⓓ
113. Ⓐ Ⓑ Ⓒ Ⓓ

**Anesthesia**
114. Ⓐ Ⓑ Ⓒ Ⓓ
115. Ⓐ Ⓑ Ⓒ Ⓓ
116. Ⓐ Ⓑ Ⓒ Ⓓ
117. Ⓐ Ⓑ Ⓒ Ⓓ
118. Ⓐ Ⓑ Ⓒ Ⓓ
119. Ⓐ Ⓑ Ⓒ Ⓓ
120. Ⓐ Ⓑ Ⓒ Ⓓ
121. Ⓐ Ⓑ Ⓒ Ⓓ

**70000 Radiology**
122. Ⓐ Ⓑ Ⓒ Ⓓ
123. Ⓐ Ⓑ Ⓒ Ⓓ
124. Ⓐ Ⓑ Ⓒ Ⓓ
125. Ⓐ Ⓑ Ⓒ Ⓓ
126. Ⓐ Ⓑ Ⓒ Ⓓ
127. Ⓐ Ⓑ Ⓒ Ⓓ
128. Ⓐ Ⓑ Ⓒ Ⓓ
129. Ⓐ Ⓑ Ⓒ Ⓓ
130. Ⓐ Ⓑ Ⓒ Ⓓ

**80000 Pathology and Laboratory**
131. Ⓐ Ⓑ Ⓒ Ⓓ
132. Ⓐ Ⓑ Ⓒ Ⓓ
133. Ⓐ Ⓑ Ⓒ Ⓓ
134. Ⓐ Ⓑ Ⓒ Ⓓ
135. Ⓐ Ⓑ Ⓒ Ⓓ
136. Ⓐ Ⓑ Ⓒ Ⓓ
137. Ⓐ Ⓑ Ⓒ Ⓓ
138. Ⓐ Ⓑ Ⓒ Ⓓ
139. Ⓐ Ⓑ Ⓒ Ⓓ
140. Ⓐ Ⓑ Ⓒ Ⓓ

**90000 Medicine**
141. Ⓐ Ⓑ Ⓒ Ⓓ
142. Ⓐ Ⓑ Ⓒ Ⓓ
143. Ⓐ Ⓑ Ⓒ Ⓓ
144. Ⓐ Ⓑ Ⓒ Ⓓ
145. Ⓐ Ⓑ Ⓒ Ⓓ
146. Ⓐ Ⓑ Ⓒ Ⓓ
147. Ⓐ Ⓑ Ⓒ Ⓓ
148. Ⓐ Ⓑ Ⓒ Ⓓ
149. Ⓐ Ⓑ Ⓒ Ⓓ
150. Ⓐ Ⓑ Ⓒ Ⓓ

# FINAL EXAMINATION

**Direction: Report only the professional component unless specifically directed to do otherwise within the question.**

## Subject Area: Medical Terminology

1. This term means the surgical removal of the fallopian tube:
   A. ligation
   B. hysterectomy
   C. salpingostomy
   D. salpingectomy

2. This combining form means "thirst":
   A. dips/o
   B. acr/o
   C. cortic/o
   D. somat/o

3. This term is also known as a homograft:
   A. autograft
   B. allograft
   C. xenograft
   D. zenograft

4. Which of the following terms means "taste"?
   A. Meissner
   B. pacinian
   C. gustatory
   D. astrocytes

5. This suffix means "removal":
   A. -penia
   B. -ectomy
   C. -itis
   D. -pexy

6. Which of the following terms does NOT describe a receptor of the body?
   A. mechanoreceptor
   B. proprioceptor
   C. thermoreceptor
   D. endoreceptor

7. This term means abnormal thickening of the skin:
   A. ductus
   B. dermatofibroma
   C. dermatitis
   D. pachyderma

8. The term that defines the relaxation phase of the heartbeat is:
   A. systole
   B. sinoatrial
   C. diastole
   D. septa

## Subject Area: Anatomy

9. This is the first portion of the small intestine:
   A. jejunum
   B. ileum
   C. duodenum
   D. cecum

10. This is a part of the inner ear:
    A. vestibule
    B. malleus
    C. incus
    D. stapes

11. This is the area behind the cornea:
    A. anterior chamber
    B. choroid layer
    C. ciliary body
    D. fundus

12. Which of the following is a covering of the chamber walls of the heart?
    A. endocardium
    B. myocardium
    C. pericardium
    D. epicardium

13. The shaft of a long bone:
    A. diaphysis
    B. epiphysis
    C. metaphysis
    D. periosteum

14. The act of turning upward, such as the hand turned palm upward:
    A. supination
    B. adduction
    C. pronation
    D. circumduction

15. The middle layer of the skin, also known as the corium or true skin, is the:
    A. epidermis.
    B. stratum corneum.
    C. dermis.
    D. subcutaneous.

16. This is the collarbone:
    A. patella
    B. tibia
    C. scapula
    D. clavicle

## Subject Area: ICD-9-CM

17. Three-week-old female with obstructive apnea.
    A. 770.8
    B. 770.82
    C. 769
    D. 770.83

18. Mild intellectual disabilities due to congenital iodine-deficiency hypothyroidism.
    A. 243, 317
    B. 244.8, 317
    C. 243, 318.0
    D. 317, 243

19. Admission for hemodialysis because of acute renal failure.
    A. V56.31, 584.9
    B. V56, 584
    C. V56.0, 584.9
    D. 584.9, V56.0

20. Glomerulonephritis due to viral hepatitis.
    A. 580.9, 070
    B. 070, 580.9
    C. 580.81, 070.9
    D. 070.9, 580.81

21. Initial encounter to repair a laceration of left hand.
    A. 882.0
    B. 883.0
    C. 887.2
    D. 882.2

22. Mr. Hallberger is 62 and has multiple problems. I am examining him in the intensive critical care unit. I understand he has fluid overload with acute renal failure and was started on ultrafiltration by the nephrologist on duty. He has an abnormal chest x-ray. He has preexisting type II diabetes mellitus and sepsis. We are left with a patient now who is still sedated and on a ventilator because of acute respiratory failure. Code the diagnoses only.
    A. 782.3, 585.9, 792, 250.40, 039.9, 518.81
    B. 789.59, 584.7, 793.19, 250.4, 039.9, 518.81
    C. 276.50, 587, 793.19, 250.00, 038.9, 518.81, 99223
    D. 038.9, 995.92, 584.9, 518.81, 250.00, 793.19

23. Bloody stool.
    A. 772.4
    B. 792.1
    C. 578.1
    D. 578.0

24. A lethargic patient presents with vomiting and severe cramping, and the physician determines during the initial encounter that the condition was caused by the ingestion of five tablets of Tylenol With Codeine and half a bottle of whiskey.
    A. 965.01, 965.4, 980.0, 780.79, 787.03, 789.00, E980.0, E980
    B. 965.09, 965.61, 980.0, 780.79, 787.03, 789.00, E980.0
    C. 966.09, 965.4, 980.0, 780.71, 787.03, 789.00, E980.4, E980.9
    D. 965.09, 965.4, 980.0, 780.79, 787.03, 789.00, E980.0, E980.9

25. Initial encounter to treat a fracture of the right patella with abrasion.
    A. 822.0, 916.0
    B. 822.0
    C. 916.0, 822.1
    D. 823.00

26. Sarcoidosis with cardiomyopathy.
    A. 135, 517.8
    B. 135, 425.8
    C. 425.8, 135
    D. 135, 425.8, V71.7

## Subject Area: HCPCS

27. A patient is issued a 22-inch seat cushion for his wheelchair.
    A. E2601
    B. E0950
    C. E0190
    D. E2602

28. A patient with chronic lumbar pain previously purchased a TENS and now needs replacement batteries.
    A. E1592
    B. A5082
    C. A4772
    D. A4630

29. A patient presents for trimming of 10 dystrophic toenails.
    A. G0127 × 2, 703.8
    B. G0127, G0127 × 9, 703.0
    C. G0127, 703.8
    D. G0127 × 5, G0127 × 5, 703.9

30. A patient with chronic obstructive pulmonary disease is issued a medically necessary nebulizer with a compressor and humidifier for extensive use with oxygen delivery.
    A. E0570, E0550
    B. E0555, E0571
    C. E0580, E0550
    D. E0575, E0550

31. Which HCPCS modifier indicates the great toe of the right foot?
    A. T1
    B. T3
    C. T4
    D. T5

## Subject Area: Practice Management

32. This entity develops and publishes an annual plan that outlines the Medicare monitoring program.
    A. MACs
    B. FIs
    C. OIG
    D. CMS

33. This program was developed by CMS to promote national correct coding methods and to control inappropriate payment of Part B claims and hospital outpatient claims.
    A. NCCI
    B. NFS
    C. HIPAA
    D. MA-PA

34. What is an NPI?
    A. National Payer Incentive
    B. National Provider Identification
    C. National Provider Index
    D. National Payer Identification

35. The RBRVS is a
    A. payment reform implemented in 1992
    B. listing of the customary charge for services
    C. payment list that indicates the prevailing charge in a locality
    D. listing of the physician's individual charges for a service

36. Which of the following is NOT considered fraud or abuse?
    A. Lack of documentation of medical necessity for services reported
    B. Accepting a $20 gift card from a shoe repair representative for each Medicare patient referred to his store
    C. Referring patients to a radiology center in which your physician is a partner
    D. Going to lunch with a pharmaceutical representative

37. This document is a notification in advance of services that Medicare probably will not pay for and the estimated cost to the patient.
    A. Wavier of Liability
    B. Coordination of Benefits
    C. Advanced Beneficiary Notice
    D. UPIN

## Subject Area: Coding Guidelines

38. Which punctuation mark between codes in the index of the CPT manual indicates a range of codes is available?
    A. period
    B. comma
    C. semicolon
    D. hyphen

39. Which of the following most accurately describes the designation "(Separate procedure)"? The procedure is:
    A. incidental to another procedure.
    B. reported if it is the only procedure performed.
    C. reported if the procedure is unrelated to a more major procedure performed at the same time on the same site.
    D. All of the above

40. Specific coding guidelines in the CPT manual are located in:
    A. the index.
    B. the introduction.
    C. the beginning of each section.
    D. Appendix A.

41. The symbol that indicates an add-on code in the CPT manual is:
    A. ▲
    B. ●
    C. +
    D. ►◄

42. When you see the symbol "⊘" next to a code in the CPT manual, you know that:
    A. the code is a new code.
    B. the code contains new or revised text.
    C. the code is a modifier -51 exempt code.
    D. FDA approval is pending.

43. The term that indicates this is the type of code for which the full code description can be known only if the common part of the code (the description preceding the semicolon) of a preceding entry is referenced:
    A. stand-alone
    B. indented
    C. independent
    D. add-on

## Subject Area: 10000 Integumentary System

### 44. OPERATIVE REPORT

**OPERATIVE PROCEDURE:** Excision of back lesion.

**INDICATIONS FOR SURGERY:** The patient has an enlarging lesion on the upper midback.

**FINDINGS AT SURGERY:** There was a 5-cm, upper midback lesion.

**OPERATIVE PROCEDURE:** With the patient prone, the back was prepped and draped in the usual sterile fashion. The skin and underlying tissues were anesthetized with 30 mL of 1% lidocaine with epinephrine.

Through a 5-cm transverse skin incision, the lesion was excised. Hemostasis was ensured. The incision was closed using 3-0 Vicryl for the deep layers and running 3-0 Prolene subcuticular stitch with Steri-Strips for the skin.

The patient was returned to the same-day surgery center in stable postoperative condition. All sponge, needle, and instrument counts were correct. Estimated blood loss is 0 mL.

**PATHOLOGY REPORT LATER INDICATED:** Dermatofibroma, skin of back. Assign code(s) for the physician service only.
A. 11406, 12002, 216.5
B. 11424, 215.7
C. 11406, 12032, 216.5
D. 11606, 232.5

45. What CPT and ICD-9-CM codes would be used to code a subsequent encounter in which a split-thickness skin graft, both thighs to the abdomen, measuring 45 × 21 cm, is performed on a patient who has third-degree burns of the abdomen? Documentation stated 20% of the body surface was burned, with 9% third degree. The patient also sustained second-degree burns of the upper back.
A. 15100 × 2, 949.3, 949.2, 948.00
B. 15100, 15101 × 9, 942.33, 942.24, 948.20
C. 15100, 15101-51 × 9, 946.3, 949.2, 948.02
D. 15100, 15101 × 8, 948.01, 942.29

46. **EMERGENCY DEPARTMENT REPORT CHIEF COMPLAINT:** Nasal bridge laceration.

**SUBJECTIVE:** The patient is a 74-year-old male who presents to the emergency department with a laceration to the bridge of his nose. He fell in the bathroom tonight. He recalls the incident. He just sort of lost his balance. He denies any vertigo. He denies any chest pain or shortness of breath. He denies any head pain or neck pain. There was no loss of consciousness. He slipped on a wet floor in the bathroom and lost his balance; that is how it happened. He has not had any blood from the nose or mouth.

**PAST MEDICAL HISTORY:**
1. Parkinson's.
2. Back pain.
3. Constipation.

**MEDICATIONS:** See the patient record for a complete list of medications.

**ALLERGIES:** NKDA.

**REVIEW OF SYSTEMS:** Per HPI. Otherwise, negative.

**PHYSICAL EXAMINATION:** The exam showed a 74-year-old male in no acute distress. Examination of the HEAD showed no obvious trauma other than the bridge of the nose, where there is approximately a 1.5- to 2-cm laceration. He had no bony tenderness under this. Pupils were equal, round, and reactive. EARS and NOSE: OROPHARYNX was unremarkable. NECK was soft and supple. HEART was regular. LUNGS were clear but slightly diminished in the bases.

**PROCEDURE:** The wound was draped in a sterile fashion and anesthetized with 1% Xylocaine with sodium bicarbonate. It was cleansed with sterile saline and then repaired using interrupted 6-0 Ethilon sutures (Dr. Barney Teller, first-year resident, assisted with the suturing).

**ASSESSMENT:** Nasal bridge laceration, status post fall.

**PLAN:** Keep clean. Sutures out in 5 to 7 days. Watch for signs of infection.
A. 12051, 873.20, E885.9
B. 12011, 873.20, E885.9
C. 12011, 873.32, E888.8
D. 12011, 11000, 873.32, E929.9

47. The patient is brought to surgery for repair of an accidentally inflicted open wound of the left thigh, the total extent measuring approximately 40 × 35 cm.

**DESCRIPTION OF PROCEDURE:** The legs were prepped with Betadine scrub and solution and then draped in a routine sterile fashion. Split-thickness skin grafts measuring about a 10,000th inch thick were taken from both thighs, meshed with a 3:1 ratio mesher, and stapled to the wounds. The donor sites were dressed with scarlet red, and the recipient sites were dressed with Xeroform, Kerlix fluffs, and Kerlix roll, and a few ABD pads were used for absorption. Estimated blood loss was negligible. The patient tolerated the procedure well and left surgery in good condition.
A. 15120, 15121 × 12, 891.0, E929.9
B. 15100, 15101, 11010, 891.0, E928.9
C. 15220, 15221 × 13, 890.0, E928.9
D. 15100, 15101 × 13, 890.0, E928.9

48. What CPT and ICD-9-CM codes would be used to code the destruction of a malignant lesion on the skin of the female genitalia measuring 1.6 cm using cryosurgery?
A. 17272, 184.4
B. 11602, 199.0
C. 11420, 198.82
D. 11622, 184.4

49. **SAME-DAY SURGERY**

**DIAGNOSIS:** Inverted nipple with mammary duct ectasia, left.

**OPERATION:** Excision of mass deep to left nipple.
   With the patient under general anesthesia, a circumareolar incision was made with sharp dissection and carried down into the breast tissue. The nipple complex was raised up using a small retractor. We gently dissected underneath to free up the nipple entirely. Once this was done, we had the nipple fully unfolded, and there was some evident mammary duct ectasia. An area 3 × 4 cm was excised using electrocautery. Hemostasis was maintained with the electrocautery, and then the breast tissue deep to the nipple was reconstructed using sutures of 3-0 chromic. Subcutaneous tissue was closed using 3-0 chromic, and then the skin was closed using 4-0 Vicryl. Steri-Strips were applied. The patient tolerated the procedure well and was returned to the recovery area in stable condition. At the end of the procedure, all sponges and instruments were accounted for.
A. 19120-RT, 610.4
B. 11404-LT, 611.1
C. 19112, 610.4
D. 19120-LT, 610.4

50. This patient returns today for palliative care to her feet. Her toenails have become elongated and thickened, and she is unable to trim them on her own. She states that she has had no problems and no acute signs of any infection or otherwise to her feet. She returns today strictly for trimming of her toenails.

    **EXAMINATION:** Her pedal pulses are palpable bilaterally. The nails are mycotic, 1 through 4 on the left, and 1 through 3 on the right.

    **ASSESSMENT:** Onychomycosis, 1 through 4 on the left and 1 through 3 on the right.

    **PLAN:** Mild debridement of mycotic nails × 7. This patient is to return to the clinic in 3 to 4 months for follow-up palliative care.
    A. 11721 × 7, 117.9
    B. 99212, 11721, 110.1
    C. 11719, 110.1
    D. 11721, 110.1

51. **OPERATIVE REPORT**
    With the patient having had a wire localization performed by radiology, she was taken to the operating room and, under local anesthesia of the left breast, was prepped and draped in a sterile manner. A breast line incision was made through the entry point of the wire, and a core of tissue surrounding the wire (approximately 1 × 2 cm) was removed using electrocautery for hemostasis. The specimen, including the wire, was then submitted to radiology, and the presence of the lesion within the specimen was confirmed. The wound was checked for hemostasis, and this was maintained with electrocautery. The breast tissue was reapproximated using 2-0 and 3-0 chromic. The skin was closed using 4-0 Vicryl in a subcuticular manner. Steri-Strips were applied. The patient tolerated the procedure well and was discharged from the operating room in stable condition. At the end of the procedure, all sponges and instruments were accounted for. Pathology report later indicated: Benign tissue, breast.
    A. 11602-LT, 238.3
    B. 11400-LT, 174.9
    C. 19125-LT, 217
    D. 19125-LT, 239.3

52. What CPT and ICD-9-CM codes would be assigned to report an initial encounter for treatment of a 40 sq cm debridement of an open anterior abdominal laceration, including subcutaneous tissue and muscle, with grit and rubble? The patient fell while speed walking and landed on a sharp rock, injuring the epigastric region of the abdomen.
    A. 11000, 879.2, E880.1, E920.8
    B. 11010, 879.6, E880.1
    C. 11042, 11045, 879.2
    D. 11043, 11046, 879.3, E888.0, E920.8, E001.0

53. What code(s) is used by the radiologist when performing preoperative placement of a needle localization wire of a single lesion of the breast? The patient was diagnosed with adenocarcinoma of the upper outer quadrant of the right breast, primary site.
    A. 19290, 19125, 174.5
    B. 19125, 174.4
    C. 19290, 174.4
    D. 19295, 174.5

## Subject Area: 20000 Musculoskeletal System

54. A small incision was made over the left proximal tibia, and a traction pin was inserted through the bone to the opposite side. Weights were then affixed to the pins to stabilize the closed tibial fracture temporarily until fracture repair could be performed. Assign codes for the physician service.
    A. 20650-LT, 823.00
    B. 20663-LT, 823.92
    C. 20690-LT, 823.40
    D. 20692-LT, 823.92

55. **OPERATIVE REPORT**

    **PREOPERATIVE DIAGNOSIS:** Left thigh abscess.

    **PROCEDURE PERFORMED:** Incision and drainage of left thigh abscess.

    **OPERATIVE NOTE:** With the patient under general anesthesia, he was placed in the lithotomy position. The area around the anus was carefully inspected, and we saw no evidence of communication with the perirectal space. This appears to have risen in the crease at the top of the leg, extending from the posterior buttocks region up toward the side of the base of the penis. In any event, the area was prepped and draped in a sterile manner. Then we incised the area in fluctuation. We obtained a lot of very foul-smelling, almost stool-like material (it was not stool, but it was brown and very foul-smelling material). This was not the typical pus one sees with a *Staphylococcus aureus*–type infection. The incision was widened to allow us to probe the cavity fully. Again, I could see no evidence of communication to the rectum, but there was extension down the thigh and extension up into the groin crease. The fascia was darkened from the purulent material. I opened some of the fascia to make sure the underlying muscle was viable. This appeared viable. No gas was present. There was nothing to suggest a necrotizing fasciitis. The patient did have a very extensive inflammation within this abscess cavity. The abscess cavity was irrigated with peroxide and saline and packed with gauze vaginal packing. The patient tolerated the procedure well and was discharged from the operating room in stable condition.
    A. 26990-LT, 682.6
    B. 27301-LT, 682.6
    C. 27301-LT, 682.60
    D. 27025-LT, 682.6

56. **OPERATIVE REPORT**

**PREOPERATIVE DIAGNOSIS:** Compound fracture, left humerus, with possible loss of left radial pulse.

**PROCEDURE PERFORMED:** Open reduction internal fixation, left compound humerus fracture.

**PROCEDURE:** While under a general anesthetic, the patient's left arm was prepped with Betadine and draped in sterile fashion. We then created a longitudinal incision over the anterolateral aspect of his left arm and carried the dissection through the subcutaneous tissue. We attempted to identify the lateral intermuscular septum and progressed to the fracture site, which was actually fairly easy to do because there was some significant tearing and rupturing of the biceps and brachialis muscles. These were partial ruptures, but the bone was relatively easy to expose through this. We then identified the fracture site and thoroughly irrigated it with several liters of saline. We also noted that the radial nerve was easily visible, crossing along the posterolateral aspect of the fracture site. It was intact. We carefully detected it throughout the remainder of the procedure. We then were able to strip the periosteum away from the lateral side of the shaft of the humerus both proximally and distally from the fracture site. We did this just enough to apply a 6-hole plate, which we eventually held in place with six cortical screws. We did attempt to compress the fracture site. Due to some comminution, the fracture was not quite anatomically aligned, but certainly it was felt to be very acceptable.

Once we had applied the plate, we then checked the radial pulse with a Doppler. We found that the radial pulse was present using the Doppler, but not with palpation. We then applied Xeroform dressings to the wounds and the incision. After padding the arm thoroughly, we applied a long-arm splint with the elbow flexed about 75 degrees. He tolerated the procedure well, and the radial pulse was again present on Doppler examination at the end of the procedure.

A. 24515-RT, 812.30, E887
B. 24500-LT, 812.20, E888.9
C. 24515-LT, 812.31, E887
D. 24505-LT, 812.20, E888.9

57. John, an 84-year-old male, tripped while on his morning walk. He stated he was thinking about something else when he inadvertently tripped over the sidewalk curb and fell to his knees. X-ray indicated a fracture of his right patella. With the patient under general anesthesia, the area was opened and extensively irrigated. The left aspect of the patella was severely fragmented, and a portion of the patella was subsequently removed. The remaining patella fragments were wired. The surrounding tissue was repaired, thoroughly irrigated, and closed in the usual manner.

A. 27524-RT, 822.0, E880.1
B. 27520-RT, 822.0, E880.1
C. 27524-RT, 822.1, E888.9
D. 27524-RT, 822.0, E888.9

58. Libby was thrown from a horse while riding along the side of the road; a truck that honked the horn as it passed her startled her horse. The horse reared up, and Libby was thrown to the ground. The condyle of her left tibia was fractured and required insertion of multiple pins to stabilize the defect area. A Monticelli multiplane external fixation system was then attached to the pins. Code the placement of the fixation device and diagnosis(es) only.
    A. 20661-LT, 823.82, E828.9
    B. 20692-LT, 823.00, E828.2
    C. 20692-LT, 823.82, E828.2
    D. 20690-LT, 823.00, E828.2

59. Maryann received a blow to her right tibial shaft while moving a large stuffed chair up a flight of stairs when the person in front of the chair slipped and released his hold on the chair. The full weight of the chair was pushed against her; when she was unable to hold the chair in place, both she and the chair fell to the landing a dozen steps below. The chair tipped on its side and landed on her tibia. On x-ray, the right tibia shaft was fractured in three places. Screws and pins were placed through the skin to secure the fracture sites.
    A. 27750-RT, 823.80, E917.3
    B. 27756-RT, 823.80, E917.3
    C. 27756-RT, 823.20, E917.3
    D. 27750-RT, 823.20, E917.3

60. The physician applies a Minerva-type fiberglass body cast from the hips to the shoulders and to the head. Before application, a stockinette is stretched over the patient's torso, and further padding of the bony areas with felt padding was done. The patient was diagnosed with Morquio-Brailsford kyphosis. Assign codes for the physician service only.
    A. 29040, 277.5, 737.41
    B. 29590, 737.41
    C. 29025, 737.41, 277.5
    D. 29000, 737.10, 277.5

61. Mary tells her physician that she has been having pain in her left wrist for several weeks. The physician examines the area and palpates a ganglion cyst of the tendon sheath. He marks the injection sites, sterilizes the area, and injects corticosteroid into two areas.
    A. 20550-LT × 2, 727.42
    B. 20551-LT, 727.41
    C. 20551-LT × 2, 727.43
    D. 20612-LT, 727.42

62. Darin was a passenger in an automobile rollover accident and was not wearing a seat belt at the time. He was thrown from the automobile and was pinned under the rear of the overturned vehicle. He sustained craniofacial separation, Le Forte III fracture that required complicated internal and external fixation using an open approach to repair the extensive damage. A halo device was used to hold the head immobile.
    A. 21435, 20661
    B. 21435
    C. 21432
    D. 21436, 20661

63. Carl Ostrick, a 21-year-old male, slipped on a patch of ice on his sidewalk while shoveling snow. When he fell, his left hand was wedged under his body and his carpometacarpal joint was dislocated. After manipulating the joint back into normal alignment, the surgeon on the following day fixed the dislocation by placing a wire through the skin at the tip of the finger and on through the carpometacarpal joint to maintain alignment. Code the subsequent procedure and diagnoses.

A. 26608-F1, 833.01, E886.0
B. 26650-FA, 833.14, E888.9
C. 26706-LT, 833.00, E885.9
D. 26676-LT, 833.04, E885.9

## Subject Area: 30000 Respiratory and Cardiovascular System

64. **OPERATIVE PROCEDURE**

**PREOPERATIVE DIAGNOSIS:** 68-year-old male in a coma.

**POSTOPERATIVE DIAGNOSIS:** 68-year-old male in a coma.

**PROCEDURE PERFORMED:** Placement of a triple lumen central line in right subclavian vein.

With the usual Betadine scrub to the right subclavian vein area and with a second attempt, the subclavian vein was cannulated and the wire was threaded. The first time the wire did not thread right, and so the attempt was aborted to make sure we had good identification of structures. Once the wire was in place, the needle was removed and a tissue dilator was pushed into position over the wire. Once that was removed, then the central lumen catheter was pushed into position at 17 cm and the wire removed. All three ports were flushed. The catheter was sewn into position, and a dressing applied.

A. 36011, 780.09
B. 36011, 780.01
C. 36556, 780.09
D. 36556, 780.01

65. What CPT and ICD-9-CM codes report a percutaneous insertion of a dual-lead pacemaker by means of the subclavian vein? The diagnosis is sick sinus syndrome, tachy-brady.

A. 33249, 427.0, 427.81
B. 33217, 427.81
C. 33208, 427.81
D. 33240, 426.12, 427.0

66. **OPERATIVE REPORT**

**PREOPERATIVE DIAGNOSIS:** Atelectasis of the left lower lobe.

**PROCEDURE PERFORMED:** Fiberoptic bronchoscopy with brushings and cell washings.

**PROCEDURE:** The patient was already sedated, on a ventilator, and intubated; so his bronchoscopy was done through the ET tube. It was passed easily down to the carina. About 2 to 2.5 cm above the carina, we could see the trachea, which appeared good, as was the carina. In the right lung, all segments were patent and entered, and no masses were seen. The left lung, however, had petechial ecchymotic areas scattered throughout the airways. The tissue was friable and swollen, but no mucous plugs were noted, and all the airways were open, just somewhat swollen. No abnormal secretions were noted at all. Brushings were taken as well as washings, including some with Mucomyst to see whether we could get some distal mucous plug, but nothing really significant was returned. The specimens were sent to appropriate cytological and bacteriological studies. The patient tolerated the procedure fairly well.

A. 31622, 31623-51, 518.0
B. 31623, 770.4
C. 31622-RT, 31623-51-LT, 518.0
D. 31624, 770.4

## 67. OPERATIVE REPORT

**PREOPERATIVE DIAGNOSIS:**
1. Hypoxia.
2. Pneumothorax.

**POSTOPERATIVE DIAGNOSIS:**
1. Hypoxia.
2. Pneumothorax.

**PROCEDURE:** Chest tube placement.

**DESCRIPTION OF PROCEDURE:** The patient was previously sedated with Versed and paralyzed with Nimbex. Lidocaine was used to numb the incision area in the midlateral left chest at about nipple level. After the lidocaine, an incision was made, and we bluntly dissected to the area of the pleural space, making sure we were superior to the rib. On entrance to the pleural space, there was immediate release of air noted. An 18-gauge chest tube was subsequently placed and sutured to the skin. There were no complications for the procedure, and blood loss was minimal.

**DISPOSITION:** Follow-up, single-view, chest x-ray showed significant resolution of the pneumothorax except for a small apical pneumothorax that was noted.

A. 32422, 799.02, 512.89
B. 32551, 71010, 799.00, 512.89
C. 32551, 512.89, 799.02
D. 32422, 799.00, 512.0

## 68. OPERATIVE REPORT

**PREOPERATIVE DIAGNOSIS:** Atherosclerotic heart disease.

**POSTOPERATIVE DIAGNOSIS:** Atherosclerotic heart disease.

**OPERATIVE PROCEDURE:** Coronary bypass grafts × 2 with a single graft from the aorta to the distal left anterior descending and from the aorta to the distal right coronary artery.

**PROCEDURE:** The patient was brought to the operating room and placed in a supine position. Under general intubation anesthesia, the anterior chest and legs were prepped and draped in the usual manner. A segment of greater saphenous vein was harvested from the left thigh, utilizing the endoscopic vein harvesting technique, and prepared for grafting. The sternum was opened in the usual fashion, and the left internal mammary artery was taken down and prepared for grafting. The flow through the internal mammary artery was very poor. The patient did have a 25-mm difference in arterial pressure between the right and left arms, the right arm being higher. The left internal mammary artery was therefore not used. The pericardium was incised sharply and a pericardial well created. The patient was systemically heparinized and placed on bicaval to aortic cardiopulmonary bypass with the stump in the main pulmonary artery for cardiac decompression. The patient was cooled to 26°C, and on fibrillation an aortic cross-clamp was applied and potassium-rich cold crystalline cardioplegic solution was administered through the aortic root with satisfactory cardiac arrest. Subsequent doses were given down the vein grafts as the anastomoses were completed and via the coronary sinus in a retrograde fashion. Attention was directed to the right coronary artery. The end of the greater saphenous vein was then anastomosed thereto with 7-0 continuous Prolene distally. The remaining graft material was then grafted to the left anterior descending at the junction of the middle and distal third. The aortic cross-clamp was removed after 149 minutes with spontaneous cardioversion. The usual maneuvers to remove air from the left heart were then carried out using transesophageal echocardiographic technique. After all the air was removed and the patient had returned to a satisfactory temperature, he was weaned from cardiopulmonary bypass after 213 minutes utilizing 5 g per kilogram per minute of dopamine. The chest was closed in the usual fashion. A sterile compression dressing was applied, and the patient returned to the surgical intensive care unit in satisfactory condition.

A. 33511, 33517, 440.9
B. 33511, 33508, 414.01
C. 33534, 33508, 414.00
D. 33511, 33517, 414.01

69. **OPERATIVE REPORT:** The patient is in for a bone marrow biopsy. The patient was sterilized by standard procedure. Bone marrow core biopsies were obtained from the left posterior iliac crest with minimal discomfort. At the end of the procedure, the patient denied discomfort, without evidence of complications. The patient has diffuse, malignant lymphoma. Assign codes for the physician service only.

A. 20225, 229.0
B. 38221, 202.80
C. 38230, 200.10
D. 38220, 202.80

70. Patient is a 40-year-old male who was involved in a motor vehicle crash. He is having some pulmonary insufficiency.

**PROCEDURE:** Bronchoscope was inserted through the accessory point on the end of the ET tube and was then advanced through the ET tube. The ET tube came pretty close down to the carina. We selectively intubated the right mainstem bronchus with the bronchoscope. There were some secretions here, and these were aspirated. We then advanced this selectively into first the lower and then the middle and upper lobes. Secretions were present, more so in the middle and lower lobes. No mucous plug was identified. We then went into the left mainstem and looked at the upper and lower lobes. There was really not much in the way of secretions present. We did inject some saline and aspirated this out. We then removed the bronchoscope and put the patient back on the supplemental $O_2$. We waited a few minutes. The oxygen level actually stayed pretty good during this time. We then reinserted the bronchoscope and went down to the right side again. We aspirated out all secretions and made sure everything was clear. We then removed the bronchoscope and pulled back on the ET tube about 1.5 cm. We then again placed the patient on supplemental oxygenation.

**FINDINGS:** No mucous plug was identified. Secretions were found mainly in the right lung and were aspirated. The left side looked pretty clear.
A. 31646, 518.52, E819.9
B. 32654, 518.82, E812
C. 31645-50, 518.52, E819.9
D. 31645-RT, 31622-51-LT, 518.52, E988.5

71. This 52-year-old male has undergone several attempts at extubation, all of which failed. He also has morbid obesity and significant subcutaneous fat in his neck. The patient is now in for a flap tracheostomy and cervical lipectomy. The cervical lipectomy is necessary for adequate exposure and access to the trachea and also to secure tracheotomy tube placement. Assign code(s) for the physician service only.
A. 31610, 15839-51
B. 31610
C. 31610, 15838
D. 31603, 15839-51

72. Connie was brought to the operating room for repair of an acute, traumatic diaphragmatic hernia.
A. 39540, 862.0
B. 39503, 756.6
C. 39541, 862.0
D. 39540, 756.6

73. This patient returns to the operating room for placement of an additional chest tube for an anterior pneumothorax due to a contusion lung injury. The same physician had just placed a chest tube 4 days earlier.
A. 32551, 860.0
B. 32420, 861.21
C. 32551-58, 861.21
D. 32551, 861.3

## Subject Area: 40000 Digestive System

74. What CPT code would you use if the physician performs a pyloroplasty and vagotomy in the same surgical session?
A. 43865
B. 50400
C. 43635
D. 43640

75. This 43-year-old female comes in with a peritonsillar abscess. The patient is brought to same-day surgery and given general anesthetic. On examination of the peritonsillar abscess, an incision was made and fluid was drained. The area was examined again, saline was applied, and then the area was packed with gauze. The patient tolerated the procedure well.
A. 42825, 475
B. 42700, 475
C. 42825, 463
D. 42700, 474.0

76. **OPERATIVE REPORT**

    **PREOPERATIVE DIAGNOSIS:** Abdominal pain.

    **POSTOPERATIVE DIAGNOSIS:** Normal endoscopy.

    **PROCEDURE:** The video therapeutic endoscope was passed without difficulty into the oropharynx. The gastroesophageal junction was seen at 40 cm. Inspection of the esophagus revealed no erythema, ulceration, varices, or other mucosal abnormalities. The stomach was entered and the endoscope advanced to the second duodenum. Inspection of the second duodenum, first duodenum, duodenal bulb, and pylorus revealed no abnormalities. Retroflexion revealed no lesions along the curvature. Inspection of the antrum, body, and fundus of the stomach revealed no abnormalities. The patient tolerated the procedure well. The patient complained of abdominal pain and weight loss.
    A. 45378, 789.00, 783.21
    B. 43235, 789.00, 783.21
    C. 49320, 783.0, 789.00
    D. 43255, 278.01, 789.01

77. This 70-year-old male is brought to the operating room for a biopsy of the pancreas. A wedge biopsy is taken and sent to pathology. The report comes back immediately indicating that primary malignant cells were present in the specimen. The decision was made to perform a total pancreatectomy. Code the operative procedure(s) and diagnosis only.
    A. 48100, 197.8
    B. 48155, 157.8
    C. 48155, 48100-51, 157.9
    D. 48155, 48100-51, 88309, 157.9

78. This patient is taken to the operating room from the intensive care unit (ICU). The area of the stoma appears to be necrotic, and on this basis the surgeon indicates that the patient has been taken back to the operating room. The stoma was originally created 4 months ago by her previous surgeon.

    **PROCEDURE PERFORMED:** Revision ileostomy stoma.

    **OPERATIVE NOTE:** With the patient moved onto the operating table, the abdomen was prepped and draped. The segment of bowel that was serving as the ileostomy was freed up. Going in through this large open wound, we were able to identify which segment of bowel this was. We resected the end of the bowel that was necrotic and freed up enough of the distal small bowel so that we could bring it out through a new stoma that was placed lateral to the original stoma. The stoma was created, the bowel was brought out, and the mucosa was sewn onto the skin. With this accomplished, we appeared to have a viable stoma. The patient tolerated this procedure and was returned to the ICU in stable condition.
    A. 44310, 560.1, E878.1
    B. 45136, 009.0, E878.0
    C. 44312, 569.62, 557.0, E878.3
    D. 44314, 557.0

79. This patient is brought back to the operating room during the postoperative period by the same physician to repair an esophagogastrostomy leak, transthoracic approach, done 2 days ago. The patient is status post esophagectomy for esophageal cancer, and is still undergoing chemotherapy. Code the procedure and the diagnosis for the complication.
   A. 43320-78, 530.10
   B. 43340-78, 578.9
   C. 43341, 997.49, 239.0
   D. 43415-78, 997.49, 150.9

80. The patient was taken to the operating room for a repair of a strangulated inguinal hernia. This hernia was previously repaired 4 months ago.
   A. 49521, 550.11
   B. 49520, 550.10
   C. 49492, 550.90
   D. 49521-78, 550.93

81. The physician is using an abdominal approach to perform a proctopexy combined with a sigmoid resection; the patient was diagnosed with colon cancer, primary site sigmoid flexure of the colon:
   A. 45540, 153.3
   B. 45541, 153.7
   C. 45550, 153.3
   D. 45345, 154.0

82. What code would you use to report a rigid proctosigmoidoscopy with removal of two nonadenomatous polyps of the rectum by snare technique?
   A. 45320, 569.0
   B. 45383, 211.3
   C. 45309 × 2, M8210/0
   D. 45315, 569.0

83. **OPERATIVE REPORT**

   **PREOPERATIVE DIAGNOSIS:** Leaking from intestinal anastomosis.

   **POSTOPERATIVE DIAGNOSIS:** Leaking from intestinal anastomosis.

   **PROCEDURE PERFORMED:** Proximal ileostomy for diversion of colon. Oversew of right colonic fistula.

   **OPERATIVE NOTE:** This patient was taken back to the operating room from the intensive care unit. She was having acute signs of leakage from an anastomosis I performed 3 days previously. We took down some of the sutures holding the wound together. We basically exposed all of this patient's intestine. It was evident that she was leaking from the small bowel as well as from the right colon. I thought the only thing we could do would be to repair the right colon. This was done in two layers, and then we freed up enough bowel to try to make an ileostomy proximal to the area of leakage. We were able to do this with great difficulty, and there was only a small amount of bowel to be brought out. We brought this out as an ileostomy stoma, realizing that it was of questionable viability and that it should be watched closely. With that accomplished, we then packed the wound and returned the patient to the intensive care unit.
   A. 44310, 998.31
   B. 44310-78, 997.49, E878.2
   C. 45136, 996.5, E878.2
   D. 45136-78, 998.32, E879.1

## Subject Area: 50000 Urinary, Male Genital System, Female Genital System, and Maternity Care and Delivery

84. This patient is 35 years old at 36 weeks' gestation. She presented in spontaneous labor. Because of her prior cesarean section, she is taken to the operating room to have a repeat lower-segment transverse cesarean section performed. The patient also desires sterilization, and so a bilateral tubal ligation will also be performed. A single, liveborn infant was the outcome of the delivery.
    A. 59510, 58600-51, V25.2
    B. 59620, 58615-51, 644.21, V27.0
    C. 59514, 58605-51, V27.0, 644.21
    D. 59514, 58611, 654.21, 644.21, V27.0, V25.2

85. The pediatric physician takes this newborn male to the nursery to perform a clamp circumcision.
    A. 54160, V50.2
    B. 54150, V50.21
    C. 54160, V50.21
    D. 54150, V50.2

86. **OPERATIVE REPORT**

    **PREOPERATIVE DIAGNOSIS:** Possible recurrent transitional cell carcinoma of the bladder.

    **POSTOPERATIVE DIAGNOSIS:** No evidence of recurrence.

    **PROCEDURE PERFORMED:** Cystoscopy with multiple bladder biopsies.

    **PROCEDURE NOTE:** The patient was given a general mask anesthetic, prepped, and draped in the lithotomy position. The 21-French cystoscope was passed into the bladder. There was a hyperemic area on the posterior wall of the bladder, and a biopsy was taken. Random biopsies of the bladder were also performed. This area was fulgurated. A total of 7 sq cm of bladder was fulgurated. A catheter was left at the end of the procedure. The patient tolerated the procedure well and was transferred to the recovery room in good condition. The pathology report indicated no evidence of recurrence.
    A. 52224, 596.7, V10.51
    B. 51020, 52204, V16.52
    C. 52234, V10.51
    D. 52224 × 4, 236.7

87. This 1-year-old boy has a midshaft hypospadias with a very mild degree of chordee. He also has a persistent right hydrocele. The surgeon brought the boy to surgery to perform a right hydrocele repair and one-stage repair of hypospadias with preputial onlay flap.
    A. 54322, 55040, 752.61, 752.63
    B. 54322, 55041-51, 752.61, 752.63, 603.9
    C. 54324, 55060-51, 752.61, 752.63, 603.9
    D. 54324, 55060, 752.63, 603.9

88. This gentleman has worsening bilateral hydronephrosis. He did not have much of a post void residual on bladder scan. He is taken to the operating room to have a bilateral cystoscopy and retrograde pyelogram. The results come back as gross prostatic hyperplasia as the cause of the hydronephrosis.
    A. 52005, 600.3
    B. 52000, 591, 600.9
    C. 52005-50, 600.91, 591
    D. 52000-50, 591, 600.9

89. This patient is a 42-year-old female who has been having prolonged and heavy bleeding during menstruation.

    **SURGICAL FINDINGS:** On pelvic exam under anesthesia, the uterus was normal size and firm. The examination revealed no masses. She had a few small endometrial polyps in the lower uterine segment.

    **DESCRIPTION OF PROCEDURE:** After induction of general anesthesia, the patient was placed in the dorsolithotomy position, after which the perineum and vagina were prepped, the bladder straight catheterized, and the patient draped. After bimanual exam was performed, a weighted speculum was placed in the vagina and the anterior lip of the cervix was grasped with a single tooth tenaculum. An endocervical curettage was then done with a Kevorkian curet. The uterus was then sounded to 8.5 cm. The endocervical canal was dilated to 7 mm with Hegar dilators. A 5.5-mm Olympus hysteroscope was introduced using a distention medium. The cavity was systematically inspected, and the preceding findings noted. The hysteroscope was withdrawn and the cervix further dilated to 10 mm. Polyp forceps was introduced, and a few small polyps were removed. These were sent separately. Sharp endometrial curettage was then done. The hysteroscope was then reinserted, and the polyps had essentially been removed. The patient tolerated the procedure well and was returned to the recovery room in stable condition. Pathology confirmed benign endometrial polyps.
    A. 58558, 57460-51, 626.2, 621.0
    B. 58558, 626.2, 621.0
    C. 58558, 57558-51, 626.2, 621.0
    D. 58558, 626.6, 239.5

90. **OPERATIVE REPORT**

    **PREOPERATIVE DIAGNOSIS:** Missed abortion with fetal demise, 11 weeks.

    **POSTOPERATIVE DIAGNOSIS:** Missed abortion with fetal demise, 11 weeks.

    **PROCEDURE:** Suction D&C.

    The patient was prepped and draped in a lithotomy position under general mask anesthesia, and the bladder was straight catheterized; a weighted speculum was placed in the vagina. The anterior lip of the cervix was grasped with a single-tooth tenaculum. The uterus was then sounded to a depth of 8 cm. The cervical os was then serially dilated to allow passage of a size 10 curved suction curette. A size 10 curved suction curette was then used to evacuate the intrauterine contents. Sharp curette was used to gently palpate the uterine wall with negative return of tissue, and the suction curette was again used with negative return of tissue. The tenaculum was removed from the cervix. The speculum was removed from the vagina.

All sponges and needles were accounted for at completion of the procedure. The patient left the operating room in apparent good condition having tolerated the procedure well.

A. 59812, 634.92

B. 59812, 638.90

C. 59820, 632

D. 59856, 632

91. **OPERATIVE REPORT**

**PREOPERATIVE DIAGNOSIS:** Right ureteral stricture.

**POSTOPERATIVE DIAGNOSIS:** Right ureteral stricture.

**PROCEDURE PERFORMED:** Cystoscopy, right ureteral stent change.

**PROCEDURE NOTE:** The patient was placed in the lithotomy position after receiving IV sedation. He was prepped and draped in the lithotomy position. The 21-French cystoscope was passed into the bladder, and urine was collected for culture. Inspection of the bladder demonstrated findings consistent with radiation cystitis, which has been previously diagnosed. There is no frank neoplasia. The right ureteral stent was grasped and removed through the urethral meatus; under fluoroscopic control, a guidewire was advanced up the stent, and the stent was exchanged for a 7-French 26-cm stent under fluoroscopic control in the usual fashion. The patient tolerated the procedure well.

A. 51702-LT, 593.3

B. 52005-RT, 595.9

C. 52332-RT, 595.9

D. 52332-RT, 593.3

92. This 41-year-old female presented with a right labial lesion. A biopsy was taken, and the results were reported as VIN III, cannot rule out invasion. The decision was therefore made to proceed with wide local excision of the right vulva.

**PROCEDURE:** The patient was taken to the operating room, and general anesthesia was administered. The patient was then prepped and draped in the usual manner in lithotomy position, and the bladder was emptied with a straight catheter. The vulva was then inspected. On the right labium minora at approximately the 11 o'clock position, there was a multifocal lesion. A marking pen was then used to mark out an elliptical incision, leaving a 1-cm border on all sides. The skin ellipse was then excised using a knife. Bleeders were cauterized with electrocautery. A running locked suture of 2-0 Vicryl was then placed in the deeper tissue. The skin was finally reapproximated with 4-0 Vicryl in an interrupted fashion. Good hemostasis was thereby achieved. The patient tolerated this procedure well. There were no complications.

A. 56605, 184.4

B. 56625, 233.32

C. 56620, 233.32

D. 11620, 184.4

93. This 32-year-old female presents with an ectopic pregnancy. The physician elects to remove the entire fallopian tube with the products of conception laparoscopically.
    A. 59120, 633.90
    B. 59151, 633.90
    C. 58943, 633.10
    D. 59120, 633.80

# Subject Area: 60000 Endocrine System, Nervous System, Eye and Ocular Adnexa

94. **OPERATIVE REPORT**

    **PREOPERATIVE DIAGNOSIS:** FUO.

    **PROCEDURE PERFORMED:** Lumbar puncture.

    **DESCRIPTION OF PROCEDURE:** The patient was placed in the lateral decubitus position with the left side up. The legs and hips were flexed into the fetal position. The lumbosacral area was sterilely prepped. It was then numbed with 1% Xylocaine. I then placed a 22-gauge spinal needle on the first pass into the intrathecal space between the L4 and L5 spinous processes. The fluid was minimally xanthochromic. I sent the fluid for cell count for differential, protein, glucose, Gram stain, and culture. The patient tolerated the procedure well without apparent complication. The needle was removed at the end of the procedure. The area was cleansed, and a Band-Aid was placed.
    A. 62272, 780.91
    B. 62268, 780.60
    C. 62272, 782.3, 780.60
    D. 62270, 780.60

95. **OPERATIVE REPORT**

    **PREOPERATIVE DIAGNOSIS:** Mechanical ectropion, left lower eye.

    **PROCEDURE PERFORMED:** Medial tarsorrhaphy, left lower eye.

    In the operating room, after intravenous sedation, the patient was given a total of about 0.5 mL of local infiltrative anesthetic. The skin surfaces on the medial area of the lid, medial to the punctum, were denuded. A bolster had been prepared and double 5-0 silk suture was passed through the bolster, which was passed through the inferior skin and raw lid margin, then through the superior margin, and out through the skin. A superior bolster was then applied. The puncta were probed with wire instrument and found not to be obstructed. The suture was then fully tied and trimmed. Bacitracin ointment was placed on the surface of the skin. The patient left the operating room in stable condition, without complications, having tolerated the procedure well.
    A. 67875-LT, 374.12
    B. 67710-LT, 374.11
    C. 67882-LT, 374.10
    D. 67880-LT, 374.12

96. Marginal laceration involving the left lower eyelid and laceration of the left upper eyelid involving the tarsus. Both required full-thickness repair. Also, there were multiple stellate lacerations above the left eye, totaling 24.2 cm and requiring full-thickness layered repair. Assign code(s) for the physician service only.
    A. 67935-E2, 12017
    B. 67930-E2, 13152-51, 13153
    C. 67935-E2, 67935-E1-51, 12056-51
    D. 67935-E2, 12017-51

97. This 66-year-old male has been diagnosed with a senile cataract of the posterior subcapsular and is scheduled for a cataract extraction by phacoemulsification of the right eye. The physician has taken the patient to the operating room to perform a posterior subcapsular cataract extraction with IOL placement, diffuse of the right eye.
    A. 66982-RT, 366.09
    B. 66984-RT, 366.14
    C. 66983-RT, 366.12
    D. 66830-RT, 366.14

98. **OPERATIVE REPORT**

    **PREOPERATIVE DIAGNOSIS:** Brain tumor versus abscess.

    **PROCEDURE:** Craniotomy.

    **DESCRIPTION OF PROCEDURE:** Under general anesthesia, the patient's head was prepped and draped in the usual manner. It was placed in Mayfield pins. We then proceeded with a craniotomy. An inverted U-shaped incision was made over the posterior right occipital area. The flap was turned down. Three burr holes were made. Having done this, I then localized the tumor through the burr holes and dura. We then made an incision in the dura in an inverted U-shaped fashion. The cortex looked a little swollen but normal. We then used the localizer to locate the cavity. I separated the gyrus and got right into the cavity and saw pus, which was removed. Cultures were taken and sent for pathology report, which came back later describing the presence of clusters of gram-positive cocci, confirming that this was an abscess. We cleaned out the abscessed cavity using irrigation and suction. The bed of the abscessed cavity was cauterized. Then a small piece of Gelfoam was used for hemostasis. Satisfied that it was dry, I closed the dura. I approximated the scalp. A dressing was applied. The patient was discharged to the recovery room.
    A. 61154, 324.0
    B. 61154, 239.6
    C. 61320, 324.0, 041.89
    D. 61150, 239.6

99. This patient is in for a recurrent herniated disc at L5-S1 on the left. The procedure performed is a repeat laminotomy and foraminotomy at the L5-S1 interspace.
    A. 63030-LT, 722.10
    B. 63030-LT, 722.11
    C. 63042-LT, 722.11
    D. 63042-LT, 722.10

100. **OPERATIVE REPORT**

**PREOPERATIVE DIAGNOSIS:** Herniated disc L4-5 on the left.

**PROCEDURE PERFORMED:** Laminotomy, foraminotomy, removal of herniated disc L4-5 on the left.

**PROCEDURE:** Under general anesthesia, the patient was placed in the prone position and the back was prepped and draped in the usual manner. An incision was made in the skin extending through subcutaneous tissue. Lumbodorsal fascia was divided. The erector spinae muscles were bluntly dissected from the lamina of L4-5 on the left. The interspace was localized. I then performed a generous laminotomy and foraminotomy here, and retracted on the nerve root. It was obvious there was a herniated disc. I removed it, entered the space, and removed degenerating material, satisfied that I had decompressed the root well. There were free fragments lying around beneath the nerve root. We removed all of these. I was able to pass a hockey stick down the foramen across the midline, satisfied I had taken out the large fragments from the interspace at L4-5, and decompressed it well. I irrigated the wound well, put a Hemovac drain in the wound, and then closed the wound in layers using double-knotted 0 chromic on the lumbodorsal fascia with Vicryl 2-0 plain, in the subcutaneous tissue, and surgical staples on the skin. A dressing was applied. The patient was discharged to the recovery room.
    A. 63030-LT, 722.10
    B. 63012-LT, 722.32
    C. 63047-LT, 722.92
    D. 63047-LT, 63048-LT, 722.10

101. This patient came in with an obstructed ventriculoperitoneal shunt. The procedure performed was to be a revision of shunt. After inspecting the shunt system, the entire cerebrospinal fluid shunt system was removed and a similar replacement shunt system was placed. Patient has normal pressure hydrocephalus (NPH).
    A. 62180, 996.1, 331.3
    B. 62258, 996.2, 331.5
    C. 62256, 996.2, 331.4
    D. 62190, 996.2, 331.5

102. Burr hole for a left frontal ventricular puncture for implanting catheter, layered repair of 8-cm scalp laceration, and repair of multiple facial and eyelid lacerations with an approximate total length of 12 cm. Assign code(s) for the physician service only.
    A. 61020, 12015-51
    B. 61107, 12034-51, 12015-51
    C. 61215, 12015-51
    D. 61107, 12034-51

103. What CPT and ICD-9-CM codes would you assign to report the removal of 30% of the left thyroid lobe, with isthmusectomy? The diagnosis was benign growth of the thyroid.
    A. 60210, 226
    B. 60220, 237.4
    C. 60212, 239.7
    D. 60225, 226, 239.7

## Subject Area: Evaluation and Management (E/M)

104. Dr. Black admits a patient with an 8-day history of a low-grade fever, tachycardia, tachypnea, and possible radiologic evidence of basal consolidation of the lung and limited pleural effusion on the left side, per patient as seen at outside clinic several days prior. The patient has also been experiencing swelling of the extremities. The pulse is rapid and thready, as checked by patient on her own during the past couple days. A complete ROS of constitutional factors, ophthalmologic, otolaryngologic, cardiovascular, respiratory, gastrointestinal, genitourinary, musculoskeletal, integumentary, neurologic, psychiatric, endocrine, hematologic, lymphatic, allergic, and immunologic was performed and negative except for the symptoms described above. Past history includes tachycardia and pneumonia. Family history includes heart disease, hypertension, and high cholesterol in both parents. The patient drinks only occasionally and quit smoking 4 years ago. The comprehensive examination was performed and diminished bowel sounds were noted. The physician orders laboratory tests and radiographic studies, including a follow-up chest x-ray, as he considers the extensive diagnostic options, the medical decision-making complexity is high for this patient.
    A. 99233, 780.60, 785.0, 786.06, 511.9, 787.5, V15.82
    B. 99233, 780.60, 427.0, 786.06, 486, 511.9
    C. 99223, 780.60, 785.0, 786.06
    D. 99223, 780.60, 785.0, 786.06, 511.9, 787.5, V15.85, V17.49

105. Bill, a retired U.S. Air Force pilot, was on observation status 12 hours to assess the outcome of a fall from the back of a parked pickup truck into a gravel pit.

    History of Present Illness: The patient is a 42-year-old gentleman who works at the local garden shop. He explained that yesterday he fell from his pickup truck as he was loading gravel for a landscaping project. He lost his footing when attempting to climb from the pickup bed and fell approximately 4 feet and landed on a rock that was protruding from the ground 4 inches, striking his head on the rock. He did not lose consciousness, but was dizzy. He subsequently developed a throbbing headache (8/10) and swelling at the point of impact. The duration of the dizziness was approximately 10 minutes. The headache persisted for 26 hours after the fall. He did take ibuprofen without significant improvement in the pain level. Review of Systems: Constitutional, eyes, ears, nose, throat, lungs, cardiovascular, gastrointestinal, skin, neurologic, lymphatic, and immunologic negative except for HPI statements. PFSH: He is married and has 2 children. He has been working at the garden shop for 4 years. He currently smokes one pack of cigarettes a day and has smoked for 10 years. His father died of heart disease when he was 52. He has one brother with ankylosing spondylitis and one sister who is healthy as far as he knows. His mother died when he was 14 years old. He is currently on no prescribed medications. A comprehensive exam is documented and rendered. The medical decision making is of low complexity.

    The physician discharged Bill from observation that same day after 10 hours, after determining that no further monitoring of his condition was necessary. The physician provided a detailed examination and indicated that the medical decision making was of low complexity.
    A. 99218, 784.0, E888.8
    B. 99234, V71.4, E884.9
    C. 99217, V71.4, E888.8
    D. 99234, 99217, 784.0, E884.9

106. A gynecologist admits an established patient, a 35-year-old female with dysfunctional uterine bleeding, after seeing her in the clinic that day. During the course of the history, the physician notes that the patient has a history of infrequent periods of heavy flow. She has had irregular heavy periods and intermittent spotting for 4 years. The patient has been on a 3-month course of oral contraceptives for symptoms with no relief. The patient states that she has occasional headaches. A complete ROS was performed, consisting of constitutional factors, ophthalmologic, otolaryngologic, cardiovascular, respiratory, gastrointestinal, genitourinary, musculoskeletal, integumentary, neurologic, psychiatric, endocrine, hematologic, lymphatic, allergic, and immunologic which were all negative, except for the symptoms described above. The family history is positive for endometrial cancer, with mother, two aunts, and two sisters who had endometrial cancer. The patient has a personal history of cervical and endometrial polyp removal 3 years prior to admission. The patients states that she does not smoke and only drinks socially. As a part of the comprehensive examination, the physician notes the patient has a large amount of blood in the vault and an enlarged uterus. The prolonged hemorrhaging has resulted in a very thin and friable endometrial lining. The physician orders the patient to be started on intravenous Premarin and orders a full laboratory workup. The medical decision making is of moderate complexity.
    A. 99215, 99222, V13.29, V16.49
    B. 99222, 626.8, V13.29, V16.49
    C. 99215, 99222, 623.8, V13.29, V16.4
    D. 99222, 626.1, V16.49

107. Karra Hendricks, a 37-year-old female, is an established patient who presents to the office with right lower quadrant abdominal pain with fever. The patient states she has had the pain for 3 days. She has taken Tylenol for her fever with some relief. The patient does have occasional diarrhea and headaches. She smokes approximately 5-10 cigarettes a day and drinks socially. The physician performs a detailed examination. The medical decision making is noted to be of a moderate complexity.
    A. 99203, 789.03
    B. 99213, 789.04, 780.60
    C. 99214, 789.03, 780.60
    D. 99221, 789.05, 780.60

108. A neurological consultation in the emergency department of the local hospital is requested by the ED physician for a 25-year-old male with suspected closed head trauma. The neurologist saw the patient in the ED. The patient had a loss of consciousness this morning after receiving a blow to the head in a basketball game. He presents to the emergency department with a headache, dizziness, and confusion. During the course of the history, the patient relates that he has been very irritable, confused, and has had a bit of nausea since the incident. All other systems reviewed and are negative: Constitutional, ophthalmologic, otolaryngologic, cardiovascular, respiratory, genitourinary, musculoskeletal, integumentary, psychiatric, endocrine, hematologic, lymphatic, allergic, and immunologic. The patient states that he does have a history of headaches and that both parents have hypertension, also a grandfather with heart disease. He also states that he does drink beer on the weekends and does not smoke. Physical examination reveals the patient to be unsteady and exhibiting difficulty in concentration when stating months in reverse. The pupils dilate unequally

(anisocoria). The physician continues with a complete comprehensive examination involving an extensive review of neurological function. The neurologist orders a stat CT and MRI. The physician suspects a subdural hematoma or an epidural hematoma and the medical decision-making complexity is high. The neurologist admits the patient to the hospital. Assign codes for the neurologist's services only.
A. 99285, 780.09, 780.4, 784.0
B. 99253, 784.0, 780.09, 780.4
C. 99255, 379.41, 784.0, 298.9, 780.4, E917.0, E007.6
D. 99245, 784.0, 780.09, 780.4, E917.0, E007.6

109. Dr. Stephanopolis makes subsequent hospital visits to Salanda Ortez, who has been in the hospital for primary viral pneumonia. She was experiencing severe dyspnea, rales, fever, and chest pain for over a week. The patient states that this morning she had nausea and her heart was racing while she was experiencing some dyspnea and SOB. The chest radiography showed patchy bilateral infiltrates and basilar streaking. Sputum microbiology was positive for a secondary bacterial pneumonia. An expanded problem-focused physical examination was performed. The medical decision making was moderate. The patient was given intravenous antibiotic as treatment for the bacterial pneumonia.
A. 99233, 786.09, 786.7, 780.60, 729.1, 786.50, 793.19, 795.39
B. 99232, 482.9, 480.9
C. 99221, 786.09, 786.7, 780.60, 729.1, 786.50, 793.19, 795.39
D. 99234, 482.89

110. An obstetrician is requested to provide an office consultation to a 23-year-old female with first-trimester bleeding from Dr A. The patient presents with a history of brownish discharge and occasional pinkish discharge. During the history, the patient relates that she has had suprapubic pain in the past week and cramping. She states her pain is 8/10. She has felt nausea and has vomited on three occasions. On one occasion, the nausea was accompanied by dizziness and vertigo. All other systems are negative at this time and included: Constitutional factors, ophthalmologic, otolaryngologic, cardiovascular, respiratory, musculoskeletal, integumentary, neurologic, psychiatric, endocrine, hematologic, lymphatic, allergic, and immunologic. The PFSH included patient history of tonsillectomy with family history of breast cancer on her mother's side. The patient does not smoke or drink. The physician conducts a comprehensive examination focused on the chief complaint and related systems. The uterus is found to be soft and involuted. There is cervical motion tenderness and significant abdominal tenderness on palpation. A left pelvic mass is palpated in the left quadrant. The physician orders a pelvic ultrasound, a complete CBC, and differential. Considering the range of possible diagnoses, the medical decision-making complexity is high.
A. 99255, 634.91, 719.65
B. 99242, 634.90, 719.65
C. 99245, 640.93, 789.34
D. 99245, 649.53, 789.34

111. Dr. Martin admits a 65-year-old female patient to the hospital to rule out acute pericarditis following a severe viral infection. The patient has complained of retrosternal, sharp, intermittent pain of 2 days' duration that is reduced by sitting up and leaning forward, accompanied by tachypnea. ROS: She does not currently have chest pain but is complaining of

shortness of breath. She states that her legs and feet have been swollen of late. She reports no change in her vision or her hearing, and she has not had a rash. No dyspnea stated. PFSH: She states that she has had an echocardiogram in the past when she complained of chest tightness and her family physician gave her some medication, but she is not certain what it was. She has three adult children, all healthy. Her husband is deceased. She does not smoke or consume alcohol. Her father died at age 69 from congestive heart failure and her mother died of influenza at 70. Refer to the admission form for a list of current medications. The examination was detailed. The medical decision making was of high complexity.

A. 99236, 786.51, 786.06, 786.05
B. 99223, 420.91, 411.1, 442.9, 415.19, 530.9
C. 99245, 420.91, 411.1, 442.9, 415.19, 530.9
D. 99221, 786.51, 786.06, 786.05

112. A 57-year-old male was sent by his family physician to a urologist for an office consultation due to hematuria. The patient has had bright red blood in his urine sporadically for the past 3 weeks. His family physician gave him a dose of antibiotic therapy for urinary tract infection; however, the symptom still persists. The patient states that he does experience some lower back discomfort when urinating, with no fever, chills, or nausea. The patient is currently taking Lotrel 10/20 for his hypertension, which is stable at this time, and has allergies to Sulfa. The urologist performs a detailed history and physical examination. The urologist recommends a cystoscopy to be scheduled for the following day and discusses the procedure and risks with the patient. The urologist also contacted the family physician with the recommendations and is requested to proceed with the cystoscopy and any further follow-up required. The medical decision making is of moderate complexity. A report was sent to attending physician. Report only the office service.

A. 99243, 599.70, 724.2
B. 99244-57, 52000, 599.0, 724.2
C. 99253, 599.9, 724.2
D. 99221, 599.70, 724.2

113. A 56-year-old established male patient presents to his family physician for a preventive checkup at the local outpatient clinic. The physician conducts a multisystem history and physical examination, and the checkup takes 45 minutes.

A. 99214, V70.4
B. 99403, V70.7
C. 99386, V70.0
D. 99396, V70.0

## Subject Area: Anesthesia

114. Which HCPCS modifier indicates an anesthesia service in which the anesthesiologist medically directs one CRNA?

A. -QX
B. -QY
C. -QZ
D. -QK

115. This is the anesthesia formula:
    A. B + M + P
    B. B + P + M
    C. B + T + M
    D. B + T + N

116. Anesthesia service for a pneumocentesis for lung aspiration, 32420.
    A. 00522
    B. 00500
    C. 00520
    D. 00524

117. If the anesthesia service were provided to a patient who had severe systemic disease, what would the physical status modifier be?
    A. P1
    B. P2
    C. P3
    D. P4

118. This type of anesthesia is also known as a nerve block.
    A. Local
    B. Epidural
    C. Regional
    D. MAC

119. The following is the anesthesia formula:
    A. BTC
    B. TBC
    C. BTQ
    D. BTM

120. Anesthesia service includes the following care:
    A. Preoperative, intraoperative
    B. Preoperative, intraoperative, postoperative
    C. Intraoperative, postoperative
    D. Preoperative, postoperative

121. What qualifying circumstances code would be used to identify the administration of anesthesia that is complicated by an emergency condition?
    A. 99100
    B. 99116
    C. 99135
    D. 99140

## Subject Area: 70000 Radiology

122. **EXAMINATION OF:** Right hip.

    **DIAGNOSIS:** Primary unilateral osteoarthritis right hip.

    **ONE-VIEW RIGHT HIP:** A single frontal view is obtained of the right hip. No previous studies are available for comparison. Right hip arthroplasty is seen. Alignment appears grossly unremarkable on this single view. There are skin staples present. Air is seen in the soft tissues, likely due to recent surgery. There appear to be two drains present. The tip of one overlies the soft tissues superolateral to the greater trochanter. The second one is more inferior. The tip overlies the right proximal femoral prosthesis.

**IMPRESSION:** Single view of the right hip with findings consistent with recent right total hip arthroplasty.
A. 72100, 719
B. 73500-RT, 715.95
C. 72100-26, 715.9
D. 73500-26-RT, 715.95, V43.64

123. **EXAMINATION OF:** Cervical spine.

**CLINICAL SYMPTOMS:** Herniated disc.

**FINDINGS:** A single spot fluoroscopic film from the operating room is submitted for interpretation. The cervical spine is not well demonstrated above the level of the inferior aspect of C6. There is a metallic surgical plate seen anterior to the cervical spine. The cephalic portion of the plate is at the level of C6 at its superior endplate. That extends in an inferior direction, presumably anterior to C7; however, there is not adequate visualization of C7 to confirm location. Density overlies the C6-7 intervertebral disc space, suggesting the presence of a bone plug in this area; however, again visualization is not adequate in this area. Further evaluation with plain radiographs is recommended.
A. 72100-26, 722.10
B. 72020-26, 722.0
C. 72100-52-26, 722.0
D. 72020-52-26, 722.11

124. This patient undergoes a gallbladder sonogram due to epigastric pain. The report indicates that the visualized portions of the liver are normal. No free fluid noted within Morison's pouch. The gallbladder is identified and is empty. No evidence of wall thickening or surrounding fluid is seen. There is no ductal dilatation. The common hepatic duct and common bile duct measure 0.4 and 0.8 cm, respectively. The common bile duct measurement is at the upper limits of normal.
A. 76700-26, 789.07
B. 76705-26, 789.06
C. 76775-26, 789.05
D. 76705, 789.07

125. **EXAMINATION OF:** Chest.

**CLINICAL SYMPTOMS:** Pneumonia.

**PA AND LATERAL CHEST X-RAY WITH FLUOROSCOPY.**

**CONCLUSION:** Ventilation within the lung fields has improved compared with previous study.
A. 71020-26, 482.89
B. 71034, 482.83
C. 71023-26, 486
D. 71023, 486

126. **EXAMINATION OF:** Abdomen and pelvis.

    **CLINICAL SYMPTOMS:** Ascites.

    **CT OF ABDOMEN AND PELVIS:** Technique: CT of the abdomen and pelvis was performed without oral or IV contrast material per physician request. No previous CT scans for comparison.

    **FINDINGS:** No ascites. Moderate-sized pleural effusion on the right.
    A. 74160-26, 789.59
    B. 74176-26, 511.9
    C. 74150, 511.9
    D. 74160, 789.59

127. Report the professional component of the following service: This 68-year-old male is seen in Radiation Oncology Department for prostate cancer. The oncologist performs a complex clinical treatment planning, approves a dosimetry calculation, manages a complex isodose plan and orders treatment devices which include blocks, special shields, and wedges. He also performs treatment management. The patient had 5 days of radiation treatments for 2 weeks, a total of 10 days of treatment.
    A. 77263, 77300-26, 77315-26, 77334, 185
    B. 77300, 77315, 77334, 77427 × 2, 185
    C. 77263, 77300-26, 77315-26, 77334-26, 77427 × 2, 185
    D. 77263, 77427 × 2, 185

128. This 69-year-old female is in for a magnetic resonance examination of the brain because of new seizure activity. After imaging without contrast, contrast was administered and further sequences were performed. Examination results indicated no apparent neoplasm or vascular malformation.
    A. 70543-26, 780.31
    B. 70543-26, 780.39
    C. 70553-26, 780.39
    D. 70553, 345.90

129. **EXAMINATION OF:** Brain.

    **CLINICAL FINDING:** Acute onset, severe headache.

    **COMPUTED TOMOGRAPHY OF THE BRAIN** was performed without contrast material.

    **FINDINGS:** There is blood within the third ventricle. The lateral ventricles show mild dilatation with small amounts of blood.

    **IMPRESSION:** Acute subarachnoid hemorrhage.
    A. 70460-26, 784.0
    B. 70250, 784.0
    C. 70450-26, 430
    D. 70450-26, 784.0

130. This patient is suffering from primary lung cancer and is in for a follow-up CT scan of the thorax with contrast material. Code the physician component only.
    A. 71250-26, 197.0
    B. 71260, 162.9
    C. 71260-26, 162.9
    D. 71270-26, 239.1

## Subject Area: 80000 Pathology and Laboratory

131. This 69-year-old female presents to the laboratory after her physician ordered quantitative and qualitative assays for troponin to assist in the diagnosis of her chief complaint of acute onset of chest pain.
    A. 84484, 80299, 786.51
    B. 84512, 84484, 80299, 786.59
    C. 84484, 84512, 786.50
    D. 84484, 84512, 786.59

132. **Report the global service.**

    **CLINICAL HISTORY:** Mass, left atrium.

    **SPECIMEN RECEIVED:** Left atrium.

    **GROSS DESCRIPTION:** The specimen is labeled with patient's name and "left atrial myxoma" and consists of a 4 × 4 × 2-cm ovoid mass with a partially calcified hemorrhagic white-tan tissue.

    **INTRAOPERATIVE FROZEN SECTION DIAGNOSIS:** Myxoma

    **MICROSCOPIC DESCRIPTION:** Sections show a well-circumscribed mass consisting of fibromyxoid tissue showing numerous vascular channels. Areas of superficial ulceration and chronic inflammatory infiltrate are noted. Areas of calcification are also present.

    **DIAGNOSIS:** Myxoma, benign, left atrium.
    A. 88305, 239.89
    B. 88307-26, 88331-26, 212.7
    C. 88307, 88331-26, 212.7
    D. 88305, 212.7

133. **CLINICAL HISTORY:** Boil, left groin.

    **SPECIMEN RECEIVED:** Necrotic fascia left groin and leg (anterior and posterior).

    **GROSS DESCRIPTION:** The specimen is labeled with the patient's name and "fascia left groin and leg" and consists of multiple segments of skin and soft tissue measuring up to 30 cm in greatest dimension. The skin is unremarkable, with the soft tissue being hemorrhagic and friable and foul smelling.

    **MICROSCOPIC DESCRIPTION:** Sections of skin and soft tissue show coagulative necrosis with neutrophilic exudates.

    **DIAGNOSIS:** Skin and soft tissue, left groin and leg, anterior and posterior showing coagulative necrosis and acute inflammation.
    A. 88304, 680.9
    B. 88305-26, 709.8
    C. 88304-26, 709.8, 680.2
    D. 88305, 682.2

134. This 34-year-old established female patient is in for her yearly physical and lab. The physician orders a comprehensive metabolic panel, automated hemogram and manual differential WBC count (CBC), and a thyroid-stimulating hormone. Code the lab only.
    A. 99395, 80050
    B. 80050-52
    C. 80069, 80050
    D. 80050

135. **CLINICAL HISTORY:** Necrotic soleus muscle, right leg.

    **SPECIMEN RECEIVED:** Soleus muscle, right leg.

    **GROSS DESCRIPTION:** Submitted in formalin, labeled with the patient's name and "soleus muscle right leg," are multiple irregular fragments of tan, gray, and brown soft tissue measuring $8 \times 8 \times 2.5$ cm in aggregate. Multiple representative fragments are submitted in four cassettes.

    **MICROSCOPIC DESCRIPTION:** The slides show multiple sections of skeletal muscle showing severe coagulative and liquefactive necrosis. Patchy neutrophilic infiltrates are present within the necrotic tissue.

    **DIAGNOSIS:** Soft tissue, soleus muscle, right leg debridement; necrosis and patchy acute inflammation, skeletal muscle—infective myositis.
    A. 88305-26, 728.2
    B. 88304-26, 728.0
    C. 88307-26, 785.4
    D. 88304-26, 728.2

136. This patient is in for a kidney biopsy (50200) because a mass was identified by ultrasound. The specimen is sent to pathology for gross and microscopic examination. Report the technical and professional components for this service. The results are pending.
    A. 88305-26, 593.9
    B. 88307-26, 593.89
    C. 88307, 593.9
    D. 88305, 593.9

137. This patient presented to the laboratory yesterday to have blood drawn for a creatine measurement. The results came back at higher than normal levels; therefore, the patient was asked to return to the laboratory today for a repeat creatine blood test before the nephrologist is consulted. Report the second day of test only.
    A. $82540 \times 2$, 790.6
    B. 82550, 790.6
    C. 82550, 790.91
    D. 82540, 790.6

138. Code a pregnancy test, urine.
    A. 84702
    B. 84703
    C. 81025
    D. $84702 \times 2$

139. This is a patient with atrial fibrillation who comes to the clinic laboratory routinely for a quantitative digoxin level. This test was performed today.
    A. 80101, 80102, 428.0
    B. 81001, V58.83, V58.69, 427.41
    C. 80162, V58.83, V58.69, 427.31
    D. 80162, 785.0

140. What CPT code would you use to report a bilirubin, total (transcutaneous)?
    A. 82252
    B. 82247
    C. 82248
    D. 88720

## Subject Area: 90000 Medicine

141. What CPT code would be used to code the technical aspect of an evaluation of swallowing by video recording using a flexible fiberoptic endoscope?
    A. 92611
    B. 92612
    C. 92610
    D. 92613

142. The patient presented for a spontaneous nystagmus test that included gaze, fixation, and recording and used vertical electrodes. Assign code(s) for the physician service only.
    A. 92541
    B. 92547
    C. 92541, 92544, 92547
    D. 92541, 92547

143. How would you report a screening hearing test in which no abnormalities are reported?
    A. 92551, V72.19
    B. 92555, V72.19
    C. 92553, V72.19
    D. 92620, V80.3

144. This 40-year-old patient who is a type II diabetic is seen in an inpatient setting for psychotherapy. The doctor spends 50 minutes face to face with the patient. The patient is seen for depression.
    A. 90818, 311, 250.90
    B. 90817, 311, 250.90
    C. 90818, 311
    D. 90817, 311

145. A patient presents for a pleural cavity chemotherapy session with 10 mg doxorubicin HCl that requires a thoracentesis to be performed.
    A. 96446, J9000
    B. 96440, 32421, J9000
    C. 96440, J9000
    D. 96446, 32421, J9000

146. What CPT code would be used to report a home visit for a respiratory patient to care for the mechanical ventilation?
   A. 99503
   B. 99504
   C. 99505
   D. 99509

147. Which code would be used to report an EEG (electroencephalogram) provided during carotid surgery?
   A. 95816
   B. 95819
   C. 95822
   D. 95955

148. **INDICATION:** Pulmonary hypertension secondary to newly diagnosed acute myocardial infarction.

   **PROCEDURE PERFORMED:** Insertion of Swan-Ganz catheter.

   **DESCRIPTION OF PROCEDURE:** The right internal jugular and subclavian area was prepped with antiseptic solution. Sterile drapes were applied. Under usual sterile precautions, the right internal jugular vein was cannulated. A 9-French introducer was inserted, and a 7-French Swan-Ganz catheter was inserted without difficulty. Right atrial pressures were 2 to 3, right ventricular pressures 24/0, and pulmonary artery 26/9 with a wedge pressure of 5. This is a Trendelenburg position. The patient tolerated the procedure well.
   A. 93451, 93503-51, 410.91
   B. 93451, 416.8
   C. 93503, 93452, 410.91
   D. 93503, 410.91, 416.8

149. **DIALYSIS INPATIENT NOTE:** This 24-year-old male patient is on continuous ambulatory peritoneal dialysis (CAPD) using 1.5%. He drains more than 600 mL. He is tolerating dialysis well. He continues to have some abdominal pain, but his abdomen is not distended. He has some diarrhea. His abdomen does not look like acute abdomen. His vitals, other than blood pressure in the 190s over 100s, are fine. He is afebrile.

   At this time, I will continue with 1.5% dialysate. Because of diarrhea, I am going to check stool for white cells, culture. Next we will see what the primary physician says today. His HIDA scan was normal. The patient suffers from ESRD and has had 6 encounters this month. Code this service.
   A. 90947, 90960, 585.6, 787.91, V45.11
   B. 90945, 585.6, 787.91, V45.11
   C. 90960, 585.6, V45.11
   D. 90945, 585.6

150. **DIAGNOSIS:** Atrial flutter.

**PROCEDURE PERFORMED:** Electrical cardioversion.

**DESCRIPTION OF PROCEDURE:** The patient was sedated with Versed and morphine. She was given a total of 5 mg of Versed. She was cardioverted with 50 joules into sinus tachycardia.

The patient was given a 20-mg Cardizem IV push. Her heart rate went down to the 110s, and she was definitely in sinus tachycardia.

**CONCLUSION:** Successful electrical cardioversion of atrial flutter into sinus tachycardia.
A. 92961, 427.61
B. 92960, 427.32
C. 92960, 92973, 427.32
D. 92960, 427.89

# Resources

The most current coding guidelines and code system updates are posted to the Evolve website at **http://evolve.elsevier.com/Buck/cpc.**

Once registered for your free Evolve resources, go to the ***Course Documents*** section, then select ***Coding Updates, Tips, and Links*** to reference the following:

- *Official Guidelines for Coding and Reporting*
- 1995 Guidelines for E/M Services
- 1997 Documentation Guidelines for Evaluation and Management Services

- CPT Updates
- ICD-9-CM Updates
- ICD-10-CM Updates
- HCPCS Updates

- Study Tips
- Weblinks

# Medical Terminology

| | |
|---|---|
| ablation | removal or destruction by cutting, chemicals, or electrocautery |
| abortion | termination of pregnancy |
| absence | without |
| actinotherapy | treatment of acne using ultraviolet rays |
| adenoidectomy | removal of adenoids |
| adipose | fatty |
| adrenals | glands, located at the top of the kidneys, that produce steroid hormones |
| albinism | lack of color pigment |
| allograft | homograft, same species graft |
| alopecia | condition in which hair falls out |
| amniocentesis | percutaneous aspiration of amniotic fluid |
| amniotic sac | sac containing the fetus and amniotic fluid |
| A-mode | one-dimensional ultrasonic display reflecting the time it takes a sound wave to reach a structure and reflect back; maps the structure's outline |
| anastomosis | surgical connection of two tubular structures, such as two pieces of the intestine |
| aneurysm | abnormal dilation of vessels, usually an artery |
| angina | sudden pain |
| angiography | radiography of the blood vessels |
| angioplasty | procedure in a vessel to dilate the vessel opening |
| anhidrosis | deficiency of sweat |
| anomaloscope | instrument used to test color vision |
| anoscopy | procedure that uses a scope to examine the anus |
| antepartum | before childbirth |
| anterior (ventral) | in front of |
| anterior segment | those parts of the eye in the front of and including the lens, orbit, extraocular muscles, and eyelid |

| | |
|---|---|
| anteroposterior | from front to back |
| antigen | a substance that produces a specific response |
| aortography | radiographic recording of the aorta |
| apex cardiography | recording of the movement of the chest wall over the end of the heart |
| aphakia | absence of the lens of the eye |
| apicectomy | excision of a portion of the temporal bone |
| apnea | cessation of breathing |
| arthrocentesis | injection and/or aspiration of joint |
| arthrodesis | surgical immobilization of joint |
| arthrography | radiography of joint |
| arthroplasty | reshaping or reconstruction of joint |
| arthroscopy | use of scope to view inside joint |
| arthrotomy | incision into a joint |
| articular | pertains to joint |
| asphyxia | lack of oxygen |
| aspiration | use of a needle and a syringe to withdraw fluid |
| assignment | Medicare's payment for the service, which participating physicians agree to accept as payment in full |
| asthma | shortage of breath caused by contraction of bronchi |
| astigmatism | condition in which the refractive surfaces of the eye are unequal |
| atelectasis | incomplete expansion of lung, collapse |
| atherectomy | removal of plaque by percutaneous method |
| atrophy | wasting away |
| audiometry | hearing test |
| aural atresia | congenital absence of the external auditory canal |
| auscultation | listening to sounds within the body |
| autograft | from patient's own body |
| avulsion | ripping or tearing away of part either surgically or accidentally |
| axillary nodes | lymph nodes located in the armpit |
| bacilli | plural of bacillus, a rod-shaped bacterium |
| barium enema | radiographic contrast medium |
| beneficiary | person who benefits from health or life insurance |
| bifocal | two focuses in eyeglasses, one usually for close work and the other for improvement of distance vision |
| bilaminate skin | skin substitute usually made of silicone-covered nylon mesh |
| bilateral | occurring on two sides |
| biliary | refers to gallbladder, bile, or bile duct |
| bilobectomy | surgical removal of two lobes of a lung |
| biofeedback | process of giving a person self-information |

| | |
|---|---|
| biometry | application of a statistical measure to a biologic fact |
| biopsy | removal of a small piece of living tissue for diagnostic purposes |
| block | frozen piece of a sample |
| brachytherapy | therapy using radioactive sources that are placed inside the body |
| bronchiole | smaller division of bronchial tree |
| bronchography | radiographic recording of the lungs |
| bronchoplasty | surgical repair of the bronchi |
| bronchoscopy | inspection of the bronchial tree using a bronchoscope |
| B-scan | two-dimensional display of tissues and organs |
| bulbocavernosus | muscle that constricts the vagina in a female and the urethra in a male |
| bulbourethral | gland with duct leading to the urethra |
| bundle of His | muscular cardiac fibers that provide the heart rhythm to the ventricles; blockage of this rhythm produces heart block |
| bundled codes | one code that represents a package of services |
| bunion | hallux valgus, abnormal increase in size of metatarsal head that results in displacement of the great toe |
| burr | drill used to create an entry into the cranium |
| bursa | fluid-filled sac that absorbs friction |
| bursitis | inflammation of bursa (joint sac) |
| bypass | to go around |
| calcaneal | pertaining to the heel bone |
| calculus | concretion of mineral salts, also called a stone |
| calycoplasty | surgical reconstruction of a recess of the renal pelvis |
| calyx | recess of the renal pelvis |
| cancellous | lattice-type structure, usually of bone |
| cardiopulmonary | refers to the heart and lungs |
| cardiopulmonary bypass | blood bypasses the heart through a heart-lung machine |
| cardioversion | electrical shock to the heart to restore normal rhythm |
| cardioverter-defibrillator | surgically placed device that directs an electrical shock to the heart to restore rhythm |
| carotid body | located on each side of the common carotid artery, often a site of tumor |
| cartilage | connective tissue |
| cataract | opaque covering on or in the lens |
| catheter | tube placed into the body to put fluid in or take fluid out |
| caudal | same as inferior; away from the head, or the lower part of the body |

| | |
|---|---|
| causalgia | burning pain |
| cauterization | destruction of tissue by the use of cautery |
| cavernosa | connection between the cavity of the penis and a vein |
| cavernosography | radiographic recording of a cavity, e.g., the pulmonary cavity or the main part of the penis |
| cavernosometry | measurement of the pressure in a cavity, e.g., the penis |
| central nervous system | brain and spinal cord |
| cervical | pertaining to the neck or to the cervix of the uterus |
| cervix uteri | rounded, cone-shaped neck of the uterus |
| cesarean | surgical opening through abdominal wall for delivery |
| cholangiography | radiographic recording of the bile ducts |
| cholangiopancreatography | ERCP, radiographic recording of the biliary system or pancreas |
| cholecystectomy | surgical removal of the gallbladder |
| cholecystoenterostomy | creation of a connection between the gallbladder and intestine |
| cholecystography | radiographic recording of the gallbladder |
| cholesteatoma | tumor that forms in middle ear |
| chondral | referring to the cartilage |
| chordee | condition resulting in the penis being bent downward |
| chorionic villus sampling | CVS, biopsy of the outermost part of the placenta |
| circumflex | a coronary artery that circles the heart |
| Cloquet's node | also called a gland; it is the highest of the deep groin lymph nodes |
| closed fracture repair | not surgically opened with/without manipulation and with/without traction |
| closed treatment | fracture site that is not surgically opened and visualized |
| coccyx | caudal extremity of vertebral column |
| collagen | protein substance of skin |
| Colles' fracture | fracture at lower end of radius that displaces the bone posteriorly |
| colonoscopy | fiberscopic examination of the entire colon that may include part of the terminal ileum |
| colostomy | artificial opening between the colon and the abdominal wall |
| component | part |
| computed axial tomography | CAT or CT, procedure by which selected planes of tissue are pinpointed through computer enhancement, and images may be reconstructed by analysis of variance in absorption of the tissue |
| conjunctiva | the lining of the eyelids and the covering of the sclera |
| contraction | drawn together |

| | |
|---|---|
| contralateral | opposite side |
| cordectomy | surgical removal of the vocal cord(s) |
| cordocentesis | procedure to obtain a fetal blood sample; also called a percutaneous umbilical blood sampling |
| corneosclera | cornea and sclera of the eye |
| corpectomy | removal of vertebrae |
| corpora cavernosa | the two cavities of the penis |
| corpus uteri | uterus |
| crackles | abnormal sounds when breathing (heard on auscultation) |
| craniectomy | permanent, partial removal of skull |
| craniotomy | opening of the skull |
| cranium | that part of the skeleton that encloses the brain |
| curettage | scraping of a cavity using a spoon-shaped instrument |
| curette | spoon-shaped instrument used to scrape a cavity |
| cutdown | incision into a vessel for placement of a catheter |
| cyanosis | bluish discoloration |
| cystocele | herniation of the bladder into the vagina |
| cystography | radiographic recording of the urinary bladder |
| cystolithectomy | removal of a calculus (stone) from the urinary bladder |
| cystolithotomy | cystolithectomy |
| cystometrogram | CMG, measurement of the pressures and capacity of the urinary bladder |
| cystoplasty | surgical reconstruction of the bladder |
| cystorrhaphy | suture of the bladder |
| cystoscopy | use of a scope to view the bladder |
| cystostomy | surgical creation of an opening into the bladder |
| cystotomy | incision into the bladder |
| cystourethroplasty | surgical reconstruction of the bladder and urethra |
| cystourethroscopy | use of a scope to view the bladder and urethra |
| dacryocystography | radiographic recording of the lacrimal sac or tear duct sac |
| dacryostenosis | narrowing of the lacrimal duct |
| debridement | cleansing of or removal of dead tissue from a wound |
| deductible | amount the patient is liable for before the payer begins to pay for covered services |
| delayed flap | pedicle of skin with blood supply that is separated from origin over time |
| delivery | childbirth |
| dermabrasion | planing of the skin by means of sander, brush, or sandpaper |

| | |
|---|---|
| dermatologist | physician who treats conditions of the skin |
| dermatoplasty | surgical repair of skin |
| dialysis | filtration of blood |
| dilation | expansion |
| discectomy | removal of a vertebral disc |
| discography | radiographic recording of an intervertebral joint |
| dislocation | placement in a location other than the original location |
| distal | farther from the point of attachment or origin |
| diverticulum | protrusion in the wall of an organ |
| Doppler | ultrasonic measure of blood movement |
| dosimetry | scientific calculation of radiation emitted from various radioactive sources |
| drainage | free flow or withdrawal of fluids from a wound or cavity |
| duodenography | radiographic recording of the duodenum or first part of the small intestine |
| dysphagia | difficulty swallowing |
| dysphonia | speech impairment |
| dyspnea | shortness of breath, difficult breathing |
| dysuria | painful urination |
| echocardiography | radiographic recording of the heart or heart walls or surrounding tissues |
| echoencephalography | ultrasound of the brain |
| echography | ultrasound procedure in which sound waves are bounced off an internal organ and the resulting image is recorded |
| ectopic | pregnancy outside the uterus (i.e., in the fallopian tube) |
| edema | swelling due to abnormal fluid collection in the tissue spaces |
| elective surgery | nonemergency procedure |
| electrocardiogram | ECG, written record of the electrical action of the heart |
| electrocautery | cauterization by means of heated instrument |
| electrocochleography | test to measure the eighth cranial nerve (hearing test) |
| electrode | lead attached to a generator that carries the electrical current from the generator to the atria or ventricles |
| electroencephalogram | EEG, written record of the electrical action of the brain |
| electromyogram | EMG, written record of the electrical activity of the skeletal muscles |
| electronic claim submission | claims prepared and submitted via a computer |
| electronic signature | identification system of a computer |
| electro-oculogram | EOG, written record of the electrical activity of the eye |

| | |
|---|---|
| electrophysiology | study of the electrical system of the heart, including the study of arrhythmias |
| embolectomy | removal of blockage (embolism) from vessel |
| emphysema | air accumulated in organ or tissue |
| encephalography | radiographic recording of the subarachnoid space and ventricles of the brain |
| endarterectomy | incision into an artery to remove the inner lining so as to eliminate disease or blockage |
| endomyocardial | pertaining to the inner and middle layers of the heart |
| endopyelotomy | procedure involving the bladder and ureters, including the insertion of a stent into the renal pelvis |
| endoscopy | inspection of body organs or cavities using a lighted scope that may be inserted through an existing opening or through a small incision |
| enterolysis | releasing of adhesions of intestine |
| enucleation | removal of an organ or organs from a body cavity |
| epicardial | over the heart |
| epidermolysis | loosening of the epidermis |
| epidermomycosis | superficial fungal infection |
| epididymectomy | surgical removal of the epididymis |
| epididymis | tube located at the top of the testes that stores sperm |
| epididymography | radiographic recording of the epididymis |
| epididymovasostomy | creation of a new connection between the vas deferens and epididymis |
| epiglottidectomy | excision of the covering of the larynx |
| episclera | connective covering of sclera |
| epistaxis | nose bleed |
| epithelium | surface covering of internal and external organs of the body |
| erythema | redness of skin |
| escharotomy | surgical incision into necrotic (dead) tissue |
| eventration | protrusion of the bowel through an opening in the abdomen |
| evisceration | pulling the viscera outside of the body through an incision |
| evocative | tests that are administered to evoke a predetermined response |
| exenteration | removal of an organ all in one piece |
| exophthalmos | protrusion of the eyeball |
| exostosis | bony growth |
| exstrophy | condition in which an organ is turned inside out |
| extracorporeal | occurring outside of the body |
| false aneurysm | sac of clotted blood that has completely destroyed the vessel and is being contained by the tissue that surrounds the vessel |

| | |
|---|---|
| fasciectomy | removal of a band of fibrous tissue |
| *Federal Register* | official publication of all "Presidential Documents," "Rules and Regulations," "Proposed Rules," and "Notices"; government-instituted national changes are published in the *Federal Register* |
| fee schedule | services and payment allowed for each service |
| femoral | pertaining to the bone from the pelvis to knee |
| fenestration | creation of a new opening in the inner wall of the middle ear |
| fissure | cleft or groove |
| fistula | abnormal opening from one area to another area or to the outside of the body |
| fluoroscopy | procedure for viewing the interior of the body using x-rays and projecting the image onto a television screen |
| fracture | break in a bone |
| free full-thickness graft | graft of epidermis and dermis that is completely removed from donor area |
| fulguration | use of electrical current to destroy tissue |
| fundoplasty | repair of the bottom of the bladder |
| furuncle | nodule in the skin caused by *Staphylococcus* entering through hair follicle |
| ganglion | knot |
| gastrointestinal | pertaining to the stomach and intestine |
| gastroplasty | operation on the stomach for repair or reconfiguration |
| gastrostomy | artificial opening between the stomach and the abdominal wall |
| gatekeeper | a physician who manages a patient's access to health care |
| glaucoma | eye diseases that are characterized by an increase of intraocular pressure |
| globe | eyeball |
| glottis | true vocal cords |
| gonioscopy | use of a scope to examine the angles of the eye |
| Group Practice Model | an organization of physicians who contract with a Health Maintenance Organization to provide services to the enrollees of the HMO |
| grouper | computer used to input the principal diagnosis and other critical information about a patient and then provide the correct DRG code |
| Health Maintenance Organization | HMO, a healthcare delivery system in which an enrollee is assigned a primary care physician who manages all the healthcare needs of the enrollee |
| hematoma | mass of blood that forms outside the vessel |
| hemodialysis | cleansing of the blood outside of the body |
| hemolysis | breakdown of red blood cells |

| | |
|---|---|
| hemoptysis | bloody sputum |
| hepatography | radiographic recording of the liver |
| hernia | organ or tissue protruding through the wall or cavity that usually contains it |
| histology | study of structure of tissue and cells |
| homograft | allograft, same species graft |
| hormone | chemical substance produced by the body's endocrine glands |
| hydrocele | sac of fluid |
| hyperopia | farsightedness, eyeball is too short from front to back |
| hypogastric | lowest middle abdominal area |
| hyposensitization | decreased sensitivity |
| hypothermia | low body temperature; sometimes induced during surgical procedures |
| hypoxemia | low level of oxygen in the blood |
| hypoxia | low level of oxygen in the tissue |
| hysterectomy | surgical removal of the uterus |
| hysterorrhaphy | suturing of the uterus |
| hysterosalpingography | radiographic recording of the uterine cavity and fallopian tubes |
| hysteroscopy | visualization of the canal and cavity of the uterus using a scope placed through the vagina |
| ichthyosis | skin disorder characterized by scaling |
| ileostomy | artificial opening between the ileum and the abdominal wall |
| ilium | portion of hip |
| imbrication | overlapping |
| immunotherapy | therapy to increase immunity |
| incarcerated | regarding hernias, a constricted, irreducible hernia that may cause obstruction of an intestine |
| incise | to cut into |
| Individual Practice Association | IPA, an organization of physicians who provide services for a set fee; Health Maintenance Organizations often contract with the IPA for services to their enrollees |
| inferior | away from the head or the lower part of the body; also known as caudalingual |
| inguinofemoral | referring to the groin and thigh |
| inofemoral | referring to the groin and thigh |
| internal/external fixation | application of pins, wires, and/or screws placed externally or internally to immobilize a body part |
| intracardiac | inside the heart |

| | |
|---|---|
| intramural | within the organ wall |
| intramuscular | into a muscle |
| intrauterine | inside the uterus |
| intravenous | into a vein |
| intravenous pyelography | IVP, radiographic recording of the urinary system |
| introitus | opening or entrance to the vagina from the uterus |
| intubation | insertion of a tube |
| intussusception | slipping of one part of the intestine into another part |
| invasive | entering the body, breaking skin |
| iontophoresis | introduction of ions into the body |
| ischemia | deficient blood supply due to obstruction of the circulatory system |
| island pedicle flap | contains a single artery and vein that remains attached to origin temporarily or permanently |
| isthmus | connection of two regions or structures |
| isthmus, thyroid | tissue connection between right and left thyroid lobes |
| isthmusectomy | surgical removal of the isthmus |
| jejunostomy | artificial opening between the jejunum and the abdominal wall |
| jugular nodes | lymph nodes located next to the large vein in the neck |
| keratomalacia | softening of the cornea associated with a deficiency of vitamin A |
| keratoplasty | surgical repair of the cornea |
| Kock pouch | surgical creation of a urinary bladder from a segment of the ileum |
| kyphosis | humpback |
| labyrinth | inner connecting cavities, such as the internal ear |
| labyrinthitis | inner ear inflammation |
| lacrimal | related to tears |
| lamina | flat plate |
| laminectomy | surgical excision of the lamina |
| laparoscopy | exploration of the abdomen and pelvic cavities using a scope placed through a small incision in the abdominal wall |
| laryngeal web | congenital abnormality of connective tissue between the vocal cords |
| laryngectomy | surgical removal of the larynx |
| laryngography | radiographic recording of the larynx |
| laryngoplasty | surgical repair of the larynx |
| laryngoscope | fiberoptic scope used to view the inside of the larynx |

| | |
|---|---|
| laryngoscopy | direct visualization and examination of the interior of larynx with a laryngoscope |
| laryngotomy | incision into the larynx |
| lateral | away from the midline of the body (to the side) |
| lavage | washing out |
| leukoderma | depigmentation of skin |
| leukoplakia | white patch on mucous membrane |
| ligament | fibrous band of tissue that connects cartilage or bone |
| ligation | binding or tying off, as in constricting the blood flow of a vessel or binding fallopian tubes for sterilization |
| lipocyte | fat cell |
| lipoma | fatty tumor |
| lithotomy | incision into an organ or a duct for the purpose of removing a stone |
| lithotripsy | crushing of a stone by sound waves or force |
| lobectomy | surgical excision of lobe of the lung |
| lordosis | anterior curve of the spine |
| lumbodynia | pain in the lumbar area |
| lunate | one of the wrist (carpal) bones |
| lymph node | station along the lymphatic system |
| lymphadenectomy | excision of a lymph node or nodes |
| lymphadenitis | inflammation of a lymph node |
| lymphangiography | radiographic recording of the lymphatic vessels and nodes |
| lymphangiotomy | incision into a lymphatic vessel |
| lysis | releasing |
| magnetic resonance imaging | MRI, procedure that uses nonionizing radiation to view the body in a cross-sectional view |
| Major Diagnostic Categories | MDC, the division of all principal diagnoses into 25 mutually exclusive principal diagnosis areas within the DRG system |
| mammography | radiographic recording of the breasts |
| Managed Care Organization | MCO, a group that is responsible for the health care services offered to an enrolled group of persons |
| manipulation | movement by hand |
| manipulation or reduction | alignment of a fracture or joint dislocation to its normal position |
| mastoidectomy | removal of the mastoid bone |
| Maximum Actual Allowable Charge | MAAC, limitation on the total amount that can be charged by physicians who are not participants in Medicare |
| meatotomy | surgical enlargement of the opening of the urinary meatus |

| | |
|---|---|
| medial | toward the midline of the body |
| Medical Volume Performance Standards | MVPS, government's estimate of how much growth is appropriate for nationwide physician expenditures paid by the Part B Medicare program |
| Medicare Economic Index | MEI, government mandated index that ties increases in the Medicare prevailing charges to economic indicators |
| Medicare Fee Schedule | MFS, schedule that listed the allowable charges for Medicare services; was replaced by the Medicare reasonable charge payment system |
| Medicare Risk HMO | a Medicare-funded alternative to the standard Medicare supplemental coverage |
| melanin | dark pigment of skin |
| melanoma | tumor of epidermis, malignant and black in color |
| Ménière's disease | condition that causes dizziness, ringing in the ears, and deafness |
| M-mode | one-dimensional display of movement of structures |
| modality | treatment method |
| Mohs surgery or Mohs micrographic surgery | removal of skin cancer in layers by a surgeon who also acts as pathologist during surgery |
| monofocal | eyeglasses with one vision correction |
| multipara | more than one pregnancy |
| muscle | organ of contraction for movement |
| muscle flap | transfer of muscle from origin to recipient site |
| myasthenia gravis | syndrome characterized by muscle weakness |
| myelography | radiographic recording of the subarachnoid space of the spine |
| myopia | nearsightedness, eyeball too long from front to back |
| myringotomy | incision into tympanic membrane |
| nasal button | synthetic circular disk used to cover a hole in the nasal septum |
| nasopharyngoscopy | use of a scope to visualize the nose and pharynx |
| National Provider Identifier | NPI, a 10-digit number assigned to a physician by Medicare |
| nephrectomy, paraperitoneal | kidney transplant |
| nephrocutaneous fistula | a channel from the kidney to the skin |
| nephrolithotomy | removal of a kidney stone through an incision made into the kidney |
| nephrorrhaphy | suturing of the kidney |
| nephrostolithotomy | creation of an artificial channel to the kidney |
| nephrostolithotomy, percutaneous | procedure to establish an artificial channel between the skin and the kidney |
| nephrostomy | creation of a channel into the renal pelvis of the kidney |
| nephrostomy, percutaneous | creation of a channel from the skin to the renal pelvis |

| | |
|---|---|
| nephrotomy | incision into the kidney |
| neurovascular flap | contains artery, vein, and nerve |
| noninvasive | not entering the body, not breaking skin |
| nuclear cardiology | diagnostic specialty that uses radiologic procedures to aid in diagnosis of cardiologic conditions |
| nystagmus | rapid involuntary eye movements |
| ocular adnexa | orbit, extraocular muscles, and eyelid |
| olecranon | elbow bone |
| Omnibus Budget Reconciliation Act of 1989 | OBRA, act that established new rules for Medicare reimbursement |
| oophorectomy | surgical removal of the ovary(ies) |
| opacification | area that has become opaque (milky) |
| open fracture repair | surgical opening (incision) over or remote opening as access to a fracture site |
| open treatment | fracture site that is surgically opened and visualized |
| ophthalmodynamometry | test of the blood pressure of the eye |
| ophthalmology | body of knowledge regarding the eyes |
| ophthalmoscopy | examination of the interior of the eye by means of a scope, also known as funduscopy |
| optokinetic | movement of the eyes to objects moving in the visual field |
| orchiectomy | castration, removal of the testes |
| orchiopexy | surgical procedure to release undescended testes and fixate them within the scrotum |
| order | shows subordination of one thing to another; family or class |
| orthopnea | difficulty in breathing, needing to be in erect position to breathe |
| orthoptic | corrective; in the correct place |
| osteoarthritis | degenerative condition of articular cartilage |
| osteoclast | absorbs or removes bone |
| osteotomy | cutting into bone |
| otitis media | noninfectious inflammation of the middle ear; serous otitis media produces liquid drainage (not purulent) and suppurative otitis media produces purulent (pus) matter |
| otoscope | instrument used to examine the internal and external ear |
| oviduct | fallopian tube |
| papilledema | swelling of the optic disc (papilla) |
| paraesophageal hiatus hernia | hernia that is near the esophagus |
| parathyroid | produces a hormone to mobilize calcium from the bones to the blood |
| paronychia | infection around nail |

| | |
|---|---|
| Part A | Medicare's Hospital Insurance; covers hospital/facility care |
| Part B | Medicare's Supplemental Medical Insurance; covers physician services and durable medical equipment that are not paid for under Part A |
| participating provider program | Medicare providers who have agreed in advance to accept assignment on all Medicare claims, now termed Quality Improvement Organizations (QIO) |
| patella | knee cap |
| pedicle | growth attached with a stem |
| Peer Review Organizations | PROs, groups established to review hospital admission and care |
| pelviolithotomy | pyeloplasty |
| penoscrotal | referring to the penis and scrotum |
| percussion | tapping with sharp blows as a diagnostic technique |
| percutaneous | through the skin |
| percutaneous fracture repair | repair of a fracture by means of pins and wires inserted through the fracture site |
| percutaneous skeletal fixation | considered neither open nor closed; the fracture is not visualized, but fixation is placed across the fracture site under x-ray imaging |
| pericardiocentesis | procedure in which a surgeon withdraws fluid from the pericardial space by means of a needle inserted percutaneously |
| pericardium | membranous sac enclosing heart and ends of great vessels |
| perineum | area between the vulva and anus; also known as the pelvic floor |
| peripheral nerves | 12 pairs of cranial nerves, 31 pairs of spinal nerves, and autonomic nervous system; connects peripheral receptors to the brain and spinal cord |
| peritoneal | within the lining of the abdominal cavity |
| peritoneoscopy | visualization of the abdominal cavity using one scope placed through a small incision in the abdominal wall and another scope placed in the vagina |
| pharyngolaryngectomy | surgical removal of the pharynx and larynx |
| phlebotomy | cutting into a vein |
| phonocardiogram | recording of heart sounds |
| photochemotherapy | treatment by means of drugs that react to ultraviolet radiation or sunlight |
| physics | scientific study of energy |
| pilosebaceous | pertains to hair follicles and sebaceous glands |
| placenta | a structure that connects the fetus and mother during pregnancy |
| plethysmography | determining the changes in volume of an organ part or body |
| pleura | covers the lungs and lines the thoracic cavity |
| pleurectomy | surgical excision of the pleura |

| | |
|---|---|
| pleuritis | inflammation of the pleura |
| pneumonocentesis | surgical puncturing of a lung to withdraw fluid |
| pneumonolysis | surgical separation of the lung from the chest wall to allow the lung to collapse |
| pneumonostomy | surgical procedure in which the chest cavity is exposed and the lung is incised |
| pneumonotomy | incision of the lung |
| pneumoplethysmography | determining the changes in the volume of the lung |
| posterior (dorsal) | in back of |
| posterior segment | those parts of the eye behind the lens |
| posteroanterior | from back to front |
| postpartum | after childbirth |
| Preferred Provider Organization | PPO, a group of providers who form a network and who have agreed to provide services to enrollees at a discounted rate |
| priapism | painful condition in which the penis is constantly erect |
| primary care physician | PCP, physician who oversees a patient's care within a managed care organization |
| primary diagnosis | chief complaint of a patient in outpatient setting |
| primipara | first pregnancy |
| prior approval | also known as a prior authorization, the payer's approval of care |
| proctosigmoidoscopy | fiberscopic examination of the sigmoid colon and rectum |
| Professional Standards Review Organization | PSRO, voluntary physicians' organization designed to monitor the necessity of hospital admissions, treatment costs, and medical records of hospitals |
| prognosis | probable outcome of an illness |
| prostatotomy | incision into the prostate |
| Provider Identification Number | PIN, assigned to physicians by payers for use in claims submission |
| pyelography | radiographic recording of the kidneys, renal pelvis, ureters, and bladder |
| qualitative | measuring the presence or absence of |
| Quality Improvement Organizations | QIO, consists of a national network of 53 entities that work with consumers, physicians, hospitals, and caregivers to refine care delivery systems |
| quantitative | measuring the presence or absence of and the amount of |
| rad | radiation-absorbed dose, the energy deposited in patient's tissues |
| radiation oncology | branch of medicine concerned with the application of radiation to a tumor site for treatment (destruction) of cancerous tumors |
| radiograph | film on which an image is produced through exposure to x-radiation |

| | |
|---|---|
| radiologist | physician who specializes in the use of radioactive materials in the diagnosis and treatment of disease and illness |
| radiology | branch of medicine concerned with the use of radioactive substances for diagnosis and therapy |
| rales | coarse sounds on inspiration, also known as crackles (heard on auscultation) |
| real time | two-dimensional display of both the structures and the motion of tissues and organs, with the length of time also recorded as part of the study |
| reduction | replacement to normal position |
| Relative Value Unit | RVU, unit value that has been assigned for each service |
| Resource-Based Relative Value Scale | RBRVS, scale designed to decrease Medicare expenditures, redistribute physician payment, and ensure quality health care at reasonable rates |
| resource intensity | refers to the relative volume and type of diagnostic, therapeutic, and bed services used in the management of a particular illness |
| retrograde | moving backward or against the usual direction of flow |
| rhinoplasty | surgical repair of nose |
| rhinorrhea | nasal mucous discharge |
| salpingectomy | surgical removal of the uterine tube |
| salpingostomy | creation of a fistula into the uterine tube |
| scan | mapping of emissions of radioactive substances after they have been introduced into the body; the density can determine normal or abnormal conditions |
| sclera | outer covering of the eye |
| scoliosis | lateral curve of the spine |
| sebaceous gland | secretes sebum |
| seborrhea | excess sebum secretion |
| sebum | oily substance |
| section | slice of a frozen block |
| segmentectomy | surgical removal of a portion of a lung |
| septoplasty | surgical repair of the nasal septum |
| serum | blood from which the fibrinogen has been removed |
| severity of illness | refers to the levels of loss of function and mortality that may be experienced by patients with a particular disease |
| shunt | an artificial passage |
| sialography | radiographic recording of the salivary duct and branches |
| sialolithotomy | surgical removal of a stone of the salivary gland or duct |
| sinography | radiographic recording of the sinus or sinus tract |
| sinusotomy | surgical incision into a sinus |

| | |
|---|---|
| skeletal traction | application of pressure to the bone by means of pins and/or wires inserted into the bone |
| skin traction | application of pressure to the bone by means of tape applied to the skin |
| skull | entire skeletal framework of the head |
| somatic nerve | sensory or motor nerve |
| specimen | sample of tissue or fluid |
| spirometry | measurement of breathing capacity |
| splenectomy | excision of the spleen |
| splenography | radiographic recording of the spleen |
| splenoportography | radiographic procedure to allow visualization of the splenic and portal veins of the spleen |
| split-thickness graft | all epidermis and some of dermis |
| spondylitis | inflammation of vertebrae |
| Staff Model | a Health Maintenance Organization that directly employs the physicians who provide services to enrollees |
| steatoma | fat mass in sebaceous gland |
| stem cell | immature blood cell |
| stereotaxis | method of identifying a specific area or point in the brain |
| strabismus | extraocular muscle deviation resulting in unequal visual axes |
| stratified | layered |
| stratum (strata) | layer |
| subcutaneous | tissue below the dermis, primarily fat cells that insulate the body |
| subluxation | partial dislocation |
| subungual | beneath the nail |
| superior | toward the head or the upper part of the body; also known as cephalic |
| supination | supine position |
| supine | lying on the back |
| Swan-Ganz catheter | a catheter that measures pressure in the heart |
| sympathetic nerve | part of the peripheral nervous system that controls automatic body function and sympathetic nerves activated under stress |
| symphysis | natural junction |
| synchondrosis | union between two bones (connected by cartilage) |
| tachypnea | quick, shallow breathing |
| tarsorrhaphy | suturing together of the eyelids |
| Tax Equity and Fiscal Responsibility Act | TEFRA, act that contains language to reward cost-conscious healthcare providers |

| | |
|---|---|
| tendon | attaches a muscle to a bone |
| tenodesis | suturing of a tendon to a bone |
| tenorrhaphy | suture repair of tendon |
| thermogram | written record of temperature variation |
| third-party payer | insurance company or entity that is liable for another's healthcare services |
| thoracentesis | surgical puncture of the thoracic cavity, usually using a needle, to remove fluids |
| thoracic duct | collection and distribution point for lymph, and the largest lymph vessel located in the chest |
| thoracoplasty | surgical procedure that removes rib(s) and thereby allows the collapse of a lung |
| thoracoscopy | use of a lighted endoscope to view the pleural spaces and thoracic cavity or to perform surgical procedures |
| thoracostomy | incision into the chest wall and insertion of a chest tube |
| thoracotomy | surgical incision into the chest wall |
| thromboendarterectomy | procedure to remove plaque or clot formations from a vessel by percutaneous method |
| thymectomy | surgical removal of the thymus |
| thymus | gland that produces hormones important to the immune response |
| thyroglossal duct | connection between the thyroid and the tongue |
| thyroid | part of the endocrine system that produces hormones that regulate metabolism |
| thyroidectomy | surgical removal of the thyroid |
| tinnitus | ringing in the ears |
| titer | measure of a laboratory analysis |
| tocolysis | repression of uterine contractions |
| tomography | procedure that allows viewing of a single plane of the body by blurring out all but that particular level |
| tonography | recording of changes in intraocular pressure in response to sustained pressure on the eyeball |
| tonometry | measurement of pressure or tension |
| total pneumonectomy | surgical removal of an entire lung |
| tracheostomy | creation of an opening into trachea |
| tracheotomy | incision into trachea |
| traction | application of pressure to maintain normal alignment |
| transcutaneous | entering by way of the skin |
| transesophageal echocardiogram | TEE, echocardiogram performed by placing a probe down the esophagus and sending out sound waves to obtain images of the heart and its movement |

| | |
|---|---|
| transmastoid | creates an opening in the mastoid for drainage antrostomy |
| transplantation | grafting of tissue from one source to another |
| transseptal | through the septum |
| transtracheal | across the trachea |
| transureteroureterostomy | surgical connection of one ureter to the other ureter |
| transurethral resection, prostate | procedure performed through the urethra by means of a cystoscopy to remove part or all of the prostate |
| transvenous | through a vein |
| transvesical ureterolithotomy | removal of a ureter stone (calculus) through the bladder |
| trephination | surgical removal of a disc of bone |
| trocar needle | needle with a tube on the end; used to puncture and withdraw fluid from a cavity |
| tubercle | lesion caused by infection of tuberculosis |
| tumescence | state of being swollen |
| tunica vaginalis | covering of the testes |
| tympanolysis | freeing of adhesions of the tympanic membrane |
| tympanometry | test of the inner ear using air pressure |
| tympanostomy | insertion of ventilation tube into tympanum |
| ultrasound | technique using sound waves to determine the density of the outline of tissue |
| unbundling | reporting with multiple codes that which can be reported with one code |
| unilateral | occurring on one side |
| uptake | absorption of a radioactive substance by body tissues; recorded for diagnostic purposes in conditions such as thyroid disease |
| ureterectomy | surgical removal of a ureter, either totally or partially |
| ureterocolon | pertaining to the ureter and colon |
| ureterocutaneous fistula | channel from the ureter to exterior skin |
| ureteroenterostomy | creation of a connection between the intestine and the ureter |
| ureterolithotomy | removal of a stone from the ureter |
| ureterolysis | freeing of adhesions of the ureter |
| ureteroneocystostomy | surgical connection of the ureter to a new site on the bladder |
| ureteropyelography | ureter and bladder radiography |
| ureterotomy | incision into the ureter |
| urethrocystography | radiography of the bladder and urethra |
| urethromeatoplasty | surgical repair of the urethra and meatus |
| urethropexy | fixation of the urethra by means of surgery |
| urethroplasty | surgical repair of the urethra |

| | |
|---|---|
| urethrorrhaphy | suturing of the urethra |
| urethroscopy | use of a scope to view the urethra |
| urography | same as pyelography; radiographic recording of the kidneys, renal pelvis, ureters, and bladder |
| uveal | vascular tissue of the choroid, ciliary body, and iris |
| varices | varicose veins |
| varicocele | swelling of a scrotal vein |
| vas deferens | tube that carries sperm from the epididymis to the urethra |
| vasectomy | removal of segment of vas deferens |
| vasogram | recording of the flow in the vas deferens |
| vasotomy | incision in the vas deferens |
| vasorrhaphy | suturing of the vas deferens |
| vasovasostomy | reversal of a vasectomy |
| vectorcardiogram | VCG, continuous recording of electrical direction and magnitude of the heart |
| venography | radiographic recording of the veins and tributaries |
| vertebrectomy | removal of vertebra |
| vertigo | dizziness |
| vesicostomy | surgical creation of a connection of the viscera of the bladder to the skin |
| vesicovaginal fistula | creation of a tube between the vagina and the bladder |
| vesiculectomy | excision of the seminal vesicle |
| vesiculography | radiographic recording of the seminal vesicles |
| vesiculotomy | incision into the seminal vesicle |
| viscera | an organ in one of the large cavities of the body |
| volvulus | twisted section of the intestine |
| vomer | flat bones of the nasal septum |
| xanthoma | tumor composed of cells containing lipid material, yellow in color |
| xenograft | different species graft |
| xeroderma | dry, discolored, scaly skin |
| xeroradiography | photoelectric process of radiographs |

# Combining Forms

| | |
|---|---|
| abdomin/o | abdomen |
| acetabul/o | hip socket |
| acr/o | height/extremities |
| aden/o | in relationship to a gland |
| adenoid/o | adenoids |
| adip/o | fat |
| adren/o, adrenal/o | adrenal gland |
| albin/o | white |
| albumin/o | albumin |
| alveol/o | alveolus |
| ambly/o | dim |
| amni/o | amnion |
| an/o | anus |
| andr/o | male |
| andren/o | adrenal gland |
| andrenal/o | adrenal gland |
| angi/o | vessel |
| ankyl/o | bent, fused |
| aort/o | aorta |
| aponeur/o | tendon type |
| appendic/o | appendix |
| aque/o | water |
| arche/o | first |
| arter/o, arteri/o | artery |
| arthr/o | joint |
| atel/o | incomplete |
| ather/o | plaque |
| atri/o | atrium |

| | |
|---|---|
| audi/o | hearing |
| aut/o | self |
| axill/o | armpit |
| azot/o | urea |
| balan/o | glans penis |
| bi/o | life |
| bil/i | bile |
| bilirubin/o | bile pigment |
| blephar/o | eyelid |
| brachi/o | arm |
| bronch/o | bronchus |
| bronchi/o | bronchus |
| bronchiol/o | bronchiole |
| burs/o | fluid-filled sac in a joint |
| calc/o, calc/i | calcium |
| cardi/o | heart |
| carp/o | carpals (wrist bones) |
| cauter/o | burn |
| cec/o | cecum |
| celi/o | abdomen |
| cephal/o | head |
| cerebell/o | cerebellum |
| cerebr/o | cerebrum |
| cervic/o | neck/cervix |
| chol/e | gall/bile |
| cholangio/o | bile duct |
| cholecyst/o | gallbladder |
| choledoch/o | common bile duct |
| cholester/o | cholesterol |
| chondr/o | cartilage |
| chori/o | chorion |
| clavic/o, clavicul/o | clavicle (collar bone) |
| col/o | colon |
| colp/o | vagina |
| coni/o | dust |
| conjunctiv/o | conjunctiva |

| | |
|---|---|
| cor/o, core/o | pupil |
| corne/o | cornea |
| coron/o | heart |
| cortic/o | cortex |
| cost/o | rib |
| crani/o | cranium (skull) |
| crin/o | secrete |
| crypt/o | hidden |
| culd/o | cul-de-sac |
| cutane/o | skin |
| cyan/o | blue |
| cycl/o | ciliary body |
| cyst/o | bladder |
| dacry/o | tear |
| dacryocyst/o | pertaining to the lacrimal sac |
| dent/i | tooth |
| derm/o, dermat/o | skin |
| diaphragmat/o | diaphragm |
| dips/o | thirst |
| disc/o | intervertebral disc |
| diverticul/o | diverticulum |
| duoden/o | duodenum |
| dur/o | dura mater |
| encephal/o | brain |
| enter/o | small intestine |
| eosin/o | rosy |
| epididym/o | epididymis |
| epiglott/o | epiglottis |
| episi/o | vulva |
| erythr/o, erythem/o | red |
| esophag/o | esophagus |
| essi/o, esthesi/o | sensation |
| estr/o | female |
| femor/o | thighbone |
| fet/o | fetus |
| fibul/o | fibula |

| | |
|---|---|
| galact/o | milk |
| gangli/o | ganglion |
| ganglion/o | ganglion |
| gastr/o | stomach |
| gingiv/o | gum |
| glomerul/o | glomerulus |
| gloss/o | tongue |
| gluc/o | sugar |
| glyc/o | sugar |
| glycos/o | sugar |
| gonad/o | ovaries and testes |
| gyn/o | female |
| gynec/o | female |
| hepat/o | liver |
| herni/o | hernia |
| heter/o | different |
| hidr/o | sweat |
| home/o | same |
| hormon/o | hormone |
| humer/o | humerus (upper arm bone) |
| hydr/o | water |
| hymen/o | hymen |
| hyster/o | uterus |
| ichthy/o | dry/scaly |
| ile/o | ileus |
| ili/o | ilium (upper pelvic bone) |
| immun/o | immune |
| inguin/o | groin |
| ir/o | iris |
| irid/o | iris |
| ischi/o | ischium (posterior pelvic bone) |
| jaund/o | yellow |
| jejun/o | jejunum |
| kal/i | potassium |
| kerat/o | hard, cornea |

| | |
|---|---|
| kinesi/o | movement |
| kyph/o | hump |
| lacrim/o | tear |
| lact/o | milk |
| lamin/o | lamina |
| lapar/o | abdomen |
| laryng/o | larynx |
| lingu/o | tongue |
| lip/o | fat |
| lith/o | stone |
| lob/o | lobe |
| lord/o | curve |
| lumb/o | lower back |
| lute/o | yellow |
| lymph/o | lymph |
| lymphaden/o | lymph gland |
| mamm/o | breast |
| mandibul/o | mandible (lower jawbone) |
| mast/o | breast |
| maxill/o | maxilla (upper jawbone) |
| meat/o | meatus |
| melan/o | black |
| men/o | menstruation, month |
| mening/o, meningi/o | meninges |
| menisc/o, menisci/o | meniscus |
| ment/o | mind |
| metacarp/o | metacarpals (hand) |
| metatars/o | metatarsals (foot) |
| metr/o | uterus, measure |
| metr/i | uterus |
| mon/o | one |
| muc/o | mucus |
| my/o, muscul/o | muscle |
| myc/o | fungus |

| | |
|---|---|
| myel/o | bone marrow, spinal cord |
| myring/o | ear drum |
| myx/o | mucus |
| nas/o | nose |
| nat/a, nat/i | birth |
| natr/o | sodium |
| necr/o | death |
| nephr/o | kidney |
| neur/o | nerve |
| noct/i | night |
| ocul/o | eye |
| olecran/o | olecranon (elbow) |
| olig/o | scant, few |
| onych/o | nail |
| oo/o | egg |
| oophor/o | ovary |
| ophthalm/o | eye |
| opt/o | eye, vision |
| optic/o | eye |
| or/o | mouth |
| orch/i, orch/o, orchi/o, orchid/o | testicle |
| orth/o | straight |
| oste/o | bone |
| ot/o | ear |
| ov/o | egg |
| ovari/o | ovary |
| ovul/o | ovulation |
| ox/i, ox/o | oxygen |
| oxy/o | oxygen |
| pachy/o | thick |
| palat/o | palate |
| palpebr/o | eyelid |
| pancreat/o | pancreas |

| | |
|---|---|
| papill/o | optic nerve |
| patell/o | patella (kneecap) |
| pelv/i | pelvis (hip) |
| pericardi/o | pericardium |
| perine/o | perineum |
| peritone/o | peritoneum |
| petr/o | stone |
| phac/o | eye lens |
| phak/o | eye lens |
| phalang/o | phalanges (finger or toe) |
| pharyng/o | pharynx |
| phas/o | speech |
| phleb/o | vein |
| phren/o | mind, diaphragm |
| phys/o | growing |
| pil/o | hair |
| pituitar/o | pituitary gland |
| pleur/o | pleura |
| pneumat/o | lung/air |
| pneumon/o | lung/air |
| poli/o | gray matter |
| polyp/o | polyp |
| pont/o | pons |
| proct/o | rectum |
| prostat/o | prostate gland |
| psych/o | mind |
| pub/o | pubis |
| pulmon/o | lung |
| pupill/o | pupil |
| py/o | pus |
| pyel/o | renal pelvis |
| pylor/o | pylorus |
| quadr/i | four |
| rachi/o | spine |
| radi/o | radius (lower arm) |
| radic/o, radicul/o | nerve root |
| rect/o | rectum |

| | |
|---|---|
| ren/o | kidney |
| retin/o | retina |
| rhin/o | nose |
| rhiz/o | nerve root |
| rhytid/o | wrinkle |
| rube/o | red |
| sacr/o | sacrum |
| salping/o | uterine tube, fallopian tube |
| scapul/o | scapula (shoulder) |
| scler/o | sclera |
| scoli/o | bent |
| seb/o | sebum/oil |
| semin/i | semen |
| sept/o | septum |
| sial/o | saliva |
| sigmoid/o | sigmoid colon |
| sinus/o | sinus |
| somat/o | body |
| son/o | sound |
| sperm/o, spermat/o | sperm |
| sphygm/o | pulse |
| spir/o | breath |
| splen/o | spleen |
| spondyl/o | vertebra |
| staped/o | middle ear, stapes |
| staphyl/o | clusters |
| steat/o | fat |
| ster/o, stere/o | solid, having three dimensions |
| stern/o | sternum (breast bone) |
| steth/o | chest |
| stomat/o | mouth |
| strept/o | twisted chain |
| synovi/o | synovial joint membrane |
| tars/o | tarsal (ankle) |
| ten/o | tendon |

| | |
|---|---|
| tend/o, tendin/o | tendon (connective tissue) |
| test/o | testicle |
| thorac/o | thorax |
| thromb/o | clot |
| thym/o | thymus gland |
| thyr/o, thyroid/o | thyroid gland |
| tibi/o | shin bone |
| toc/o | childbirth |
| tonsill/o | tonsil |
| top/o | place |
| tox/o, toxic/o | poison |
| trache/o | trachea |
| trich/o | hair |
| tympan/o | eardrum |
| uln/o | ulna (lower arm bone) |
| ungu/o | nail |
| ur/o | urine |
| ureter/o | ureter |
| urethr/o | urethra |
| urin/o | urine |
| uter/o | uterus |
| uve/o | uvea |
| uvul/o | uvula |
| vagin/o | vagina |
| valv/o, valvul/o | valve |
| vas/o, vascul/o | vessel |
| ven/o | vein |
| ventricul/o | ventricle |
| vertebr/o | vertebra |
| vesic/o | bladder |
| vesicul/o | seminal vesicles |
| vitre/o | glass/glassy |
| vulv/o | vulva |
| xanth/o | yellow |
| xer/o | dry |

# Prefixes

| | |
|---|---|
| a- | not |
| an- | not |
| ante- | before |
| audi- | hearing |
| bi- | two |
| brady- | slow |
| de- | lack of |
| dys- | difficult, painful |
| ecto- | outside |
| endo- | in |
| epi- | on/upon |
| eso- | inward |
| eu- | good/normal |
| exo- | outward |
| extra- | outside |
| hemi- | half |
| hyper- | excess, over |
| hypo- | under |
| in- | into |
| inter- | between |
| intra- | within |
| meta- | change, after |
| multi- | many |
| neo- | new |
| nulli-, nulti- | none |
| oxy- | sharp, oxygen |
| pan- | all |
| para- | beside |

| | |
|---|---|
| per- | through |
| peri- | surrounding |
| poly- | many |
| post- | after |
| primi- | first |
| pseudo- | false |
| quadri- | four |
| retro- | behind |
| sub- | under |
| supra- | above |
| sym- | together |
| syn- | together |
| tachy- | fast |
| tetra- | four |
| tri- | three |
| tropin- | act upon |
| uni- | one |

# Suffixes

| | |
|---|---|
| -agon | assemble |
| -algesia | pain sensation |
| -algia | pain |
| -ar | pertaining to |
| -arche | beginning |
| -ary | pertaining to |
| -asthenia | weakness |
| -blast | embryonic |
| -capnia | carbon dioxide |
| -cele | hernia |
| -centesis | puncture to remove (drain) |
| -chezia | defecation |
| -clast, -clasia, -clasis | break |
| -coccus | spherical bacterium |
| -cyesis | pregnancy |
| -desis | fusion |
| -dilation | widening, expanding |
| -drome | run |
| -dynia | pain |
| -eal | pertaining to |
| -ectasis | stretching |
| -ectomy | removal |
| -edema | swelling |
| -emia | blood |
| -esthesis | feeling |
| -gram | record |
| -graph | recording instrument |
| -graphy | recording process |

| -gravida | pregnancy |
| -ia | condition |
| -iatrist | physician specialist |
| -iatry | medical treatment |
| -ical | pertaining to |
| -ictal | pertaining to |
| -in | a substance |
| -ine | a substance |
| -itis | inflammation |
| -listhesis | slipping |
| -lithiasis | condition of stones |
| -lysis | separation |
| -malacia | softening |
| -megaly | enlargement |
| -meta | change |
| -meter | measurement; instrument that measures |
| -metry | measurement of |
| -oid | resembling |
| -oma | tumor |
| -omia | smell |
| -one | hormone |
| -opia | vision |
| -opsy | view of |
| -orrhexis | rupture |
| -osis | condition |
| -oxia | oxygen |
| -para | woman who has given birth |
| -paresis | incomplete paralysis |
| -parous | to bear |
| -penia | deficient |
| -pexy | fixation |
| -phagia | eating |
| -phonia | sound |
| -phylaxis | protection |
| -physis | to grow |
| -plasty | repair |
| -plegia | paralysis |

| | |
|---|---|
| -pnea | breathing |
| -poiesis | production |
| -poly | many |
| -porosis | passage |
| -retro | behind |
| -rrhagia | bursting of blood |
| -rrhaphy | suture |
| -rrhea | discharge |
| -schisis | split |
| -sclerosis | hardening |
| -scopy | to examine |
| -spasm | contraction of muscle |
| -steat/o | fat |
| -stenosis | blockage, narrowing |
| -stomy | opening |
| -thorax | chest |
| -tocia | labor |
| -tom/o | to cut |
| -tome | an instrument that cuts |
| -tomy | cutting, incision |
| -tripsy | crush |
| -tropia | to turn |
| -tropin | act upon |
| -uria | urine |
| -version | turning |

# Abbreviations

| | |
|---|---|
| ABG | arterial blood gas |
| ABN | Advanced Beneficiary Notice; used by CMS to notify beneficiary of payment of provider services |
| ACL | anterior cruciate ligament |
| AD | right ear |
| AFB | acid-fast bacillus |
| AFI | amniotic fluid index |
| AGA | appropriate for gestational age |
| AGCUS | atypical glandular cells of undetermined significance |
| AKA | above-knee amputation |
| ANS | autonomic nervous system |
| APCs | Ambulatory Payment Classifications, patient classification that provides a payment system for outpatients |
| ARDS | adult respiratory distress syndrome |
| ARF | acute renal failure |
| ARM | artificial rupture of membrane |
| AS | left ear |
| ASCUS | atypical squamous cells of undetermined significance |
| ASCVD | arteriosclerotic cardiovascular disease |
| ASD | atrial septal defect |
| ASHD | arteriosclerotic heart disease |
| AU | both ears |
| AV | atrioventricular |
| BCC | benign cellular changes |
| BiPAP | bi-level positive airway pressure |
| BKA | below-knee amputation |
| BP | blood pressure |
| BPD | biparietal diameter |

| | |
|---|---|
| BPH | benign prostatic hypertrophy |
| BPP | biophysical profile |
| BUN | blood urea nitrogen |
| BV | bacterial vaginosis |
| bx | biopsy |
| C1-C7 | cervical vertebrae |
| ca | cancer |
| CABG | coronary artery bypass graft |
| CBC | complete blood (cell) count |
| CF | conversion factor, national dollar amount that is applied to all services paid on the Medicare Fee Schedule basis |
| CHF | congestive heart failure |
| CHL | crown-to-heel length |
| CK | creatine kinase |
| CMS | Centers for Medicare and Medicaid Services, formerly HCFA, Health Care Financing Administration |
| CNM | certified nurse midwife |
| CNS | central nervous system |
| COB | coordination of benefits, management of payment between two or more third-party payers for a service |
| COPD | chronic obstructive pulmonary disease |
| CPAP | continuous positive airway pressure |
| CPD | cephalopelvic disproportion |
| CPK | creatine phosphokinase |
| CPP | chronic pelvic pain |
| CSF | cerebrospinal fluid |
| CTS | carpal tunnel syndrome |
| CVA | stroke/cerebrovascular accident |
| CVI | cerebrovascular insufficiency |
| D&C | dilation and curettage |
| D&E | dilation and evacuation |
| derm | dermatology |
| DHHS | Department of Health and Human Services |
| DLCO | diffuse capacity of lungs for carbon monoxide |
| DRGs | Diagnosis Related Groups, disease classification system that relates the type of inpatients a hospital treats (case mix) to the costs incurred by the hospital |
| DSE | dobutamine stress echocardiography |

| DUB | dysfunctional uterine bleeding |
| ECC | endocervical curettage |
| EDC | estimated date of confinement |
| EDD | estimated date of delivery |
| EDI | electronic data interchange, exchange of data between multiple computer terminals |
| EEG | electroencephalogram |
| EFM | electronic fetal monitoring |
| EFW | estimated fetal weight |
| EGA | estimated gestational age |
| EGD | esophagogastroduodenoscopy |
| EGJ | esophagogastric junction |
| EMC | endometrial curettage |
| EOB | explanation of benefits, remittance advice |
| EPO | Exclusive Provider Organization, similar to a Health Maintenance Organization except that the providers of the services are not prepaid, but rather are paid on a fee-for-service basis |
| EPSDT | Early and Periodic Screening, Diagnosis, and Treatment |
| ERCP | endoscopic retrograde cholangiopancreatography |
| ERT | estrogen replacement therapy |
| ESRD | end-stage renal disease |
| FAS | fetal alcohol syndrome |
| FEF | forced expiratory flow |
| $FEV_1$ | forced expiratory volume in 1 second |
| $FEV_1:FVC$ | maximum amount of forced expiratory volume in 1 second |
| FHR | fetal heart rate |
| FI | fiscal intermediary, financial agent acting on behalf of a third-party payer |
| FRC | functional residual capacity |
| FSH | follicle-stimulating hormone |
| FVC | forced vital capacity |
| fx | fracture |
| GERD | gastroesophageal reflux disease |
| GI | gastrointestinal |
| H or E | hemorrhage or exudate |
| HCFA | Health Care Financing Administration, now known as Centers for Medicare and Medicaid Services (CMS) |
| HCVD | hypertensive cardiovascular disease |
| HD | hemodialysis |

| | |
|---|---|
| HDL | high-density lipoprotein |
| HEA | hemorrhage, exudate, aneurysm |
| HHN | hand-held nebulizer |
| HJR | hepatojugular reflux |
| H&P | history and physical |
| HPV | human papillomavirus |
| HSG | hysterosalpingogram |
| HSV | herpes simplex virus |
| I&D | incision and drainage |
| IO | intraocular |
| IOL | intraocular lens |
| IPAP | inspiratory positive airway pressure |
| IRDS | infant respiratory distress syndrome |
| IVF | in vitro fertilization |
| IVP | intravenous pyelogram |
| JBP | jugular blood pressure |
| KUB | kidneys, ureter, bladder |
| L1-L5 | lumbar vertebrae |
| LBBB | left bundle branch block |
| LEEP | loop electrosurgical excision procedure |
| LGA | large for gestational age |
| LLQ | left lower quadrant |
| LP | lumbar puncture |
| LUQ | left upper quadrant |
| LVH | left ventricular hypertrophy |
| MAT | multifocal atrial tachycardia |
| MDI | metered dose inhaler |
| MI | myocardial infarction |
| MRI | magnetic resonance imaging |
| MSLT | multiple sleep latency testing |
| MVV | maximum voluntary ventilation |
| NCPAP | nasal continuous positive airway pressure |
| NSR | normal sinus rhythm |
| OA | osteoarthritis |
| OD | right eye |
| OS | left eye |
| OU | each eye |

| | |
|---|---|
| PAC | premature atrial contraction |
| PAT | paroxysmal atrial tachycardia |
| PAWP | pulmonary artery wedge pressure |
| PCWP | pulmonary capillary wedge pressure |
| PEAP | positive end-airway pressure |
| PEEP | positive end-expiratory pressure |
| PEG | percutaneous endoscopic gastrostomy |
| PERL | pupils equal and reactive to light |
| PERRL | pupils equal, round, and reactive to light |
| PERRLA | pupils equal, round, and reactive to light and accommodation |
| PFT | pulmonary function test |
| pH | symbol for acid/base level |
| PICC | peripherally inserted central catheter |
| PID | pelvic inflammatory disease |
| PND | paroxysmal nocturnal dyspnea |
| PNS | peripheral nervous system |
| PROM | premature rupture of membranes |
| PSA | prostate-specific antigen |
| PST | paroxysmal supraventricular tachycardia |
| PSVT | paroxysmal supraventricular tachycardia |
| PT | prothrombin time |
| PTCA | percutaneous transluminal coronary angioplasty |
| PTT | partial thromboplastin time |
| PVC | premature ventricular contraction |
| RA | remittance advice, explanation of services |
| RA | rheumatoid arthritis |
| RBBB | right bundle branch block |
| RDS | respiratory distress syndrome |
| REM | rapid eye movement |
| RLQ | right lower quadrant |
| RSR | regular sinus rhythm |
| RUQ | right upper quadrant |
| RV | respiratory volume |
| RVG | *Relative Value Guide* |
| RVH | right ventricular hypertrophy |
| RVS | relative value studies, list of procedures with unit values assigned to each |
| RV:TLC | ratio of respiratory volume to total lung capacity |

| | |
|---|---|
| SHG | sonohysterogram |
| sp gr | specific gravity |
| SROM | spontaneous rupture of membranes |
| subcu, subq, SC, SQ | subcutaneous |
| SUI | stress urinary incontinence |
| SVT | supraventricular tachycardia |
| T1-T12 | thoracic vertebrae |
| TAH | total abdominal hysterectomy |
| TEE | transesophageal echocardiography |
| TENS | transcutaneous electrical nerve stimulation |
| TIA | transient ischemic attack |
| TLC | total lung capacity |
| TLV | total lung volume |
| TM | tympanic membrane |
| TMJ | temporomandibular joint |
| TPA | tissue plasminogen activator |
| TSH | thyroid-stimulating hormone |
| TST | treadmill stress test |
| TURBT | transurethral resection of bladder tumor |
| TURP | transurethral resection of prostate |
| UA | urinalysis |
| UCR | usual, customary, and reasonable—third-party payers' assessment of the reimbursement for health care services: usual, that which would ordinarily be charged for the service; customary, the cost of that service in that locale; and reasonable, as assessed by the payer |
| UPJ | ureteropelvic junction |
| URI | upper respiratory infection |
| UTI | urinary tract infection |
| V/Q | ventilation/perfusion scan |
| VBAC | vaginal birth after cesarean |
| WBC | white blood (cell) count |

# Further Text Resources

## ANATOMY AND PHYSIOLOGY

| Book Title | Author | Imprint | Copyright Date | ISBN-13 |
|---|---|---|---|---|
| *The Anatomy and Physiology Learning System,* 4th Edition | Applegate | Saunders | 2010 | 978-1-4377-0393-1 |
| *Gray's Anatomy for Students,* 2nd Edition | Drake, Vogl, Mitchell | Churchill Livingstone | 2010 | 978-0-443-06952-9 |
| *Anthony's Textbook of Anatomy and Physiology,* 19th Edition | Thibodeau, Patton | Mosby | 2010 | 978-0-323-05539-0 |

## CODING

| Book Title | Author | Imprint | Copyright Date | ISBN-13 |
|---|---|---|---|---|
| *Step-by-Step Medical Coding,* 2012 Edition | Buck | Saunders | 2012 | 978-1-4557-0622-8 |
| *2012 ICD-9-CM, Volumes 1 & 2* (Professional Edition) | Buck | Saunders | 2012 | 978-1-4557-0710-2 |
| *2012 ICD-9-CM, Volumes 1, 2, & 3* (Professional Edition) | Buck | Saunders | 2012 | 978-1-4557-0713-3 |
| *2012 HCPCS Level II* (Professional Edition) | Buck | Saunders | 2012 | 978-1-4557-0770-6 |
| *The Next Step, Advanced Medical Coding,* 2012 Edition | Buck | Saunders | 2012 | 978-1-4557-0646-4 |
| *The Practice Step: Facility-Based Coding Cases,* 2012 Edition | Buck | Saunders | 2012 | 978-1-4557-0752-2 |
| *The Practice Step: Physician-Based Coding Cases,* 2012 Edition | Buck | Saunders | 2012 | 978-1-4557-0753-9 |
| *CCS Coding Exam Review 2012: The Certification Step* | Buck | Saunders | 2012 | 978-1-4557-0683-9 |
| *Online Internship for Medical Coding* | Buck | Saunders | 2012 | 978-1-4557-0735-5 |
| *ICD-9-CM Coding: Theory and Practice,* 2012 Edition | Lovaasen, Schwerdtfeger | Saunders | 2012 | 978-1-4557-0545-0 |
| *ICD-10-CM/PCS Coding Theory and Practice* | Lovaasen, Schwerdtfeger | Saunders | 2012 | 978-1-4557-0795-9 |

## PATHOPHYSIOLOGY

| Book Title | Author | Imprint | Copyright Date | ISBN-13 |
|---|---|---|---|---|
| *Pathology for the Health Professions,* 3rd Edition | Damjanov | Saunders | 2006 | 978-1-4160-0031-0 |
| *Essentials of Human Diseases and Conditions,* 4th Edition | Frazier, Drzymkowski | Saunders | 2008 | 978-1-4160-4714-8 |
| *Pathophysiology for the Health Professions,* 4th Edition | Gould | Saunders | 2011 | 978-1-4377-0965-0 |
| *The Human Body in Health and Illness,* 4th Edition | Herlihy | Saunders | 2011 | 978-1-4160-6842-6 |
| *The Human Body in Health and Disease,* 5th Edition | Thibodeau, Patton | Mosby | 2010 | 978-0-323-05492-8 |

## MEDICAL TERMINOLOGY

| Book Title | Author | Imprint | Copyright Date | ISBN-13 |
|---|---|---|---|---|
| *The Language of Medicine,* 9th Edition | Chabner | Saunders | 2011 | 978-1-4377-0560-6 |
| *Jablonski's Dictionary of Medical Acronyms & Abbreviations,* 6th edition | Jablonski | Saunders | 2009 | 978-1-4160-5899-1 |
| *Exploring Medical Language,* 7th Edition | LaFleur, Brooks | Mosby | 2009 | 978-0-323-04950-4 |
| *Building a Medical Vocabulary (with Spanish Translations),* 7th Edition | Leonard | Saunders | 2009 | 978-1-4160-5627-0 |
| *Quick & Easy Medical Terminology,* 5th Edition | Leonard | Saunders | 2007 | 978-1-4160-2494-1 |
| *Mastering Healthcare Terminology,* 3rd Edition | Shiland | Mosby | 2010 | 978-0-323-05506-2 |
| *Dorland's Illustrated Medical Dictionary,* 31st Edition | | Saunders | 2007 | 978-1-4160-2364-7 |

## INTRODUCTION TO COMPUTERS

| Book Title | Author | Imprint | Copyright Date | ISBN-13 |
|---|---|---|---|---|
| *Computerized Medical Office Procedures: A Worktext,* 3rd Edition | Larsen | Saunders | 2011 | 978-1-4377-1608-5 |

## BASICS OF WRITING/MEDICAL TRANSCRIPTION

| Book Title | Author | Imprint | Copyright Date | ISBN-13 |
|---|---|---|---|---|
| *Medical Transcription Guide: Do's and Don'ts,* 3rd Edition | Diehl | Saunders | 2005 | 978-0-7216-0684-2 |
| *Medical Transcription: Techniques and Procedures,* 6th Edition | Diehl | Saunders | 2012 | 978-1-4377-0439-6 |

## COMPREHENSION BUILDING/STUDY SKILLS

| Book Title | Author | Imprint | Copyright Date | ISBN-13 |
| --- | --- | --- | --- | --- |
| *Career Development for Health Professionals: Success in School and on the Job,* 3rd Edition | Haroun | Saunders | 2010 | 978-1-4377-0673-4 |

## BASIC MATH

| Book Title | Author | Imprint | Copyright Date | ISBN-13 |
| --- | --- | --- | --- | --- |
| *Basic Mathematics for the Health-Related Professions* | Doucette | Saunders | 2000 | 978-0-7216-7938-9 |
| *Using Maths in Health Sciences* | Gunn | Churchill Livingstone | 2001 | 978-0-443-07074-7 |

## MEDICAL BILLING/INSURANCE

| Book Title | Author | Imprint | Copyright Date | ISBN-13 |
| --- | --- | --- | --- | --- |
| *Health Insurance Today: A Practical Approach,* 3rd Edition | Beik | Saunders | 2011 | 978-1-4377-1770-9 |
| *Medical Insurance Made Easy: Understanding the Claim Cycle,* 2nd Edition | Brown | Saunders | 2006 | 978-0-7216-0556-2 |
| *Insurance Handbook for the Medical Office,* 11th Edition | Fordney | Saunders | 2010 | 978-1-4377-0128-9 |
| *Electronic Health Record "Booster" Kit for the Medical Office,* 2nd Edition | Buck | Saunders | 2012 | 978-1-4557-2301-0 |
| *Practice Kit for Medical Front Office Skills,* 3rd Edition | Buck | Saunders | 2012 | 978-1-4377-2201-7 |
| *ePractice Kit for Medical Front Office Skills with MedTrack Systems* | Buck | Saunders | 2012 | 978-1-4377-2722-7 |

# Index

# Index

# ELSEVIER

## Trust Elsevier
### to Provide Your Complete Coding Advantage!

## Content

978-1-4557-0622-8     978-1-4557-0646-4

## Simulations

978-1-4557-0735-5

Create a customized portfolio to show employers

## Courses

978-1-4557-0733-1

## Study Tools

978-1-4577-0730-0     978-1-4557-0767-6

evolve
learning system

978-1-4557-0683-9     978-1-4557-0659-4

More study tools available

## Educator Support

978-1-4377-2273-4     978-1-4377-2276-5

evolve
learning system

## Learn more at Elsevieradvantage.com!